Family
Encyclopedia
of
Natural Healing

Family Encyclopedia of Natural Healing

by

John Heinerman,
and
Lendon Smith, M.D.

ISBN: 1-55517-492-2
v.1

Published by Bonneville Books

Distributed by:
925 North Main, Springville, UT 84663 • 801/489-4084

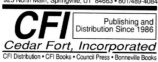

CFI   Publishing and
Distribution Since 1986

Cedar Fort, Incorporated
CFI Distribution • CFI Books • Council Press • Bonneville Books

Typeset by Virginia Reeder
Cover design by Adam Ford
Cover design © 2000 by Lyle Mortimer

Printed in the United States of America

Dedicated to
my father and brother, Jacob
and Joseph Heinerman.

INTRODUCTION

The purpose for writing this book has been two-fold: First, to prepare a reference volume of reliable information which could be trusted; and secondly, to provide consumers with reasonable options to numerous health problems besides the solutions offered through regular medical care.

In no way has it been our intention to substitute these remedies with the treatments prescribed by doctors. But rather to offer accessory care which complements rather than detracts from what your own physician might recommend. In many cases, for simpler ailments, our own alternatives might work just as effectively if not better than those solutions provided by modern medicine.

However, we have been careful to repeatedly emphasize that for *life-threatening* situations, you should *always* consult a competent and qualified doctor of your choice *first*! In some cases, this might include a chiropractor, an osteopath, a naturopath, a homeopath, an accupuncturist, an herbalist, and even a Native American shaman perhaps. For we believe that no single group holds all of the answers to the restoration of good health. But that *many* hands and minds are involved in the wellness process, even if someone's healing profession might seem to be a little unorthodox or outside the circles of accepted healing practices.

No book in print is the definitive answer to every health problem around. And no authors are capable of providing workable solutions for every single illness there is. But, hopefully, we have come as close to this ideal as is humanly possible, with only the utmost regard for the reader's personal welfare in mind.

—John Heinerman, August 2000

ABDOMINAL CRAMPS, PAIN AND SWELLING

Symptoms

Any symptoms related to the belly. Cramping is the involuntary tightening of the abdominal wall muscles, sometimes accompanied by short jabs of pain. The muscles of the abdominal wall go into spasm to protect the inflammation beneath, such as an ulcer or an inflamed appendix.

Usually food sensitivities, stress or a viral gastroenteritis (stomach flu) show themselves as intermittent cramps localized to the area of the navel. The abdominal wall, however, should be soft, pliable, and non-tender in between the cramps. In intestinal flu, the pain is temporarily relieved with the passage of a big, sloppy, watery, usually greenish movement. Albeit weak, the victim feels almost normal between the cramping. Intestinal flu has a low white blood cell count at around the 5—6,000 level; it usually means a viral infection. The usual story is vomiting and weakness for a day and then diarrhea for one day (adults call it one-day flu), but the cramps and sloppy stools usually last seven days in children.

Duodenal and most stomach ulcers are *always* relieved with food, and especially antacids. Constipation is *always* the passage of hard, often dry stools; the consistency is the criterion for constipation, not the frequency. But constipated stools are usually passed less than once every day.

Appendicitis is usually revealed by the presence of a constant pain in the right lower quadrant of the abdomen. The pain is like a severe gas pain. It doesn't go away with a bowel movement.

It is constant and the abdominal muscles over the inflamed area are spastic. Palpation is very painful; the area is exquisitely tender. One must seek the advice of a doctor. A white blood cell count is usually elevated to about 12,000. If the appendix bursts, peritonitis sets in. Peritonitis, a rare condition, causes shock, high fever, and a terrible generalized abdominal pain.

Swelling of the abdomen can be caused by intestinal gas, obesity, pregnancy, fluid accumulation, organ dysfunction (heart, lung, liver or kidneys), and even something as mundane as an ovarian cyst which has been known to reach gargantuan proportions sometimes. (Consider the bizarre case of a Florida woman who had a 400-lb. cyst removed from her ovaries by surgeons, which required four strong hospital orderlies to cart out on a stretcher sometime in late October, 1991.)

Some detective work is required to sort out the foods to which one might be sensitive. It is usually the most favored foods: milk, wheat, soy, eggs, corn, peanuts, and chocolate. But anything can do anything. It takes about four days of abstinence from any food to get relief from symptoms for gas, cramps, and sloppy bowels. However, it takes at least 21 days to get rid of all the chemicals that the dairy products have produced. Babies will have colic from cow's milk in infancy. The sensitivity moves to their ears (otitis), then the lungs (asthma), the bladder (enuresis), head (migraine), nasopharynx (sinusitis and post-nasal drip). The body is trying to tell the owner that milk is the sensitizer. Skin tests are virtually worthless for *sensitizing* foods; they only work for the discovery of food and inhalant *allergies*.

Relief Measures

Linda Holmes of Oshkosh, Wisconsin experienced belly aches every time she ate beans. So she started drinking some warm ginger root tea with them, and her cramps disappeared in no time at all. She simmered 2 level teaspoonfuls of grated ginger root in one quart of boiling water for seven minutes, and then steeped it for another 20 minutes. She strained the tea and drank about 1.5 cups whenever she ate beans again.

Peppermint tea made the same way (but without simmering) is ideal for colic. Warm slippery elm bark or marshmallow root teas are handy for peritonitis-type and inflammatory pains. Useful fruit juices would include papaya and mango.

Maurice Mességué, France's most famous folk healer who once treated Pope John XXIII and King Farouk of Egypt, advises blending "two pinches of basil (entire plant), one pinch of chamomile blossoms and one pinch of peppermint steeped in a quart of boiling water." Then "take 4 cups of this in the course of the day."

Relief Measures

Health food stores now sell a great variety of foods that are dairy, corn, soy, and wheat-free. A rice milk is very tasty. The best, low-roughage diet for the intestinal flu is the BRAT diet: bananas, rice, applesauce, and (white bread) toast. Homeopathic Nux Vomica is, standard for vomiting. Many people have found relief when given 1 cc

shots of vitamin B-12. It seems to control allergies and improve digestion and absorption. Betaine HCl will cut down the gas that comes from a high protein diet. Most digestive enzyme remedies have papain and trypsin to help with the digestion in the small intestine.

ABORTION INFECTIONS

Symptoms

A septic condition brought about by sloppy abortion procedures through unskilled surgeons in unsanitary settings. Generally marked by pus and other pathogenic organisms in the blood and female organs, resulting in localized infection, fever and so forth. More common in Third World countries than in the highly industrialized nations.

Relief Measures

Bratislvaia, Czechoslovakia is one of those places where such things are relatively common in routine abortions. Dr. Jarsolav Kresânek, an experienced clinical herbalist, recommends use of black currant "healthy young leaves (especially after the flowering period, before the fruits appear)" and blossoms because of their "silica...vitamin C [and] mineral salts." In addition, he suggests summer savory "leaves together with the flowers" on account of their "silica...and mineral salts." Both work well to fight this kind of infection, he insists.

A half handful of each herb is put into 1.5 pints of boiling water and steeped for 30 minutes, before straining. 2-3 cups in between meals is advised. Goldenseal root (3 capsules) and goldenseal root/echinacea combination (2 capsules) are useful here, too.

Food and Nutrients

This can be a life-threatening infection and needs huge doses of vitamin C, intravenously if possible. Fifty to one hundred grams daily would be close to the appropriate dose. It should be enough to soften up the bowel movements a bit. Vitamin C up to 50,000 I.U. daily for about a week is also helpful.

ABRASION

Symptoms

Abrasion is the loss of the superficial skin from friction such as a scrape from skidding on the cement. It is treated similarly to a second-degree burn.

Relief Measures

Only soap and water should be used to cleanse this. If tar or asphalt is involved, it must be removed or when the skin heals there will remain the black particles like a tattoo. Only a dry, sterile gauze dressing is applied, then more gauze, and then an Ace bandage to hold the area quiet. Antibiotic ointments, boric acid, or alcohol are not to be used as they are sensitizing and irritating.

Foods and Nutrients

Vitamin C (1000-5000 mg.), zinc (30 mg.) and vitamin A (20,000 I.U.) each day should promote healing. If one feels the

need for an ointment, calendula is safe and helpful.

ABSCESS

Symptoms

Abscess is a firm, red, swollen, tender, and hot infection on the skin surface. It usually comes from a break in the skin from a thorn, a sliver, an ingrown toenail, or human bite. Infection gets in and the germs multiply and the white blood cells come to the rescue.

Relief Measures

Here is an old trick learned years ago from a Hungarian grandmother. She would take an old sewing needle from her treadle machine drawer, hold it over the gas burner or a lit match for 30 seconds to sterilize the tip, then gently work it into and around the affected area until the foreign particle causing all of the discomfort had been removed. She would then wash the surface with some tincture of witch hazel and that would be that!

Moist heat is standard for infection, abscesses, boils, cellulites and carbuncles. It dilates the capillaries, increasing the circulation, bringing more white blood cells to the area to fight the infection. How to do the hot pack: Add one teaspoon of table salt to a quart of hot water. Put a small hand towel in this solution. Wring out the excess water and place on the infected area. Cover with plastic to make it air tight. Cover the entire area with a big dry bath towel, and hold all this in place with an elastic bandage. It will stay warm and moist for 12 hours, like overnight. Don't change it as it will cool off and interrupt the healing. It should look less red and be less tender. One should not lance a boil until it appears to be ready to erupt itself. Then wait one more day. A surgeon's advice would be prudent.

Foods and Nutrients

Anything involving the skin would be helpful—vitamin A (50,000 I.U.) and zinc (50 mg.). Infections do better if vitamin C is added in large doses (1,000 mg.)—enough to soften the bowel movements.

ACHING MUSCLES

Symptoms

Aching muscles are often due to an overexertion of physical movement of some kind. Strenuous lifting and bending will certainly affect muscles in the upper part of the arms and the lower back region. Whereas intense and rapid physical movements of the arms and legs in activities like swimming, tennis, and jogging will bring about soreness as well.

Viral infections such as influenza, for example, can also produce muscular aches and pains. Being confined to bed for lengthy periods of time will certainly make the calves, thighs, buttocks and back hurt if they stay in one position too long.

Relief Measures

One of the most efficient ways to relieve muscular soreness is with the application of heat and those aromatic herbs with volatile oils which are capable of penetrating deep into injured sore tissue mass to relieve inflammation. Any herbal salve or liniment containing eucalyptus is recommended for this. Vicks Vapo-Rub is a drugstore alternative to consider. When placing a heating aid upon an area of the body, remember to first lay a clean, white diaper cloth over the skin first. This prevents the surface from becoming overheated.

Certain products containing the chief constituent of cayenne pepper, capsaicin, are now on the market which provide speedy relief for muscular aches and pains. One of them is a roll-on called The Right Solution. It contains capsicum oleoresin (.025% capsaicin) in a base of black walnut extract, yucca tincture, alfalfa extract, wintergreen leaf extract, white willow bark extract, licorice extract, and aloe vera (see Appendix).

Peppermint oil (just a few drops) and fluid extract of capsicum (about 7-10 drops) applied on aching muscles, in that order, and gently rubbed into the skin with the palm of the hand will also work effectively.

Foods and Nutrients

Acute, sudden onset of pain from an injury can be calmed with a homeopathic preparation of arnica. For the more chronic muscle aches, most people start out with calcium (1000 mg.) and magnesium (500 mg.) each day for child and adult alike. These simple, safe minerals can be very helpful. To be more accurate, however, the results of a blood test to determine if the victim is alkaline, would be most helpful. If alkalinity is obvious, then acidifiers such as betaine HCl, ammonium chloride and even ascorbic acid would be necessary to make the minerals availabe to the enzymes in the cells. Doan's pills (magnesium salicylate) are safe and effective. Some aches in the legs are due to narrowed blood vessels and there isn't enough oxygen getting to the muscles there. Low potassium in the system can result in sore muscles. Regular exercise and massage are invaluable here. Chiropractors are specialists in the care of muscular aches and pains. Consulting one near you might not be a bad idea.

Stop ingesting any food or drink with aspartame in it. Be more conscientious about reading labels on the things you buy for personal consumption. Recent evidence indicates that aspartame (which also goes by the name of Nutra-Sweet) is a leading cause of many muscular aches and pains.

ACNE VULGARIS

Symptoms

Acne vulgaris is a simple pustular eruption of the skin, occurring primarily on the face, upper back, and chest, mainly during puberty and adolescence. Properly attributed to an overactive pilosebaceous apparatus, and perhaps affected by hormonal activity as well. Not always due to masturbation or heavy consumption of chocolate as once explained by the old school of medical thought. In our more enlightened times, it can involve certain environmental factors as well.

Comes in four basic grades, the first being a mild bout with just a few scattered whiteheads and blackheads. The fourth and most serious grade, consists of numerous whiteheads, blackheads, pustules, nodules, and cysts. Grade four acne is generally accompanied by severe inflammation that becomes red or purple. And it's usually a sign that the sufferer had better see a competent dermatologist soon.

Relief Measures

Such unsightly blemishes can be cosmetically covered up. Maurice Stein, a famous Hollywood makeup artist who has worked on such movies as "Funny Girl" and all of the entire "Planet of the Apes" series informed one of us sometime back, "John, I think if a person looks for a foundation makeup that has a high pigment level, it should help him or her a lot. In fact, the more pigment the better it is. When I cover acne on an actor's or actress' face, I look for a pigment level of 50-70%; but your normal range for most foundations is 18% or less."

Sometimes foods can cause an allergic reaction that brings on acne. Some allergists suspect that seafoods might induce this due to their high iodine content. Still others implicate dairy foods like milk, butter, cheese and even eggs in some cases. Generally speaking, it's safe to say that greasy foods (deep-fried or grilled) and sugary products (candy, soda pop, colas, dessert items) will trigger an acne outbreak if nothing else does.

And here's the rule on what and what not to squeeze: Don't squeeze any pimple with a red base, as that means it is already inflamed and even infected; let it rest. You can gently try to get rid of blackheads (oxidized oil) using the dermatologists' loop, but if you are not careful you could start an infection.

One of the best kinds of acne medications is good old pine tar soap. You have to get it from a veterinary supply house, as a rule, instead of a drugstore. Scrub the skin good with it, rinse thoroughly with cold water and then rub gently with a hand towel. Applying a little hydrogen peroxide to whiteheads that seem on the verge of bursting with a Q-tip is good to do. And when washing the face, use a wash cloth to open the pores. For excessively oily skin, cleanse the surface with a cotton ball saturated with rubbing alcohol.

Food and Nutrients

Vitamin A can help the skin fight off the infection that may lead to scarring. 10-20,000 I.U. is safe to take. Larger doses, like 50-100,000 I.U. are safe for a few days, but its use in high doses should be monitored by a knowledgeable physician. Beta-carotene (50,000 I.U.) and zinc (30 mg.) promote skin health. Zinc is needed if the subject has white spots on the nails. The taste test for zinc deficiency: if a weak solution of zinc is dropped on the tongue and the subject finds it no different than water, the subject is zinc-deficient. Vitamin B-6 (100 mg.) is helpful for some girls with acne who have flareups of it at the time of their menstrual periods.

ADDICTIONS (FOOD, DRUG & EXERCISE)

Symptoms

Simply defined, an addiction is any kind of a habitual psychological and physiological dependence on a substance or practice which is beyond voluntary control. While compulsive eating habits, alcoholism, and drug abuse have received prominent coverage in the media of late, virtually nothing has been said about the exercise craze which dominates many people's lives. These are the ones who get hooked on their own self-generated endorphins, which are abundantly produced during intensive physical activity and create a "feel good" sensation or chemical euphoria that is quite satisfying to the body.

We believe that everything ought to be done in moderation, no matter whether it entails eating, drinking, self-medicating, working, playing, exercising, loving or even sleeping. Some things, of course, are not meant to be indulged in at all, such as using cocaine or heroin.

Some addictions are obvious while others remain very subtle. Watching an overweight person chow down a greasy doughnut or sugary sweet roll, quickly lets us know that such a one is a food addict, just as a wino lying in an alleyway with an empty liquor bottle nearby indicates he's an alcoholic; or junkies with needle marks all over their forearms indicates a constant need for illicit drugs.

But what about other scenarios that seldom, if ever, come to mind, but are equally disturbing? Kids glued to TV sets all over the country for hours on end. Teenagers and college-age young people who absolutely have to have their daily doses of heavy metal rock music in order to get by. Gamblers at the gaming tables and slot machines in Las Vegas and Atlantic City, who don't know when to quit. Corporate executives driven by greed and power who want to acquire more assets than what they really need. Coaches who push their star players and teams to the point of sheer exhaustion for one more win or another trophy to add to their already expansive collections of the same. Senior citizens who gulp down more over-the-counter and prescription medications than they ought to for imagined aches and pains they really don't have. And some health enthusiasts who have carried the benefits of fasting and enemas to such extremes that they're squeaky-clean insides have actually made them quite ill.

Aren't all of these addictions, too, in some form or another? Some doctors think so and believe that they can be just as harmful to the human psyche and system as anything else that's overdone. Excesses in *anything* outside the purview of common sense should be curtailed as soon as possible. "*Moderation in ALL things*" is the yardstick by which our personal interests and habits always ought to be measured.

Relief Measures

Determining that something is going to be done with a particular excess is the *first* step in getting rid of an addiction. The *second* involves carrying that determination out by doing something about it. Often meditation, acupuncture, or bio-feedback techniques are helpful in this reorientation process. The *third* step is in receiving encour-

agement from friends and relatives or even yourself (if you're alone) for the progress made thus far. A *fourth* is a sense of accomplishment, realizing that you've finally started doing something about what once seemed an impossible situation to deal with. A *fifth* anticipation is knowing you've finally conquered the problem for good and the *sixth* is realizing there is NO turning back to former ways that were harmful or destructive. (Readers are advised to consult the index under "Addictions" in Norman Cousins' best-seller, *Head First, the Biology of Hope,* for further information.)

Food and Nutrients

One of the easiest ways to overcome food, beverage, drug and exercise addictions is to AVOID those things which are spicy and tend to excite the body or nerves in any way. Therefore, the preferred items to be consumed ought to be somewhat neutral in nature, and neither excessively acidic nor particularly alkaline. They need not be necessarily bland either, but rather modest in their flavor appeals. Avoid arousing those nerve centers within the body which can produce abnormal cravings for things which are meant to be brought under control.

Herbs which are useful in helping to curb addictions include catnip, hops, lobelia, passion flower, peppermint, saw palmetto, skullcap, spearmint, valerian and wood botony. They can be taken in capsule or tea form, whichever is preferred. The Bach Flower Remedies, which were discovered by a British doctor, Edward Bach, have also been very useful as well. Consider the case of a 42-year-old English gentleman who served a brief stint in the House of Commons in the British Parliament some years ago. Alcoholism nearly ruined his political and business careers, until he started taking the agrimony treatment. In just two months, he completely lost his taste for hard liquor and was able to once more concentrate on his political responsibilities. Cherry Plum and Impatiens are also two other handy remedies. They are just two of five remedies which constitute Dr. Bach's famous "Rescue Remedy" for emergency situations. They are all taken in droplet form beneath the base of the tongue, and are available at some health-food stores and nutrition centers nationwide.

Another fairly recent development in combatting addictions is to employ certain essential oils on the surface of the skin to produce states of physical relaxation and mental and emotional calmness and well being. Since they are too highly concentrated to be used directly on the skin, they need to be diluted in some kind of base oil such as olive or sesame oils (use 10% dilutions here) or sweet almond, apricot kernel,or sunflower seed oils (all of which can be used 100%). Make sure these base oils are cold-pressed and say so on their respective labels, since some are processed with chemical agents. Use about 20 drops of an essential oil to about 4 teaspoonfuls of a base oil.

Essential oils for overcoming addictions include: rose, sandalwood, fennel, birch, parsley, nutmeg, grapefruit, marjoram, bergamot, basil, peppermint, lavender, chamomile (Roman), valerian, lemon, and orange. They can be used in warm baths or else gently massaged into the skin after a hot shower. The best places for applying them are on the base of the neck, along the spine, on the insides of the wrists, on the solar plexus, on the ankles and the soles of the feet, as well as along the top of the forehead. Most oils can be obtained from Great Amer-

ican Natural Products in St. Petersburg, Florida (see Appendix).

Many people have noticed intermittent bouts of being spacy, anxious, nervous or sleepy. Through trial and error they have found that an alcoholic drink, a caffeine drink, a cigarette, some sugar, certain foods, or drugs will get their bodies and their minds going again. These attacks are due to low blood sugar, the reason for getting hooked on anything, food, habit, drink, or drug. The best thing for people who notice these swings in mood and energy is to eat 5-6 small meals a day. The foods must be wholesome and nourishing, and one must avoid his or her favorite food. (Common sensitizers: milk, wheat, soy, corn, eggs, nuts, and chocolate.) Remember, 80% of people with food sensitization have low blood sugar.

Calcium (1000 mg.) and magnesium (500 mg.) have a calming effect without causing drowsiness. B-6 (50-100 mg.) helps the enzymes that produce some tranquility. All addictions respond to vitamin C, especially (50-100 grams) intravenously.

ADDISON'S DISEASE

Symptoms

Addison's Disease is rare and serious as it is life threatening. It is usually due to destruction of the adrenal glands by hemorrhage or bacterial infection. It is characterized by extreme fatigue, low blood pressure, weight loss, pigmentation of the skin and mucous membranes, and loss of appetite. Adrenal gland hormone replacement is advised.

Most doctors do not believe that there is any condition between Addison's and normal adrenals, despite the work of Hans Selye, M.D. (1936) who discovered that stressors—physical, emotional, or chemical can produce milder forms of adrenal gland exhaustion: swollen adrenal glands, atrophy of the thymus and lymph tissue, and stomach hemorrhages and ulcers. The body thus stressed is susceptible to infection, autoimmune diseases and nervous and mental exhaustion.

Relief Measures

Licorice and dandelion roots (3 capsules of each daily) are top herbs for arresting this condition. Make sure the licorice is the deglycyrrhinized kind, since regular licorice root has glycyrrhizin in it, which can cause edema, hypertension and kidney damage. Four capsules of slippery elm bark each day are good when taken with 1 glass of Kyo-Green chlorophyll drink (see Appendix under Wakunaga).

Food and Nutrients

Anything loaded with sugar ought to be avoided at all costs. Read labels and look for "hidden" sugars ending in "-ose" (mannose, dextrose, sucrose, fructose) or things like corn syrup or honey.

Clinical experience has determined that *proper* protein is important in rebuilding the adrenal glands. This should come from plant foods rather than more meat. Nuts and legumes are ideal sources for this.

Vitamins and minerals are helpful, too. Vitamin A (20,000 I.U.), C (10 grams),

B-6 (100 mg.), pantothenic acid (1000 mg.), calcium (1000 mg.), and zinc (30 mg.) should all be used daily to help rebuild the adrenals. A nourishing diet eaten in six small meals a day helps sustain the blood sugar more evenly.

ADDITIVES (CHEMICAL)

Symptoms

Chemical additives are around us in the air, water and food that we breathe, drink and eat. As well as in the toiletries we use on our bodies, the clothes we wear, the furniture we sit or sleep on, the carpets we walk or lay on, and so forth. When absorbed in small amounts they can by easily discarded through the normal channels of elimination.

Short-term effects are barely noticeable. Usually it takes years before their nasty side-effects become more apparent. Still, allergies are one of the most common symptoms.

Relief Measures

To prevent an accumulation within the system, consume those foods which will flush them out. Vegetable and fruit juices, some herb teas such as chickweed or dandelion, and high-fiber foods (whole grain cereals and breads) are some of these. Do not use deodorants. Drink plenty of distilled or mineral or spring water (at least 6 glasses a day). Herbal diuretics like buchu or laxatives such as senna may be necessary at times.

Periodic sweatbaths in a hot tub, sauna or steam room is useful. Also monthly weekend fasting, subsisting only on liquid nourishment. As well as *dry* brush rubs on the skin morning and evening to circulate the blood and help wash away deposits of harmful chemicals in muscle tissue.

Food and Nutrients

Vitamin C (1000 mg.), calcium (600 mg.) and magnesium (400 mg.) will assist in flushing out harmful chemical garbage. So will potassium (1200 mg.) and phosphorus (800 mg.). Foods containing Nutra-Sweet (aspartame) should be avoided; and don't use Equal sweetener either.

ADENOID ENLARGEMENT

(See also TONSILLITIS)

Symptoms

The adenoids and tonsils are lymphoid structures concerned with the defense of the body against infection entering either by way of the nose or mouth. While the tonsils are more readily visible on either side of the back of the throat, the adenoids located in the back spaces of the nose are almost invisible except with the aid of special instruments used for detecting and examining them.

Enlargement of these adenoids can cause obstruction to breathing or even block the tubes from the ears to the mouth. Once upon a time not so long ago in modern medicine, both tonsils and adenoids were routinely removed upon the advice of most physicians who viewed them more as nuisances than as practical requirements for

a healthy body. Now, though, just the opposite view is taken by many of them.

Relief Measures

Foods that produce clogging mucus should be eliminated from the diet; these include dairy products, eggs, and refined flour items. Certain antibiotic herbs like Wakunaga goldenseal root or Kyolic aged garlic extract are especially helpful to take (see Appendix). About 2 capsules of the former and 3 capsules of the latter are recommended. We suggest the *liquid* Kyolic instead of the tablet kind, believing that in this particular instance, it can be more readily dispersed throughout the system where needed the most.

Also hot compresses of mullein herb tea applied on either side of the nose on the cheeks and also across the throat, will help immensely to reduce swelling of these glands. Warm mullein tea can also be gargled and even inhaled, if necessary, to effectively deal with such enlargements.

Food and Nutrients

The tonsils and adenoids act like sponges and soak up the mucus that many foods produce. Milk is the most common trouble-maker. Children who are heavy milk drinkers often start out with colic from this and then move to noisy breathing, stomachaches, constipation, and ear infections. If the tonsils and adenoids aren't too large, the discontinuation of cow's milk products may be curative. Soy milk and goat's milk are reasonable alternatives, but they may also be allergenic to some.

Vitamin C (1, 000 mg.) and echinacea fluid extract (10 drops) are helpful to control the infections that plague those with enlarged tonsils and adenoids. Strep sore throat is more often associated with cow's milk ingestion than anything else.

ADRENAL EXHAUSTION

Symptoms

Somewhat butterfly in shape, each of these flattened, roughly triangular bodies rests upon the upper end of each kidney. They are just one of several different ductless glands furnishing internal secretions necessary for energy and stamina.

Extreme stress and constant physical and emotional activities of an intense nature, tend to biochemically "whip" these poor glands to the point of sheer exhaustion. When this happens, irritating fatigue and an inability to respond to even the simplest stimuli become evident.

Relief Measures

Sometime in the middle of the last decade (1980's), one of us (Heinerman) went to the island of Jamaica to interview the late Mrs. Marshall, one of Kingston's most famous folk healers *and* voodoo practitioners. Mixing together a delightful blend of herbal remedies, black magic *and* orthodox Christianity, it seemed like there was virtually nothing which this woman couldn't deal with.

Her sage advice for fatigue-related problems was this: "Honey, you tell readers that all they need to do is to just get plenty of rest! That'll cure 'em of the lazy bones habit for sure!" She also suggested taking time out each day to reflect and meditate upon one's life and surrounding environs. "Honey, everybody needs a 'quiet time' to themselves, when they can sit and think a spell. It does the body good, you know."

Perhaps nothing more needs to be said than this. Other than that "...if someone is bothering any of your readers, you just have them send a photograph or lock of hair or personal effect of their enemy to me, and I guarantee I'll whip up a little spell to make their enemy think twice before ever bothering them again, honey." When she passed on to the great beyond, it is said that her funeral gathered one of the largest crowds ever known in those parts—certainly a fitting tribute to the tens of thousands she faithfully served in her long life of useful service to humanity.

Foods and Nutrients

The same nutritional recommendations given for Addison's disease apply here as well. Consult that entry for further information.

AGING

Symptoms

Currently 1.6 of every five Americans is pushing 60—the greater majority being females than males—and the end doesn't seem to be in sight as yet. In fact, since 1970, the older set have grown twice as fast as the rest of the population.

No two individuals age alike or even at the same rate. We've known college kids in their twenties, who because of riotous living and indulgences in alcohol, drugs, junk food and promiscuous sex, actually look 50, whereas some senior citizens, because of their ruddy complexions, smooth skin and healthy lifestyles, come across as being in their late 40's. One of us (Smith) is in his 70's, but has been told by many of his former patients and medical students that he actually looks 20-30 years *younger* than what he really is!

The external signs of aging are wrinkled and flabby skin, baldness or greying of the hair (or both), muscle shrinkage, diminished strength, weaker vision, and loss of hearing. Internally, we find brittle bones, memory loss, heart problems, kidney failure, urogenital system incapacities, loss of sexual prowess, and decreased immune functions.

Relief Measures

While there is no real proverbial "Fountain of Youth" such as the one explorer Ponce de Leon was searching for in the Florida wilds, to keeps us forever young and beautiful, there are some things we can do to extend our years considerably.

First of all, stop smoking. And if you don't smoke but live or work around those who do, then take immediate steps to get into a smoke-free atmosphere, because recent medical evidence shows beyond a doubt that *second-hand* smoke is just as bad for you as smoking itself.

Secondly – eat well-rounded meals that are low in animal flesh but high in plant proteins and fiber. The ancient Jewish histo-rian, Flavius Josephus in his *Antiquities of the Jews* (Chapter 3, Book I, Verse 9) gave us several very good explanations as to why the people before the Flood lived for many *centuries* before dying:

> But let no one, upon comparing the lives of the lives of the ancients with our lives, and with the few years which we now live, think that what we have said of them is false; or make the shortness of our lives at present an argument, that neither did they attain to so long a duration of life, for those ancients were beloved of God, and [lately] made by God himself; *and because their food was then fitter for the prolongation of life*, might well live so great a number of years: and besides, God afforded them a longer time of life on account of their virtue, and the good use they made of it... [italics added for emphasis].

Also the way in which food is prepared has a lot to do with whether you'll grow old fast or age gracefully. Frying, charbroiling and deep-fat frying of animal proteins produces an abundance of scavenger molecules called free radicals. Think of them as roving gangs of molecular thugs, running loose in your body wreaking havoc and hell wherever it pleases them. But steaming, baking, and boiling virtually eliminate these things from your cooked foods.

Thirdly remember to exercise regularly. Keeping fit and trim increases your resistance to disease. Something so simple as walking each day, can really help to boost your own immune strength.

Fourth—only use alcohol in moderation, *never* excessively.

Fifth—have periodic checkups from several different types of doctors. Besides a regular medical doctor, we also recommend a good Oriental physician, who is skilled in diagnosing the tongue, eyes, skin pallor and moisture content, pulse, urine color, and fecal smell, to determine what condition many of your internal organs may be in.

Sixth, remember what the late Mrs. Marshall had to say about rest, under the previous entry. Most Americans suffer from what we consider to be a hidden national malady of epidemic proportions—namely, *sleep deprivation*! There is no such thing as "catching up on lost sleep." If you believe that old fairy tale, then we have some desert cactus country up here in Portland and some lovely beach property that fronts the ocean here in Salt Lake City, that we're both interested in selling to the naive and foolish.

Seventh, don't overstay your time in the sun or cold. The ancient Maya believed that certain "wind spirits" were the cause of many pulmonary disorders in the young and old alike. Always wear protective clothing and head gear when exposed to either extreme for very long.

An eighth factor to look at is just that: *looking* around you more carefully in order to avoid bad falls or nasty tumbles. More hips are broken or injured by slips in the bathtub or trippings down the stairs in the elderly, than in any other age bracket.

A ninth consideration is to remain close to your friends and family. Strong social contacts will always eliminate depression. Loneliness kills more people than all other factors combined!

And finally, maintain a positive attitude towards life in general. Try to find the humor in something; or, as others have put it: "Learn to make lemonade out of lemons." Stop being an antisocial critter and the world's worst grouch. Stop your moaning and groaning, and constant complaining. Cease to be cantankerous. Only grizzly bears and wolverines love an ornery snarl. Enjoy what you have, irregardless of how little or how much it may be; and realize that others elsewhere can be a lot worse off than you may be.

And remember to let your heart be like an open flower—the more you open up inside, the more of your own inner beauty and good comes forth for others to see and enjoy!

Food and Nutrients

One of the authors of this book is a retired physician now in his mid-to-late 70's. Here is his own first-person account of what he has done to successfully retard the aging processes in himself.

"I feel so much better now at 70-plus years than I did as an adolescent or young adult.

"*Headaches* are non-existent now. (I used to think they were due to stressors that came with a pediatrician's life. I finally got the message they were due to the withdrawal from coffee early in the morning because I did not have any from bedtime on. A cup every hour during the day kept the vascular spasms away.)

"*Warts* are gone. (I was warty until I realized I'm a vitamin A needed. Big doses, albeit for short periods of time—100,000 to

200,000 International Units a day for 3-5 days will stop my flu or cough in just a few days. The last time I took these big doses, a plantar wart fell off my foot.)

"Hands and feet are warmer now. (I now drink two glasses of electrolytes [minerals in solution] mixed with milk each day. This has perked up my circulation, but my blood pressure stays in the normal range.)

"Blood pressure is 130/85, cholesterol is 240, but the HDL is high (High-Density Lipoproteins or "good" cholesterol). I run about five blocks every day, get a little short of breath, but am able to recite Shakespeare as I do so.

"Nocturia is under control because I take saw palmetto (3 capsules) every day which keeps my generous prostate under control.

"I laugh more than I cry; this is the single most important part of my life. I have projects, and there are people who need me.

"Life Balances is a program in which I have been involved for about eight years. It is based on the biochemical truism that our senses of smell and taste determine our vitamin and mineral needs: if something smells good, we need it. If it smells bad, we do not need it.

AGITATION

Symptoms

Marked by irregular moods, rapid or violent actions sometimes, or an excited state of mind or feelings. Anytime the system is stirred up to the point of being uncomfortable to someone else, then this is agitation.

Relief Measures

The source of the trouble should first of all be sought out and then promptly removed from mind, heart or physical premises. Secondly, the person thus agitated should learn to forgive others (if they have been the source of vexation) or himself or herself (if the individual is to blame instead). Thirdly, a more calm composure should be sought for; and this can be obtained through any number of ways: i.e., visualization, biofeedback, meditation, classical music, deep-breathing exercises, resting, strolling, massaging, etc.

One of the best ways, believe it or not, is to have your hair combed or brushed by someone else, while you are in a reclining position on a couch (assuming you still have enough hair with which to do this). The Bible informs us that every time Samson became agitated with his Philistine oppressors and went stomping off to slay a bunch of them, he afterwards headed straight for Delilah's house, where she promptly soothed his nerves and mind by repeatedly stroking his hair as his head lay in her lap. (Just don't let your hair be cut in this position is all we ask!)

While having someone close to you comb your hair while you are lying down may seem a little strange at first, upon putting this recommendation to the test you will be truely amazed at just how relaxing it can be. Almost as good as a warm oil massage is, believe it or not!

Foods and Nutrients

Most of us do not get enough calcium and magnesium in our diets. If one is sensitive, ticklish, has trouble falling asleep, and has little muscle cramps in feet and legs, and hates crowds, he/she is usually low in magnesium. 500 mg. of this a day for one week will help with your agitation. Valerian root is beneficial to most who are on the edge of discomfort. We suggest a homeopathic preparation of 10-12 drops or 3-4 pills a day.

AIDS

(ACQUIRED IMMUNE DEFI- CIENCY SYNDROME)

MEDICAL DISCLAIMER

Our publisher asked us to place a medical disclaimer by this particular entry. In doing so we wish our readers to understand that what is offered here comes from those who've specialized in the treatment of this malicious malady. In no way do we wish to convey that the few solutions offered here are absolute by any means. AIDS is an extremely complex condition which requires considerable medical attention and many diverse opinions. Ours is but just one of these.

Symptoms

The chief difficulty in detecting some of the early symptoms associated with infection by the HIV virus is that they mimic symptoms which are common to other less threatening illnesses. For instance, the fever, sore throat and lethargy common to HIV infection, also appear with the onset of influenza. And other HIV symptoms such as swollen lymph nodes, rash, depression, loss of appetite, weight loss, and eye pain are all very similar to mononucleosis or "kissing disease" (a herpes infection). But a full blood analysis will show that the white blood cell counts in those who test HIV positive, drop more significantly than they do in other illnesses with overlapping symptoms.

Herewith is a list of the most common symptoms generally reported for HIV infection, ranked in order of their frequency: fever, lethargy, malaise, sore throat, loss of appetite, muscle pain, headache, joint pain, weight loss, swollen lymph nodes, pain behind the eyeball, dehydration, nausea, depression, diarrhea, irritability, torso rash, dry cough, abdominal pain, runny nose, and dark urine.

Relief Measures

While a number of different therapies have been advocated for AIDS cases, one of the most important seems to be stimulating the production of certain "killer cells" within the immune system that can aggressively attack the AIDS virus. A colleague of ours, Laurence Badgley, M.D., who has successfully treated many such cases from his clinic in Foster City, California, believes that medicinal mushrooms from the Orient play a vital role in this.

In Chapter 11 of his book, *Healing AIDS Naturally*, Dr. Badgley cited his own test results with four AIDS patients who were placed on shiitake mushroom therapy for several months. In every case, there was a dramatic jump in their T-cell and absolute helper cell productions, resulting in a leveling off of the disease to some extent.

He also observed that Chinese herbs seem to work much better in controlling the effects of this nasty disease than do most Western herbs.

Dr. Badgley also mentioned aged garlic extract as being very effective in fighting the AIDS virus. Our own experience, together with numerous scientific reports from around the world, have shown Kyolic aged garlic extract from Japan to be the most superior form of this wonderful herb ever made. Kyolic is available in either liquid or tablet forms from most health food stores and nutrition centers nationwide (see Appendix under Wakunaga).

Besides these, there are also echinacea, licorice root, wheatgrass and algae, which Dr. Badgley has given to many of his AIDS patients in times past with very good results. The Kyo-Green mixture from Wakunaga, consisting of young barley and wheat grasses, Bulgarian chlorella, brown rice and kelp seaweed in powdered form, is in our judgement the best source of chlorophyll nutrition for rebuilding the blood supply in all AIDS cases. (See Appendix under Wakunaga for further information if your local health food store doesn't carry this product.)

Other herbs which are useful in rebuilding devastated immune systems are goldenseal root (capsule), chaparral (tea), red clover (tea), and pau d'arco (fluid extract).

NOTE : The reader is advised to consult the index of Dr. Badgley's book for most of the items cited above. (Laurence Badgley, M.D. *Healing AIDS Naturally* (San Bruno, Calif.: Human Energy Press, 1987)

Foods and Nutrients

An issue of the *Journal of Orthomolecular Medicine* (Vol. 5, no. 1, pp. 25-31) published in Canada in 1990, observed that some AIDS patients who've consumed very spicy cuisines on a frequent basis have been able to hold related infections (herpes, candida, tuberculosis) to a minimum. More specifically, those who ate "very spicy foods from one of many countries that use hot spices, such as Mexico, Brazil, Burma, China (Szechuan/Hunan), Thailand and Korea," had stronger immune systems, showed significant weight gains, and looked healthier than other AIDS patients who didn't consume such cuisines very often.

Most medical doctors who treat people with AIDS use large doses of vitamin C intravenously at least twice a week. Twenty-five to fifty grams of ascorbic acid plus calcium, magnesium, the B-complex group, and zinc can all go into this IV. The patient with AIDS must have a clean lifestyle, no booze, no smoking, no drugs, and relatively little or no sexuality, at least not the kind that is unprotected anyway. He must exercise to the limit of comfort. Fruits, vegetables, lightly cooked and lean meat, whole grains and some dairy, if tolerated, is the diet. Oral supplements include aloe vera, essential fatty acids, and all the vitamins and minerals in there most bio-available form.

(One of the authors, who is a retired physician, is connected with the Fons Vitae product that seems to show great promise in helping the truncated immune system) Sodium and calcium are the key ingredients in the blood test that can help the professionl monitor the progress of AIDS as they are the guardians of the cell walls.

AZT gets mixed reviews. It seems if people are healthy, they can tolerate the drug, but if they have any of the opportunistic infections (pneumocystis, Kaposi's sarcome, dementia, diarrhea, severe weight loss, and a low T cell count (below 100) it probably will make the disease worse and inevitably hasten death.

AIR POLLUTION

Symptoms

Air pollution comes in different forms. Smog, for which Los Angeles has become infamous, results when industrial hydrocarbons and nitrogen oxides unite in the presence of sunlight. In some places such as Kansas City, for instance, other ingredients may be present that are far more harmful to human health: an EPA inventory discovered almost 70,000 lbs. of phosgene in Kansas air. This gas was used to kill thousands of soldiers in World War I.

An even more common place to find air pollution, however, is right in our own homes, apartments or condominiums. Certain invisible gases like radon and carbon monoxide are often higher indoors wherever there are basements, gas ranges, furnaces and people who smoke. Then there is the

formaldehyde from particleboard, insulation, furniture, and carpeting; not to mention the ammonia from cleaning products and an assortment of aerosols from such things as hairspray and air freshener.

Still another potential source for foul air is in the office buildings that many of us are forced to work in from day to day. Besides the asbestos and mercury from fire-retardant or acoustic insulation and paint in them, there are contaminants present besides those previously listed: argon, cadmium, carbon monoxide, hydrogen cyanide, lead, methane, various nickel compounds, and nitrogen dioxide. Many times a variety of these different compounds will collect together in large accumulations, especially in warm weather, to produce a phenomena which the media has often referred to as "sick building syndrome." The World Health Organization estimates that over 30% of all modern buildings currently have indoor air pollution of some kind.

The most common signs of extreme air pollution sickness from home, office or the outdoors are these: throbbing headache, raw throat, eye irritation, runny nose, physical exhaustion, coughing, and tightness in the chest.

Relief Measures

Place a drop or two of lavendar or peppermint oil on a cotton ball and slowly inhale the aroma of either. A nice room spray can also be made by combining 2 drops each of the essential oils of cinnamon, cloves, lavender and lime in 2 1/2 cups of warm water and then spray a fine mist of such into the air around you. Also burning incense that has had a couple of drops of pine, cypress, cedarwood, or sandalwood oil put on it, is another way to purify the air around you.

Also drinking warm herbal teas can help release toxins from within the mucousal lining of the lungs and flush them out of the system more easily. These include chamomile, spearmint, yarrow, coltsfoot or mullein. To one pint of boiling water, add a teaspoonful of one of the above herbs; cover and steep for 30 minutes; then strain and drink while still *warm*.

In addition to the herbs, one is also encouraged to do some deep-breathing exercises in forests that are heavy with pine trees or near the seashore. Both areas tend to generate a lot of negative air ions, which can have a very positive energy influence on the entire body.

And don't forget that potted indoor plants, of the pleasant aromatic kind, help to offset some of the indoor contaminants most of us are faced with each day of our lives. So think about putting some of them in your home and office.

Foods and Nutrients

One must avoid the ingestion of any food that might contain unnatural substances: drugs, pesticides, hormones, lead, aspartame; and eat foods as little cooked as possible. Fruits, vegetables, whole grain breads and cereals, and skim or 1% milk.

Vitamin C is the chief supplement to help the liver oxidize these foreign poisons. Intravenous ascorbic acid at about the 25-50 gram level can reverse the drug or toxic symptoms in a matter of minutes. Calcium, magnesium and zinc are secondary aids.

Look for those foods highest in these nutrients and frequently include them in your diet. The September 1, 1991 issue of the *American Journal of Epidemiology* reported that red and yellow fruits and vegetables substantially reduced the risks of lung cancer in Finnish men. With what we now know about the hazards of second-hand smoke, the importance of eating more of these kinds of produce cannot be over-emphasized. One of the former directors of the National Aeronautics & Space Administration (NASA), Dr. James C. Fletcher, died of lung cancer. He was of the Mormon faith and *never* smoked a day in his life. But he worked around many people who did for years, and as a result of this contracted the disease. He was never much for fruits and vegetables as such.

Another study in support of the prophylactic health benefits of produce and grains against toxic air appeared in the October 1985 *American Journal of Clinical Nutrition*. Russian factory workers who ate a lot of rye or wheat bread, beans, green peas, potato, cabbage, tomato, and cranberries suffered *less* lung problems in poisoned air environments, than did their confederates who didn't consume so much of these things.

ALCOHOLISM

Symptoms

Most people drink to be sociable, and because alcohol tastes good, warms their tummies and relaxes them. But drinking has a dark side beyond the traditional hangover from having one too many: cirrhosis of the liver, cancer, stroke, hypertension, sugar diabetes, gout, inability to sleep, the shakes, indigestion and impotence.

Excessive consumption of alcohol is also fraught with terrible violence as well. It's estimated that at least half of nearly all murders, rapes, muggings, suicides, drownings, highway deaths, and work-related accidents are directly linked to chronic alcoholism. In fact, public intoxication accounts for close to 45% of all arrests made in the U.S. today.

The accompanying table provides an index of symptoms that are geared to the number of drinks consumed and the blood-alcohol level of the body for each of them.

Number of drinks (includes bottles of beer, glasses of wine, or shots of whiskey).	2	3	5
Blood alcohol level	50mg/100ml	80mg/100m	130mg/100ml
Effects upon the body	One feels a little impaired and the body reactions are dimmed a bit.	The mind is joyful, the stomach warm, but the judgement noticeably impaired as inhibitions start to dissapear.	At this level, a drinker's risk of having a serious accident is increased almost fourfold.

Number of drinks (includes bottles of beer, glasses of wine, or shots of whiskey)	10	12	24
Blood alcohol level	260mg/100ml	320mg/100ml	640mg/100ml
Effects upon the body	Personal aggression is greatly magnified, language efforts become slurred, and the chances of being in a terrible automobile accident increases 20 times the normal rate.	At this point, vision becomes doubled or blurred or both; and mental competance is greatly impaired.	By now the mind and body are in the Twilight Zone somewhere.

Number of drinks (includes bottles of beer, glasses of wine, or shots of whiskey)	32
Blood alcohol level	850mg/100ml (1 bottle of cheap or expensive whiskey)
Effects upon the body	The "Grim Reaper" may be calling, as the likelihood of death dramatically increases.

Relief Measures

Fructose is one form of sugar which enables the body to burn alcohol faster than it ordinarily would. An 8 fluid ounce glass with equal parts of orange and grapefruit juice in it will definitely help to speed up the removal of alcohol from the blood stream the morning following "a night out on the town with the boys."

Or consider blending equal parts of carrot juice and pineapple juice together in the same size glass and drinking this instead. Also, spreading some dark honey or black-strap molasses on some Graham crackers or ginger snaps and eating them is still another way to help get rid of whatever alcohol may be left inside the body.

A combination of three herbs will help to repair whatever damage has been done to the liver by alcohol, provided, of course, that the abuse hasn't been prolonged for too many years. Made as a tea, two cups of this mixture should be drunk twice daily in between meals. In a quart of boiling water, combine one level teaspoonful each of black haw bark, peach bark, and dandelion root; cover and simmer on low heat for 5 minutes, then steep away from the stove for another 45 minutes. Strain, sweeten with molasses or honey, and drink.

Foods and Nutrients

Diet plays a big part in alcoholism that is genetically inherited. For a genetic alcoholic, one drink is too many and a 1,000 not enough. Blue-eyed blondes, green-eyed red-heads, and American Indians are at risk to develop alcoholism. For such as these, fried and deep-fried foods and excessive consumption of refined carbohydrates can be disastrous in terms of being able to adequately cope with their alcoholism and trying to help their livers recuperate from such abuse.

Some children indicate by their behavior if they are at risk for alcoholism later in life. Children who crave sugar are more likely to have hypoglycemia. If a child's or adult's behavior can be described as "mood swings," or "Jekyll and Hyde," then they are the ones more likely to need or seek out drugs or alcohol for the quick fix later in life. It is not psychiatric; it is chemical.

Ninety percent of alcoholics have hypoglycemia to some degree. Eighty percent of those with food sensitivities have hypo-glycemia. If both parents have alcoholism, 50% of the children will become alcoholics eventually. If only one of the parents is an alcoholic, 10-20% will become alcoholic, even if the child is separated at birth from the drinking parent. After a period of drinking, an alcoholic is in a state of nutrient defi-ciency. The B-complex vitamins and magnesium are the main ones lost. These are the very nutrients that help to stabilize the metabolism.

Alcoholics need psychological support, extra vitamins and minerals, prefer-ably intravenously for a while. Fifty to one hundred milligrams of each of the Bs, and 500-700 mg. of magnesium for a couple of weeks is prudent. They must eat small amounts of good food every 2-3 hours, and stay away from sugar.

Foods such as blackstrap molasses, nuts, bran, granulated kelp (for seasoning instead of black pepper), tomato or V-8 juice with some lime juice added, brewer's yeast, and dessicated liver, are things which will supply alcoholics with many of the nutrients their bodies desperately need.

In addition, some doctors who treat alcoholism insist that replenishing amino acids plays a vital role in repairing the ravages of a hangover. They say that by consuming a small amount of carbohydrates at the same time (like pasta for instance), it will help to get these amino acids back into the bloodstream much faster.

ALLERGIES (FOOD & ENVIRONMENTAL)

Symptoms

The word allergy was coined by von Pirquet to indicate a state of altered reactivity. Allergy is a condition of sensitivity to some substance, chemically, a protein usually, which is called an allergen. The allergic person reacts in a way that others do not when they eat, inhale, or touch the allergen. Allergy is a normal protective mechanism that has gone off the rails. It's a useful defense for the nose to pour forth its watery secretion to wash out a harmful irritant or bacterial toxin, but plain maddening if it does the same thing for a grain of timothy grass pollen.

Doctors have classified allergic reactions into four major types: Type I is anaphylactic and IgE (Irmiunoglobulin E) dependent; Type II is cytotoxic; Type III is immune-complex mediated; and Type IV is cell-mediated (or delayed reaction). The development of reaginic antibodies like IgE

(or less often IgG) in sufficient quantities, usually evokes the symptoms characteristically associated with hay fever, asthma, hives, and anaphylactic shock and spasmodic breathing. Or put another way, when your body reacts in an abnormal manner to something it doesn't really like, that's an allergy. Stuffy nose, watery and itchy eyes, wheezing lungs, and raw throat are the most immediate signs to look for.

Remedial Measures

Of the three most common allergies—contact, food or inhalant—the last is the most common because we breathe air all the time. The four worst nuisances that are airborne happen to be house dust, pollen, pet dander, and mold. Knowing this can help someone suffering from an inhalant allergy to make some changes in his or her lifestyle. Such as keeping the home or apartment clean and relatively dust-free. Or not living around or being near plants or trees which make such a person routinely sneeze. And certainly keeping dogs, cats, and caged birds out of one's living quarters. As well as to frequently wash baseboards, walls and floors where mold and mildew might easily accumulate.

An air-tight home may be cozy in the winter time, but it's an unhealthy dwelling place, too. Good air-conditioning units, while generating positive air ions that can make us feel sluggish and moody sometimes, keep room humidity low enough to discourage dust mites and molds from accumulating. Keeping windows open or slightly ajar, even in the winter time, provides just enough air circulation to hold down air borne contaminants that could otherwise make us sneeze and wheeze.

Another suggestion which may sound a little silly to some but is actually quite helpful, is to wear a face mask, if necessary. Such as the kind surgeons or house painters using spray equipment might wear on their jobs. If dust mites are a real problem in your home or apartment, then encasing your mattress and pillow in plastic might just give some relief for you at night.

And, believe it or not, getting rid of wall-to-wall carpeting and substituting in its place hardwood floors with throw rugs on them, has helped more than one family who has been horrendously plagued with allergies, mostly of the inhalant kind. Granted it's expensive to do so, but certainly worth the peace of mind and sound state of health. If it isn't practical or economically feasible to do an entire house or apartment this way, then at least make *one* room a sanctuary of sorts that is dust free.

A combination of aniseed, fennel, elecampane, and mullein is very helpful in treating inhalant and food allergies (other than seafood). If an allergy to seafood exists, substitute horehound for mullein. In a quart of boiling water, add 1 teaspoonful of each herb; lower heat, cover and simmer 5 minutes. Then steep away from heat for an hour; strain, and drink 1 cup *cool* twice or thrice daily as needed.

Cold stinging nettle tea, calamine lotion, tincture of witch hazel, comfrey salve or aloe vera gel or juice, rubbed on or soaked into the skin will help bring wonderful relief to contact allergies.

Foods and Nutrients

The authors have noticed something over the many years that they either been practicing medicine, studying diseases in other cultures, lecturing around the country and in Canada or a combination of all of these. It is this: people who consume large quantities of sugary foods tend to have much greater incidents of allergies than those who hold their sugar intake to an absolute minimum. There is somehow a strange corollary between allergic reactions and sweet things, be it a jelly-filled doughnut or some organic dates from your local health food emporium.

The bottom line is that *they're both loaded with sugar* and can trigger an allergy reaction in many hypersensitive people before they know what has hit them. Whenever we've had occasion to readjust people's diets and *take them off of sugar altogether,* we've noticed a dramatic drop in allergic symptoms. Think about it the next time you chow down a candy bar, a piece of pie, a canned or bottled soda pop or cola, or even something healthier like apple or grape juice (both of which are very high in natural sugars, too).

The principal reason that sugar and sugary foods lead to allergies is that they force the blood sugar to rise and fall. When the blood sugar plummets, the body assumes a stressor is operative and the adrenal glands are stimulated to secrete extra cortisol and adrenalin. Cortisol is the hormone that can assuage allergies and inflammations. If it is used up in this inappropriate response, allergies and sensitivities will gain a foothold. The chemicals, like histamine, that are secreted by the allergic process act as stressors themselves and the adrenals become more depleted. This is a vicious cycle to overcome.

It is important to know that the adrenals contain more vitamin C per weight than any other tissues. (Northern Canadian Indians eat fresh adrenal glands in lieu of fruits they cannot get. The result is no scurvy.) People whose blood tests indicate alkalosis are likely to have allergies. Ascorbic acid is an acid and obviously could help to bring the chemistry of the body to an optimal homeostasis. Vitamin B-6 (100 mg.) helps control allergies. And calcium (1,000 mg.) is a natural antihistaminic.

Five to 10 grams of vitamin C per day will help control allergies along with rebuilding the depleted adrenal glands. Pantothenic acid is a known cortisol precursor. Five hundred to 1,000 mg. per day is usually sufficient. Ammonium chloride is a safe acidifier to counteract the alkalinity, and it also provides some nitrogen to help the body make histidine, a natural antihistamine. The diet must be free of sugar and toxins, and an effort made to search out sensitizing foods and keep them out of the diet. Six small meals daily keeps the blood sugar more evenly balanced.

ALZHEIMER'S DISEASE

Symptoms

Memory loss in Alzheimer's is irreversible, though it's benign in the early stages—when victims begin to forget appointments or friends' names. As millions of brain cells die, it worsens inexorably to a malignant state in which sufferers don't even remember that they have friends.

The most obvious symptoms of this heart-rending condition are confusion, forgetfulness and eventual dementia. Those who must live around Alzheimer's victims also experience a toll on their own mental and emotional health as well. It can be a real drain to the psyche and soul, some insist.

The number of Americans reported to have died from Alzheimer's disease jumped more than tenfold in just 8 years. Recently an unassuming little protein fragment called beta amyloid has been arousing considerable interest within the medical community. This aberrant molecule, a small piece of a normal protein called APP, always seems to be turning up in victims' brains, surrounded by masses of dead neurons.

Relief Measures

Several interesting preventive measures of late have turned up in the scientific literature relative to the near management of Alzheimer's disease. *Science News* for August 24, 1991 reported that another brain protein, called substance P, prevents further brain damage by beta amyloid. Now, a large number of scientific reports published in the past few decades have shown that the capsaicin in cayenne pepper actually stimulates the production of substance P within the body. Maybe this is why in countries like Mexico or Thailand which utilize a lot of this chili pepper, you will find very few cases of this disease.

While not conclusively proven as yet, a growing body of evidence seems to suggest that deposits of aluminum in muscle tissue may be a contributing factor to Alzheimer's. *Science News* (131:73) reported on research in Sri Lanka which showed that cooking in aluminum pots and pans with water containing fluorides increases the aluminum concentration by up to 1,000 times *more* than by cooking with *un*fluoridated water. So, installing a water purifier that can remove the fluorides from your tap water and *not* using any aluminum cookware, makes good sense.

Foods and Nutrients

Science News for September 15, 1990 reported that the trace element silicon—present in body tissues as silicic acid—binds to aluminum, reducing that metal's toxic potential. One herb which is abnormally high in silicon is horsetail or shavegrass. Also certain mucilaginous herbs like comfrey and marshmallow roots contain fair amounts of it, too. A product made for Alta Health Products of Pasadena, Calif. called Sil-X probably has one of the highest concentrations of organic silicon to be found in supplemental form. Several capsules each day with a meal is recommended. The product is available in most health food stores nationwide.

Investigators at the Medical College of Georgia evaluated the effectiveness and safety of using large doses of thiamine to treat patients suffering dementia from Alzheimer's disease. As reported in Volume 28 of the Annals of Neurology(1990), there was a substantial slowdown in the deterioration of cognitive functions.

AMNESIA

Symptoms

This is a disturbance in the memory of information stored in long-term memory, in contrast to short-term memory, commonly manifested by total or partial inability to recall past experiences.

Relief Measures

When one of the authors went to Bombay, India in January, 1990 for an important medicinal plants and folk medicine symposium, he was given a nifty Ayurvedic remedy for treating amnesia by several physicians there. A warm-to-mildly hot sesame seed oil massage is applied along the spine, around the neck, over the scalp, down to the heart and solar plexus to increase blood flow. Also, hot packs of boiled, grated ginger root are freely applied as well to some of these same areas. And cayenne pepper is recommended to increase blood circulation, too. All work well for amnesia I was told.

Food and Nutrients

Vitamin B-6 (100-200 mg.) is the chief memory vitamin. It is almost a specific for those who cannot remember their dreams. Magnesium (500 mg.) does help with memory. Manganese (5-10 mg.) may be helpful. Candidiasis can impair memory. L-glutamine has been shown to be beneficial. Acetylcholine may make a difference, too.

ANEMIA

Symptoms

Iron deficiency is one of the most common nutritional shortfalls in America today. Almost 20% of childbearing women have some form of it. And in developing countries, where meat can be scarce and iron-enriched foods difficult to procure, over 60% of the population can be iron deficient in some way.

Body cells contain iron. Much of our iron is present in hemoglobin, the stuff that makes blood red looking, and in myoglobin in muscle tissue. Iron is stored in the liver, spleen, bone marrow, and other organs. Low iron intake over many years can eventually lead to a depletion in these stores, as the body robs it from such places to replace lost blood, as in the case of menstruation, for instance.

The beginning stages of iron deficiency have no symptoms to speak of. It occurs when the body's iron stores become exhausted, a condition marked by a drop in the blood's iron levels and an increase in transferrin, that protein which transports iron throughout the circulatory system. As the iron dwindles in bone marrow, so does the marrow's ability to produce healthy red blood cells, which need iron. If the iron balance worsens, full-blown iron-deficiency anemia—marked by low hemoglobin levels—can develop. Since iron is an essential component of hemoglobin, a shortage of iron can impair the transport of oxygen from the lungs to the body's cells; as a result, work performance is often impaired. It can take months or years for actual symptoms to develop, like weakness, shortness of breath, paleness, poor appetite, and increased susceptibility to infection. But once adequate iron is consumed, all of these quickly disappear.

Relief Measures

Certain plant foods have respectable amounts of iron in them. Herbs like burdock root, yellow dock root, and red clover all contain measurable quantities of iron. Four capsules of any of these daily with meals is suggested. Likewise, beet root is high in iron, too. One level teaspoonful *each* of organic beet powder and Kyo-Green chlorophyll powder from Wakunaga (see Appendix) in 8 fl. oz. of juice or water will really boost the body's iron supply.

Food and Nutrients

About 30 mg. of a good iron supplement is suggested for those who think they may need this. In some cases, where anemia patients may not respond well to supplemental iron, a good dose of vitamin B-6 will do the trick for them. And so far as pernicious anemia goes, injections of vitamin B-12 and oral doses of folic acid will help to overcome that problem in no time at all.

The chart below gives some food sources of iron, but doesn't take into consideration just how well or poorly the iron present may be absorbed into the body. Close to 15-30% of the iron in meat, fish and poultry is absorbed a lot better, than say the 5% from fruits, vegetables, whole grains and eggs would be.

Iron Source (mg)	Amount	Iron
beef liver, sautéed	3 oz.	7.5
clams	3 oz.	5.2
oysters, raw	3 oz.	4.8
pork chop, broiled	3 oz	3.3
steak, lean, broiled	3 oz	3.0
sardines, canned	3 oz.	2.5
chicken, cooked (dark meat)	3 oz.	2.0
lamb, broiled	3 oz.	1.7
tuna, canned	3 oz.	1.6
ham	3 oz.	1.2
chicken, cooked (white meat)	3 oz.	1.0
salmon or white fish (broiled)	3 oz.	1.0
dried apricots	3 oz.	4.0
molasses, blackstrap	1 tbsp.	3.2
baked beans	.5 cup	3.0
potato, baked (with skin intact)	medium	2.8
almonds	2 oz	2.7
lima beans, dried, cooked	.5 cup	2.1
raisins	3 oz.	1.9
spaghetti, enriched, cooked	1 cup	1.4
Brewer's yeast	1 tbsp.	1.4
peas, cooked	.5 cup	1.2
breakfast cereal, fortified	1 oz.	1-10
egg	1	1.0
broccoli, cooked, chopped	.5 cup	0.9
peanut butter	3 tbsp.	0.9
bread, whole grain	1 slice	0.7

Iron deficiency anemia (iron-poor blood) is the most common nutritional deficiency in infancy, especially if the baby is on cow's milk. The iron in all mammalian milk is species specific, that is, the small amount of iron in cow's milk will be absorbed by the calf, but goes right on through the human intestine. Breast-fed babies will not get anemic if the mother is on a reasonably good diet.

Starting solid food at about 5-8 months is appropriate for the bottle baby but not appropriate for the allergy-prone or breast-fed baby. Protein, B-6, copper, folic acid, and B-12 along with iron are needed to manufacture hemoglobin and red blood cells. Vitamin C taken along with iron will boost the iron absorption about ten-fold.

ANEURYSM

Symptoms

An aneurysm is a bulging out of the wall of a vessel due to a genetic weakness or localized infection. About one in 100 of us have one of these areas of weakness. The thin wall may blow out—like an old inner tube—at anytime, bad high blood pressure would encourage the rupture. A cerebro-vascular accident (CVA) is the name given to this usually fatal catastrophe.

Early symptoms can mimic frequent migraine or cluster headaches. The bulge within blood vessel wall itself can either seep blood slowly or else burst at any given moment. This is precisely what happened to the late nutritionist, Paavo Airola of *How To Get Well* fame.

In the event an aneurysm does rupture, a stroke becomes quickly evident. Sudden, unbearable headaches, double vision, and rigid neck quickly occur, and unconsciousness soon sets in.

Relief Masures

Certain herbs are called for here. They can do internal mending and hold high blood pressure down. Yarrow tea and capsules do a nice job of mending injured tissue. So does mullein, too. About six capsules of either, daily with meals, is advised. Or two cups of tea with meals. Also think about using marshmallow root and powdered slippery elm bark as well. About four capsules of each per day is recommended here.

Kyolic aged-garlic extract is one of the very best things for holding down hypertension. The same goes with ginkgo biloba. Wakunaga of America makes a very nice combination of both in a product called Ginkgo Go. About 3 capsules is suggested. These fine products are available in most health food stores. (See Appendix for details.)

Foods and Nutrients

Vegetarians have known for centuries that they will not develop high blood pressure. The predominant fruit and vegetable diet eventually metabolizes in the body to acetic acid. Acetic acid is a specific for ridding the body of sodium. (See the entry under HYPERTENSION for more specific data.) There are few if any clues that an aneurysm is present until the balloonlike weakness erupts and the stroke appears.

Even for someone like Dr. Airola, who was a vegetarian in the latter part of his life, this preventive diet was no absolute guarantee to never getting an aneurysm. Other factors are involved besides diet, and it was one of these unknown things that claimed him quite suddenly.

ANGINA PECTORIS

Symptoms

The word angina means suffocation, for that is precisely how it feels. This is a condition in which the coronary arteries are constantly on the borderline of insufficiency. Because the heart isn't getting enough oxygen, there will be repeated attacks of the same kind of pain common to an ordinary heart attack. But with adequate rest the pain soon passes.

Mostly characterized by a gripping pain like a giant vise around the entire chest, often radiating up through the neck and down the left side of the arm, the pain is often brought on after consuming a big meal loaded with fat and sugar, considerable physical effort and anxiety combined, and just physical effort or emotional upset alone.

The people most apt to suffar angina are those working under stressful conditions, where constant demands are made upon their mental and emotional resources. Such likely occupations would include school teachers, policemen, firemen, bank tellers, airline flight attendants, ticket agents, stock brokers, sales persons, secretaries, computer programmers, professional athletes, coaches, and so forth.

Relief Measures

Breathing clean, clear air is one of the best ways to help defeat angina. Travelling to a wooded area, near the seashore or by a large waterfall, and breathing in that kind of negative air ions helps a lot. Doing some deep-breathing exercises such as is taught in yoga for up to 30 minutes a day can be very beneficial to the heart.

Taking several cups of *warm* hawthorn berry tea also relieves pressure on the heart as well. Drinking some tomato or low-sodium V-8 juice every other day with 1/2 teaspoon of cayenne pepper and a 1/4 teaspoon of lemon juice concentrate mixed into it, will certainly improve blood circulation.

Modifications in the what and the way you eat are important, too. Reduce intake of saturated fats and cholesterol and increase intakes of high-fiber vegetables like radishes, celery stalk, carrot, and green onion and whole grains such as cooked oatmeal, for instance.

Exercise is also important. The aerobic kind (bouncing on a mini-trampoline, horseback riding, bicycling, swimming, and playing tennis) seems to be the best for helping to reduce the plaque congesting the arteries of the heart.

Learning to relax more through meditation, biofeedback, visualizing, reading, listening to soothing music or rocking in a chair, reduces the incidence of pain attacks.

Foods and Nutrients

The low fat, low sugar diet is mandatory for anyone with angina due to coronary vessel narrowing. The fat is limited to 10% of the total calories. A vegetarian diet is ideal for this. Smoking isn't permitted. One to two alcoholic drinks a day are the maximum. Exercise just to the point of slight chest pain only. Vitamin B-6 (50-100 mg) has proven to slow the transition from angina to actual attack. Vitamin C (1,000 mg.) helps, as does magnesium (500 mg.) to prevent a fatal arrhythmia. Coronary by-pass surgery is the last thing on the list to consider.

ANIMAL BITES

Symptoms

Usually produced on the hands, forearms or legs by vicious dogs or angry cats. Such bites may also include lacerations made by the claws of such animals. Besides some bleeding, swelling and itching become evident very soon. And if left unattended for very long, could also result in serious inflammation, throbbing pain and fever. Whereas human bites are more likely to lead to serious infection.

Relief Measures

Thoroughly wash the afflicted areas with soap several times. Then flood with hydrogen peroxide or whiskey. After which put some tincture of mercurochrome on and leave uncovered so that the air can get to it. If pus forms beneath the skin crust, it may have to be lanced with a sewing needle that has been sterilized in the flame of a gas range, match or cigarette lighter. Then repeat above process again.

Dust the area with some powdered golden seal root. And take several capsules of Kyolic aged-garlic extract internally. Both are available under the Wakunaga label from local health food stores (see Appendix). The afflicted sites can also be washed with salt water (2 tablespoonfuls of table salt in one 8 oz. glass of water).

It may become necessary after thoroughly cleansing and gently drying the wound to place a few layers of sterile cotton bandage over it. This sterile bandage will protect the injury from infection and splints it to facilitate more rapid healing.

Foods and Nutrients

Foods rich in vitamins A, C, and E are called for here. Dark leafy greens made into salads, carrot juice, fresh citrus fruits, baked or canned fish, wheat germ, and soybeans are all useful. Additional intake of these vitamins in supplement form may be necessary as well. Zinc (100 mg.) wouldn't hurt either.

ANOREXIA NERVOSA

Symptoms

This malady begins with an innocent flirtation with not eating—usually by a 13-year-old girl who feels she has no control over any aspect of her life. Her parents are furious that she is being so obstinate. They are also concerned that she may starve herself to death. It can happen: one of the authors, who has been a pediatrician for many years has seen numerous cases fitting this typical scenario.

This anorexic girl, however, may be delighted that she has found something that she can control for a change. She may eat two tablespoons of cottage cheese and four lettuce leaves daily as her weight plunges from 100 to 80 pounds and still believe that she is too heavy!

This aversion to food and fear of obesity affects girls and young women more often than it does boys or men. If left unattended, it can prove to be life-threatening.

Relief Measures

Tranquilizing herbs such as hops, catnip, and chamomile in the forms of warm teas, are very soothing to the digestive tract and the nervous system. They help to relieve a lot of inner anxiety a girl may have about her own weight. Of course, plenty of positive support in the way of encouragement from friends and family members will greatly help. Some psychological counseling may be necessary as well.

Foods and Nutrients

Rebuilding her scrawny skeleton with fruit and vegetable juices, is one way to help an anorexic young lady who may still not enjoy eating as such. Liquid nourishment is easier to take because all she has to do is swallow and not do any chewing to speak of.

The anorexic patient becomes severely depleted in zinc as a rule. So much, in fact, that even a weak zinc solution tastes just like water to her. After a few weeks of zinc (60 mg.) and B-complex (3 high-potency tablets) supplementation, she will probably regain most of her appetite.

ANKYLOSING SPONDYLITIS

Symptoms

This is a progressive, inflammatory kind of arthritis believed to be of genetic origin, but usually triggered by sudden stress or a hidden virus. Norman Cousins was stricken with this shortly after his visit to Russia some years ago. Medical treatment barely helped him. His determination to do something about it resulted in a total remission of this disease: large doses of vitamin C (10-20 grams intravenously), and hours of viewing comedies ranging from Groucho Marx flicks to episodes of the old TV comedy, "Candid Camera."

Symptoms include nagging pain in the hips, neck, or lower or middle back, which worsen with bending. Stiffness and lower back inflammation might appear, often at the joint where the tailbone meets the pelvic bones. Spine and chest motion can be difficult and painful. Pain often comes and goes at random, so some victims are fooled into thinking they've "slipped a disc" or maybe strained their backs. In the more advanced stages, the spine becomes forwardly fixed, forcing the victim to walk with head downwards.

Relief Measures

While some of the same remedies suggested for arthritis (see under this entry) will obviously be of benefit, it seems that more mental and emotional efforts are necessary to get some real relief. Negative thoughts and feelings are more harmful in this type of degenerative disease than dietary or physical abuses might be. A definite change of attitude is needed in such instances. The sufferer should opt for more of an aggressive determination if he or she has been previously mild-mannered and passive. Faith and hope are sorely needed here, and stories of inspiration and courage will cheer the patient "onward and upward."

Foods and Nutrients

Citrus fruits and juices and dark leafy greens high in vitamin C are useful. Cousins discovered that intravenous vitamin C helped tremendously: 10 grams the first day, 12.5 the second, 15 the third, and so on until a full 25 grams was being taken by the end of the first week. His sedimentation rate (a test for inflammation) improved significantly as a result of this and lots of laughter. Also, the same nutrients used for Addison's disease and adrenal exhaustion would be appropriate here as well.

ANXIETY

Symptoms

This is an apprehension of danger and dread usually accompanied by restlessness, tension, tachycardia and shortness of breath. These are generally unattached to a clearly identifiable stimulus.

Relief Measures

When one of the authors toured the South some time ago, we came across a place where there isn't much anxiety. The place is Lynchburg, Tennessee, home of the Jack Daniels distillery, maker of fine southern whiskey. Many of the "good ole boys" were sitting around on time-worn benches in their bib overalls outside of the Hardware and General Store, whittling away on their pieces of wood with jack knifes as if nothing ever happened. "Shoot!" snorted local resident Herb Fenner, "tourists like you don't excite me none. I jest set here and keep on doin' what muh daddy and granddaddy used to do—an' that's jest whittling'."

I asked Hank, another "good ole boy" what they did when they were finished. He spat out a stream of dark tobacco juice and drawled, "Shoot! Then we jest fetch ourselves another piece and start whittlin' away on that one."

Herb spoke up and said, "Muh cousin Horace lives up north in Shee-cago, I think. An' works for one of them big corpy-rashuns. 'While back he started worryin' himself sick till he almost keeled over from a heart attack. 'An ya' know what I told him on the phone? Why, I said, 'Horace, your problem is ya' worry too much. What ya' need is to do some whittlin' and then you'll be all right. Last time I checked in with him, he was doing better tho' he told me he couldn't whittle wurth a damn!" (Chuckles and laughters from all of the "good ole boys" sitting there.)

I think what the fellows in front of the general store in Lynchburg were trying to tell me is that you need to get some kind of hobby to divert your attention away from whatever is causing your anxiety. And once that is accomplished somehow, then the mind can obtain much badly needed rest.

Foods and Nutrients

All of us are exposed to stressors of some kind. Some are so hypersensitive that they would freak out if they broke a finger-nail. Others just sail through life as risk-takers: they thrive on new, exciting adventures, and seem to be calm about near-death experiences. One of the authors, who has been a physician for many years, has dealt with many people who notice stressors easily such as going to school, work, church or shopping; in fact, every activity is a scary encounter for them.

Now this poor inability to filter out incoming stimuli is often due to a severe magnesium deficiency. Five hundred milligrams daily is the standard dose. Vitamin B-6 (100 mg.) will make the magnesium work better for them. Six small meals instead of three large ones should be consumed. And *no* sugar should be permitted. This will keep the blood sugar balance normal and reduce the anxiety common to hypoglycemia.

APPENDICITIS

Symptoms

Appendicitis is the inflammation of the appendix, an organ that is a fingerlike, finger-sized offshoot from the intestine, where the small intestine and colon join, in the lower right hand corner of the abdomen. Pain is the first sign that something is very wrong. It usually wakens the sufferer in the middle of the night, starting in the middle of the abdomen but shifting in a few hours to the right lower quadrant of the body.

Vomiting, usually only once, may then occur, or merely nausea and a distaste for food. Tenderness to pressure in one spot can be found. A slightly elevated temperature of around 100 °F. may be present and constipation is common.

A few days preceding these symptoms, however, there is usually indigestion or large discharges of gas, usually in someone not subject to such troubles. Appendicitis is most common through childhood and peaks between the ages of 15 to 30, after which there is a gradual decline.

Relief Measures

Teas made from the leaves of several berry bushes seems to be an old but effective European remedy for treating a condition such as this. Maria Treben, a very famous Austrian herbalist, mentioned an incident which took place many years ago with her seven-year-old boy.

'If a cup of freshly picked blackberry leaves tea was drunk once in a while, there never would be an irritation of the appendix.'This saying of my childhood's family doctor I remembered, when, one morning, my son awoke, looking very pale and feeling pain in the region of the appendix. I rang for the doctor and prepared a cup of blackberry leaves tea immediately and gave it to my son to drink. His colour soon returned and when the doctor arrived he could not find any sign of an irritation of the appendix.

[Also] drink one or two cups of raspberry leaf tea a day, taking care to sip it slowly. Continue to take the raspberry leaf tea until the [appendix] irritation has subsided.

One of the authors was born and reared on a farm in the early part of his life, and had all of his doctoring needs done the old-fashioned way with "granny remedies." At age eight, while living in Salem, Utah, he contracted appendicitis, but no outside medical advice was sought for. He remembers his father (who's still living by the way) giving him small half cupfuls of buckthorn bark tea every six hours or so. Within a few days, the appendicitis had resolved and he returned to school well again.

Food and Nutrients

Appendicitis is virtually unknown among primitive cultures as they consume considerable roughage in their diets. Because of such high-fiber intakes, they cannot get constipated. Most appendicitis cases are found in the chronically constipated and those who subsist mostly on refined foods.

Different methods of food preparation have to be instituted in order to avoid becoming constipated or even getting appendicitis. Instead of peeled, mashed potatoes, choose to serve and eat baked potates with the skins left intact. Rather than boil vegetables to death, just lightly steam or microwave them so that they retain a lot of their crunchiness. Opt for salads more with *raw* vegetables included, instead of the cooked or canned kinds. Eat more whole-grain bread and cereal instead of the spongy white stuff and boxed breakfast foods high in sugar content.

We feel **we must warn** readers that appendicitis is a very serious, life-threatening condition which requires *prompt and immediate medical attention!* The initial pain feels like the worst case of intestinal gas one has ever had, but passing some flatus or experiencing a bowel movement doesn't relieve it. The white blood cell count usually shoots up to about 12,000 mm3.

Sometimes a surgeon isn't sure that the symptoms, the signs, and the blood count clearly indicate the need for an operation. The surgeon may admit the patient to the hospital and have the temperature and WBC checked every 30-60 minutes. This would be the time to try some of the aforementioned remedies, but *not* before. Early appendicitis is theoretically and possibly reversible as it starts from the impaction of a small piece of hard stool or a worm. But once the wall of the appendix becomes inflamed and swollen so that the obstructive fecolith cannot get out, *surgery becomes mandatory*!

APPETITE (LACK OF)

Symptoms

Lack of appetite is usually manifested when a person has a disinclination to eat. A gradual aversion to most food forms, even including favorite dishes. This condition may be partly psychological as well as physiologically based.

Relief Measures

Setting the saliva glands in motion is one way to stimulate an appetite. Saliva seems to have in it a triggering mechanism that kicks the hunger switch on in the gut and brain. Things which stimulate saliva flow include horseradish, green onion, thyme, sage, watercress, celery, garlic, onion, and capsicum. Some can be chewed very slowly (celery) for this effect, while others (capsicum) may be added to food during the cooking process.

Foods and Nutrients

Zinc may be deficient in those who have not eaten well or wholesomely enough. When zinc levels are low, the taste buds send a distorted message to the brain (dysgeusia). Food may taste like excrement and eating is further reduced. White spots on the nails often accompany a zinc deficiency. People so affected often cannot taste a weak zinc solution, but those with normal amounts of zinc in their bodies will spit out the zinc drops because of the strong, disagreeable taste. Standard dose for this appetite deficiency is 60 mg. a day for a week, then reduced to 30 mg. daily for a month, followed by 15 mg. after that on a regular basis.

Foods rich in zinc may also help: brewer's yeast, liver, seafood, soybeans, spinach, sunflower seeds, and mushrooms.

ARRHYTHMIAS

Symptoms

These are irregular heart beats. The heart is set to a specific rhythm of beats under normal circumstances. But in some cases, an irregularity occurs. One evident sign of this is that the rate of beat is often quicker during inhalation and slower during exhalation. Sinus arrhythmia, however is considered normal.

Arrhythmias can develop because of sudden stress. Case in point is the renowned and wealthy hotel magnate, Leona Helmsley. Convinced that she could beat the charges of income tax fraud brought against her, she turned down the New York City state prosecutor's offer to accept a plea bargain and pay two million dollars in back taxes. Instead, she spent well over ten million dollars of her own money in legal fees and six long years in the courts, hoping to win.

For all of her efforts, though, she was found guilty and sentenced to prison. This so shattered her pride and nerves that upon leaving a Manhattan courthouse Wednesday, March 1 8, 1 992, the 71-year-old multi-millionaire collapsed and was quickly admitted to New York Hospital-Cornel Medical Center for arrhythmia and high-blood pressure. Coming from a woman who routinely exercised and kept herself in the best of shape, this sudden health setback surprised everyone, but was prompted by stress.

Relief Measures

One of the first things to avoid is caffeinated substances. These include coffee, colas, soft drinks, over-the-counter and prescription medications, chocolate, and health-food energy supplements containing guarana, kola nut or yerba mate.

Two medical studies have linked arrhythmias with coffee drinking. The first one, the Boston Collaborative drug Surveillance Program, showed a 60% higher risk among those who drank 6 or more cups daily, compared to nondrinkers. The second study, of male medical students at the Johns Hopkins Medical Institute, showed a two-to-three-fold greater risk of arrhythmias and heart disease among coffee drinkers.

Foods and Nutrients

Low levels of potassium in the blood stream can cause a fatal heart beat, irregularity or even stoppage. This was the case in a few score of people on a weight-reducing diet that allowed them only protein: they got no fruit or vegetables where the potassium is abundant. Low magnesium levels can allow the heart to beat irregularly. These people are usually sensitive and ticklish also.

Both minerals should be obtained from food sources as much as possible. Foods rich in potassium include blackstrap molasses, figs, raisins and certain seafoods. Those rich in magnesium include green leafy vegetables, some nuts, bran, cereal grains, and seafood. About 2,000 mg. of potassium gluconate and 600 mg. of magnesium would be the supplemental intake for this condition.

ARTERIOSCLEROSIS/ ATHEROSCLEROSIS

Symptoms

There are several basic differences between the two of these. A general thickening and hardening of the walls of the arteries is called arteriosclerosis, which occurs in two forms. The first type of hardening is caused by slow depositing of calcium in the artery walls, thereby restricting the flow of blood to body cells. A second, much more advanced type of hardening caused by a buildup of fatty plaque within these artery walls is called atherosclerosis.

Symptoms of the first often parallel some of those connected with the second, but are not as easily detected, however. They include, but aren't limited to hypertension, cramping or muscle paralysis, a sensation of heaviness or pressure in the chest area, and pains radiating from the chest to the left arm and shoulder blade. This second is also known as Coronary Arterial Disease (CAD).

Relief Measures

Slow and gradual exercise is the first thing to be done. Walking, clmnbing stairs, bicycling and dancing are some of these. Their lengths can be increased provided there are no adverse reactions and someone is monitoring the progress of improvement.

The second approach is dietary: eliminate or drastically reduce much of your fat intake. Go for "lean and mean" instead of "thick as a brick" in your steaks and ribs. Meat that is too well marbled with fine lines

of white fat may have you ending up on a slab someday. Switch to fish and lamb, for a change. We hesitate to recommend poultry because of the terrific amounts of growth hormones and chemicals in them. And also, because cultures like the Navajo Indians, who *don't* eat poultry seldom ever get cancer.

We also suggest a reduction in fatty dairy products as well, although admittedly they seem to be useful in their place for supplying the body with calcium in osteoporosis. And the medical literature supports our contention that fat and sugar do not mix well in the same meal; in fact, if anything, they only tend to accelerate the process of atherosclerosis much faster. Hence, a bad meal scenario would be something like this: fried steak and potatoes with a glass of 4% milk and apple pie ala mode for dessert.

Garlic and onions really cut cholesterol and triglyceride levels. They can be consumed in the raw form or, in the case of the former, taken as a marvelous health food supplement called Kyolic aged-garlic extract. Whole grain cereals like cooked oatmeal or shredded wheat also help to ream out artery walls. Think of them and 7-grain bread as sort of the food version of the much advertized Roto-Rooter which cleans out your clogged drains and toilets.

Watching your salt intake is important, too. Think of seasoning your food with coarsely granulated kelp (a seaweed) obtainable from any local health food store, instead of the usual table salt or black pepper. You might also think of trimming your refined carbohydrate intake, too.

Foods and Nutrients

The research that the late Nathan Pritikin, an engineer, espoused, has now been accepted as the best and safest method of getting the plaques from the walls of the vessels. His program is a 10% fat diet, plenty of fruits, vegetables and whole grains, skim milk, poulty with the skin intact, and fresh-water or salt-water fish.

According to the July 4, 1985 issue of *The New England Journal of Medicine*, autopsy findings indicated that Mr. Pritikin, who died by suicide in February of that year at age 69, had a "near absence of atheroscle-rosis" in his heart. "The near absence of its effects are remarkable," concluded the doctors who made the initial examination of his remains.

More recent research has demon-strated that serum triglycerides are more of the culprit in arteriosclerosis than even cholesterol is. Triglycerides are a combina-tion of sugar (glycerol) and certain fatty acids (stearic, oleic and palmitic), which are metabolized much like carbohydrates to produce glucose for energy. We usually ingest them in the form of all the things we love such as oil, butter, cream and fried meats. Triglycerides are also made by the liver. After eating a fatty or refined carbohydrate meal, most of the free fatty acids go to the liver and are quickly re-esterified into triglycerides.

The major function of triglycerides is to transport energy to the cells in your body. Triglycerides are the main fat found in your body. In order to be burned for energy, they must be broken down into fatty acids, then transported to muscle cells. If too little energy is expended, the free fatty acids not utilized will become part of the triglyceride and stored again for future use. So, the less active you are, the less triglycerides will be burned.

Here is a list of the "naughty" foods many of us eat on a regular basis, which are sinfully delicious but terribly artery-choking as well. Because of their high triglyceride contents, they should be avoided or greatly decreased in our diets: cocoa/chocolate; diet and regular sodas; cakes, pies, pastries, candy, cookies; white flour products; sugar, honey, etc.; jello, pudding; butter, margarine, lard, etc.; very sweet juices; poultry skin; fried and deep-fried foods; processed luncheon meats; hot dogs; cake mixes; potato chips, roasted and salted peanuts, etc.

In their places, you should consume more whole grains, fresh fruits and vegeta-bles, nuts and seeds, legumes and peas, and fish.

ARTHRITIS

Symptoms

Arthritis is earth's oldest disease. Extinct dinosaurs and mummified pharoahs have had to contend with the crippling effects of osteoarthritis. In An *X-Ray Atlas of the Royal Mummies* of Egypt, this observation is made on page 291: "The most common skeletal abnoramlity in the royal pharoahs is hyertropic or degenerative arthritis." And Science News for April 29, 1980 reported that paleontologists from Brigham Young University in Provo, Utah, unearthed the arthritic skeletal remains of an ancient dinosuar which measured over 120 feet long and wasn't yet "fully grown." They gave it the name of supersaurus.

The major types of arthritis are as follows: osteoarthritis afflicts about 16 million people, mostly of older ages; rheumatoid arthritis afflicts about 2 1/2 million annually and is an autoimmune disease (induced by an immune system gone haywire); juvenile rheumatoid arthritis afflicts about 250,000 kids a year; akylosing spondylitis afflicts about 2 1/2 million (this is the same disease which the late Norman Cousins recovered from and wrote about in his book, *Anatomy of an Illness*); gout afflicts 1.6 million; scleroderma afflicts about 300,000; and systemic lupus erythematosus afflicts close to half-a-million a year, most of them being women.

Characteristic symptoms of rheumatoid usually appear in the body joints first: gradual increasing pain, tenderness, swelling, and stiffness. Swellings are often symmetrical and spindle-shaped; the skin is smooth and shiny and the nail brittle, sometimes discolored. The onset can be more acute, when the joints are hot as well as swollen, and there is a low irregular fever, loss of weight, and general ill feeling.

Relief Measures

Slow and gentle exercise may be the key to removing much of the pain attending arthritis, according to a Houston medical researcher I know. Dr. Chiu Nan Lai, formerly with the M.D. Anderson Hospital & Tumor Institute, informed one of us (Heinerman) a few years ago (1985) that the Taoist exercise and meditation routine called tai ch'i chuan, had helped many of her own friends

and colleagues successfully conquer their arthritic pains.

"It will obviously hurt, when they attempt to stretch," she acknowledged, "but to *not* do any kind of exercise at all is even worse!" Keeping the mind in a proper perspective as one stretches restores basic health to degenerated joints, she reassured.

Two medical doctors conducted an interesting experiment with 101 arthritic patients in Southern California. Half were given yucca capsules to take and the other half lookalike placebos. Of the 50 receiving an average of 4 yucca capsules daily, 61% reported feeling less pain, stiffness and swelling in their arthritis than did those on the placebo. This test was conducted at the National Arthritis Medical Clinic in Deseret Hot Springs, Calif. and later published in the *Journal of Applied Nutrition* (Fall 1975).

Other useful modalities for remedying arthritis include: swimming; heat or ice packs; and massage.

Foods and Nutrients

Arthritic sufferers would do well to avoid bell peppers, eggplant, potatoes, tomatoes, and dairy products, since they are known to actually increase the aggravations common to this disease.

A special kind of fasting is an effective way to treat rheumatoid arthritis, according to the Oct. 12, 1991 medical journal, *The Lancet* (338(8772):899). Scientists observed 27 people on a special diet and 26 people on a regular diet at a health farm. Those on the special diet fasted for over a week, then were put on a vegetarian diet for an entire year. The diet during the fast included herbal teas, aged garlic, vegetable broth, watered-down potatoes and parsley, and juice extracts from carrots, beets and celery. During the next phase, they were then put on a gluten-free vegan diet for 3-5 months. (A vegan diet is an extreme vegetarian diet that entirely omits any type of animal protein, including fish. Gluten-free simply means that these subjects didn't consume any food containing wheat, oats, rye or barley.)

During this diet, they were asked not to eat food that contained gluten, meat, fish, eggs, dairy products, refined sugar, or citrus fruits, salt, strong spices, alcoholic beverages, tea, and coffee. The diet was then changed to a diet consisting of dairy products and vegetables (lactovegetarian diet) for the remainder of the study. After just a month at the health farm, the diet group showed significant improvement: fewer tender and swollen joints, less stiffness, and more grip strength. These benefits were still present a year later. The special-diet group also lost more weight than the regular-diet group did. But the reduction in weight explains only a small portion of the improvement, the report noted. The research said that some people's arthritis might be triggered or aggravated by hidden food allergies.

Useful foods and supplements include olive oil, carrot juice, and vitamins A, C, and D, and copper. Certain oils seem to be the best forms in which to take many of these nutrients on a daily basis: fish oil capulses (equal to 50,000 units) for the vitamin A; cod liver oil (1 tsp. or 2 capsules) for the vitamin D; wheat germ oil (1 tsp. or 2 capsules equivalent to 800 units) for the vitamin E; and olive oil (1 tbsp.). Also zinc (100 mg.), vitamin B-6 (50 mg.), niacinamide

(250 mg.) and copper from blackstrap molasses (1 tsp.) are necessary.

ASPHYXIATION

Symptoms

Asphyxia results when there is an impaired intake of adequate oxygen and a defective release of sufficient carbon dioxide waste gases from the lungs. Immediate signs are a blue discoloration of the skin and obvious breathing distresses.

Relief Measures

If this is caused by food stuck anywhere in the throat, then administration of the Heimlich maneuver from behind a person, with curled fist placed against the abdomen and just above the navel and a sudden, upward thrusting motion to expel the offending object is in order.

For the distressing tight cough that makes me feel I'm being choked, the rubbing of a very small (10 drops) amount of peppermint or eucalyptus oil extracts on the chest, throat, neck and beneath the nostrils of the person is helpful, too.

Drinking some hot peppermint or spearmint tea will also help to increase the intake of oxygen into the body.

Foods and Nutrients

Intravenous calcium and magnesium mixed with vitamin C (20 grams) from your physician will generally stop asthma mid-wheezing. Chiropractors find that a cervical adjustment will usually control many cases of asthma-induced asphyxiation. Drinking hot black or green tea is also helpful.

ASTHMA

Symptoms

This ailment is nothing to wheeze at, since close to 5,000 people die from it every year. And as the air keeps getting dirtier in many of our major metropolises, so too does the incidence of asthma keeping rising with it.

It is characterized by bouts of panting breathlessness, due to temporary closure of the smaller airways in the lung tissues where effective breathing takes place. Attacks of tightness in the throat or chest, with a feeling of suffocation, labored, wheezey breathing with special difficulty in breathing out, and paroxysms of coughing, usually set in. At first, the sputum is sticky, then comes freely and the spasm relaxes: relief but exhaustion. Attacks are common at night or the early morning hours, and can last from minutes to hours, sometimes even days as it were.

Relief Measures

We've put down a list of "don'ts," which we feel are imperative to follow if you expect to get any relief from your condition.

A. Don't smoke or be around second-hand smoke.

B. Don't keep pets in the home.

C. Stay away from central heating and air-conditioning as much as possible. Use steam radiators or wood-burning stoves to heat and circulatory fans to cool.

D. Avoid household (air freshener) and personal (hairspray) aerosols as much as you can.

E. Stay out of frigid air and do not drink ice-cold beverages, no matter how good they may taste on a hot day!

F. Avoid ALL dairy products and eggs, which produce excess mucus.

G. Stay away from sugar and ALL sugary products! We can't emphasize this enough! Our individual and collective studies have shown us that with the omission of sugar and sweet things from the diet, asthma suffering decreases by at least 50% or more!

H. Look out for food additives, such as MSG (monosodium glutamate) and sulphites, since they are known to trigger an asthma attack in no time at all. This means eliminating all cheap luncheon meats such as bologna from the diet.

I. Stay away from pizza! It wreacks havoc with asthma.

Now here's some things "to do" which should afford considerable relief for your misery and suffering:

(1). Do mild aerobic exercises: swimming, playing tennis, jumping on a mini-trampoline, ballroom dancing, horse-backing riding (but stay away from the hay), etc.

(2). Invest in a good juicer. Buy your fruits and vegetables organically-grown whenever possible. And treat yourself to a glass of carrot/pineapple or apple/mixed greens at least once a day. Drink some of the pulp, too; don't discard all of it because that is rich in fiber which the body needs for cutting down cholesterol and triglycerides.

(3). A cup of hot black coffee or green or black tea will give relief during an asthma attack.

(4). Devise your own inhalant. Make a strong tea of eucalyptus and peppermint leaves, then pour some of this solution into an empty and clean spray bottle. Hold the nozzle about an inch away from your open mouth, take a slow deep breath, and just after you start breathing in—about 2 seconds or so—push down on the spray apparatus and squirt some of the tea inside. Continue this procedure, all the while breathing, and then hold your breath for about 5 seconds. We've discovered that this tends to open up the airways rather nicely.

Foods and Nutrients

Researchers at the Columbia University College of Physicians and Surgeons discovered some time ago that 50 milligrams of vitamin B-6 judiciously administered each day to asthmatic patients, really helped to improve their breathing conditions.

Drinking or eating *hot* teas, juices, or broths is also another way to experience relief. Unless otherwise allergic to such spices, including a pinch of cayenne pepper

and a little finely minced garlic clove in such clear soups or broths wouldn't hurt either.

Intravenous injections of calcium and magnesium mixed with some vitamin C (10 grams) from your doctor or an alternative-minded physician should stop asthma midwheeze. Frequent chiropractic adjustments will usually help to control even the worst cases of asthma if preceding dietary guidelines are strictly adhered to.

ATHLETE'S FOOT

Symptoms

This skin infection is characterized by redness, itching and peeling between the toes: patches of soft white skin come off, leaving sore, raw areas instead. Usually caused by a fungus, but sometimes eczema can give a similar appearance. A contact rash will not appear on the web between the toes. The dye or fabric in the shoes is the contractant.

Relief Measures

Soaking your feet in some sea water each day for about 20 minutes, helps to remove infection, an Israeli physician at the big hospital in Tel Aviv told one of us (Heinerman) a decade ago. Or mix your own solution of equal parts (3 tablespoonfuls) of table salt and epsom salts in 1.5 quarts of lukewarm water.

And after this foot soak, thoroughly dry between the toes of both feet. Then take a soft-bristle toothbrush and brush in between them to remove any dead layers of skin. After this, dust them with a generous application of equal parts (1 teaspoonful each) of powdered golden seal root and Arm & Hammer baking soda.

Foods and Nutrients

Cut the ends off two vitamin E capsules, squeeze out the contents and mix with the powder of two crushed zinc tablets. Rub this mixture between the toes daily. Calendula ointment is safe and helpful at times.

ATROPHY (MUSCULAR)

Symptoms

Muscular atrophy is due to old age, malnutrition or debilitating diseases of some kind. It is manifested by the shrinkage of muscle tissue.

Relief Measures

Powdered slippery elm bark made into a soup (.5 teaspoonful in 1 cup hot water) or taken orally (3 capsules daily) helps a lot. Also the coarsely cut bark made into a tea (1.5 tablespoonfuls in one pint boiling water and steeped for 30 minutes) will enable diminished tissue to rebuild itself. And adding yarrow and mullein only expedites the process even more.

Food and Nutrients

Certain protein-rich plant foods are useful in the diet here. Soy-derived products such as tofu, vegetables like okra, olive oil and barley soup are all good to use.

Supplements to be taken should include vitamin E and an amino acid concentrate of some sort.

AUTISM

Symptoms

Autism is a rare condition as it affects one in every 3,000 kids. Outwardly the child looks relatively normal but doesn't behave that way. He or she doesn't respond to his or her immediate environment, fails to make eye contact, refuses affection, and repeats the same behavior again and again.

In the award-winning film, *Rainman*, actor Dustin Hoffman portrayed a man afflicted with autism but still able to do some amazing things, such as multiplying and dividing huge numbers in his mind.

Relief Measures

Rebeccah Christian of Farmington, Utah related some of the things which she did for her own ten-year-old autistic child named Roo. At age 4* when his problems first became evident, his mother started him on weekly chiropractic treatments beginning back in 1986. "After just six months of treatment," she wrote, "Roo began progressing so rapidly in school that he outgrew educational programs shortly after they were written."

In addition to this, the mother started giving her son regular massages on his neck and spine. "...He would get restless...

[so] I would try to relax him with massage and in doing so," she mentioned, "I discovered the acupressure points in his neck were raised and felt like little pearls under his skin, about an inch apart. Energy was trying to move up his spine but was getting stuck at the base of his skull. By putting one hand on the distended points and the other at the base of his spine, I tried to move the energy back down. Sometimes this worked, and sometimes it wouldn't budge. Eventually I got the idea of re-routing that energy through my own body and back into the top of his head, skipping over the part of the circuit that didn't work. As the energy flowed through me and back into him, I felt the hard points in his neck melt away under my fingertips and the muscles relax. He would take a deep breath, sigh and sleep peacefully for another two hours."

Some skeptics may scoff at this particular method of hers, but to those of us who are open-minded enough to understand what true healing is all about, the flow of energy from mother to child makes just as much physical sense as the flow of loving energy does in an emotional way.

Rebeccah admitted that her "best choices have been the intuitive ones, which have come from within me, and not from without." The drug prescription her pediatrician had originally written for her autistic child was never filled. But she didn't discard it either. Instead, she had it framed and hung on her living room wall as a reminder that sometimes the best solutions to complex health problems don't always come out of a bottle or from a doctor's prescription, but rather just from common sense and gut feeling.

Foods and Nutrients

Dr. Bernard Rimland is considered a world authority on autism. His 1964 classic, *Infantile Autism*, became a major contribution in the field of psychology. In the April 1978 issue of the *American Journal of Psychiatry*, he reported the amazing results he had with vitamin B-6 and magnesium therapy in autistic children. (The addition of the mineral is to prevent increased irritability from the B-complex member.)

When both were routinely given to autistic children, most of their behavior problems diminished considerably. And dramatic improvements were observed in social relations with other people and especially in their speech efforts.

Foods high in B-6 and magnesium should be added to an autistic child's diet. Foods rich in B-6 include: avocado, banana, blackstrap molasses, brewer's yeast, cabbage, dessicated liver, fish, green leafy vegetables, meat, organ meat, peanuts, prunes, raisins, walnuts, wheat germ, and whole grains. For instance, .5 lb. of baked trout contains 1.5 mg. of B-6, while 1 cup of fresh or frozen blueberries contains 1 mg of this vitamin.

Magnesium-rich foods include: bran honey, green vegetables, nuts, seafood, spinach, bone meal, kelp, roasted peanuts, and some dried cereals (bran or cornflakes, for instance).

AUTOIMMUNITY

Symptoms

Autoimmunity is a situation in which the bodys' immune system works against its own tissue—heart, kidneys, joints, etc. Immunologists consider this to be a state in which a person's own body tissues are subject to deleterious effects of the immune system. In other words, when someone is suffering from an autoimmune disease of some kind, it's usually that set of conditions induced by one's own immune defenses which apparently have run amok and are wreaking havoc with the body.

Put another way, "an autoimmune condition is one in which the body becomes allergic to itself," as one author wrote in a recent best-seller (*How to Double the Power of Your Immune System*). The symptoms will determine which organ or tissue has been attacked.

These are the diseases which doctors now consider to be autoimmune or body-caused: Addison's disease, ankylosing spondylitis, celiac disease, chronic ulcerative colitis, Crohn's disease, diabetes, Graves' disease (what President Bush's wife has), myasthenia gravis, pernicious anemia, psoriasis, rheumatoid arthritis, scleroderma/dermatosclerosis and systemic lupus erthythematosus.

Relief Measures/Foods & Nutrients

Since nearly all of these problems are discussed elsewhere within this book at length, we will confine ourselves for the most part to just some general recommendations which we believe apply to *ALL* autoimmune disorders.

First of all, white sugar and other hidden food sugars (sucrose, dextrose, mannose, fructose, etc.) must be eliminated from the diet completely. For some strange reason that we haven't quite figured out yet, sugary foods tend to exacerbate autoimmune symptoms a lot more.

Secondly, fried and deep-fried foods should be cut from the diet. Foods ought to be baked, steamed or boiled instead.

And thirdly, white flour products of ALL types should be curtailed. In their place, substitute whole grain cereals and breadstuffs.

Also, *ALL* caffeine and soft drink beverages should be avoided as well. In their stead, opt for fruit and vegetable juices and coffee substitutes (Pero, Ovaltine, etc.)

We are inclined to think that the above classes of foods remove from the body certain key elements which set the stage for autoimmune disorders. These nutrients include: vitamins B-Complex, C, D, and E and minerals like magnesium, manganese, copper, iron, zinc, and chromium.

BACKACHE

Symptoms

Backaches are due to a variety of factors: poor posture, improper lifting, overexercise or overwork, obesity, injury, etc. Customarily marked either by stiffness and difficulty in moving or sudden, jabbing pains that may radiate over a wide area of the back and thighs.

Relief Measures

A Spanish physician, Juan Mendoza, M.D. from the city of Seville told one of us some years ago when we were in his city of Seville, some of the things he did for treating backaches.

Bicycling in a ramrod straight military posture was one of the ways. This necessitates having the handlebars raised high enough to permit this position, however. Another was applying hot packs which had been soaked in a small solution of boiling water and a few drops of peppermint oil and eucalyptus extracts. Ice packs were a third recourse. Gathering yourself into a tight ball while sitting on the floor, and then slowly opening up and laying down in a spread-eagled position was a fourth.

Chiropractors and osteopathic physicians are the best resource for people to consult for back problems of any kind. They have been specially trained for things like this.

Foods and Nutrients

Calcium and magnesium are the main healing nutrients here. These minerals only work, however, if they are in an acidic medium. Doan's Pills (magnesium salicylate) will control pain and provide the safe amount of magnesium in an acid form to help calm the back and other muscles. Another alternative is to take a calcium-magnesium supplement (where the ratio is 2:1) with some orange, grapefruit, pineapple, or grape juice, all of which will provide the necessary acidic medium for their total assimilation into the body.

Ammonium chloride (7.5 grams) is a standard and safe acidifier. One tablet 3 times a day should help. People who are alkaline should notice that the bottle of ammonium chloride smells quite good. Some people who are alkaline because of a high sodium level in the blood will find that they love the taste of vinegar and pickles.

Apple cider vinegar is another good medium to use in conjunction with a cal-mag supplement. Foods made with apple cider vinegar can be consumed when taking this supplement. Guacamole dip, salsa, and cole slaw are just three items which can be made from this healthier vinegar.

Readers should be cautioned, though, that if none of the foregoing remedies or dietary and supplementary suggestions help very much, then a physical checkup with x-rays of the back is in order.

BAD BREATH

Symptoms

If you watch TV to any extent, you've probably seen some of those Scope mouth-wash commercials of late, in which various people who love each other dearly, refuse to be kissed or hugged until they've gotten rid of halitosis problems. Then the're ready for as much smooching and embracing as their partners are willing to give them.

Want to check your breath to see if it approximates that of a German Shepherd police dog? Simply cup your hands, take a deep breath and then exhale into them, while at the same time sniffing. If your brain bells start clanging in alarm and those red sirens of your nervous system commence screaming, then you know your in trouble for sure!

Relief Measures

A Canadian dentist one of us (Hein-erman) knows, who practices a holistic form of dentistry in Toronto, gave the following advice on getting rid of halitosis:

(1). Have your teeth checked for cavities and cleaned regularly. Be sure to brush and floss on a daily basis!

And rinse your mouth regularly with mouthwash, salt water, cold black or green tea (which are great cavity preventers by the way), or just plain cold water. (Wouldn't you know that he would suggest things like this anyway considering his profession and all?)

(2). Stay away from the deli counter and those spicy luncheon meats or sausages that taste terrific, but leave your tantalizing breath causing others to drool as you talk to them closeup.

(3). Booze breath is best avoided by leaving beer and hard liquor alone when in the company of others. Unless, of course, they happen to be party animals, too and wouldn't mind another beer or whiskey breath beside them.

(4). Learn to chew your food more carefully. Undigested meals within the gut always seem to travel back up eventually to let others know this guy or gal gobbles stuff down like the ravenous wolf did Little Red Riding Hood's grandmother.

(5). Chew fresh sprigs of parsley, fresh mint leaves or mint gum or seeds of fennel or anise or a short piece of licorice root bark after a particularly aromatic meal.

(6). Believe it or not, we'd like to add another dental tip our molar mechanic friend in Toronto forgot to add: be sure to swish your mouth out with cold water after eating something to remove debris between teeth; and always remember to brush your tongue in addition to your chompers!

Foods and Nutrients

Foods that cannot be digested down to its basic amino acids, simple carbohy-drates, and fatty acids might be absorbed through the intestinal wall, and passed on to the liver. If the liver cannot detoxify these undigested particles, they will next travel to the lungs and be exhaled for everyone around to notice. The kidneys can detoxify and excrete many poisons also, as well as the skin. When they are properly functioning, the chances of bad breath occurring are greatly reduced.

Digestive enzymes like betaine HCL and comfrey root, pepsin, bromelain, and raw duodenal concentrate will aid the intestines to break the foods down to their basic nutritive components. Some people have nauseatingly bad breath because of post-nasal drip. The most common food causing that is milk, and should, therefore, be omitted from the diet.

Certain foods, which contain some of the above enzymes that are helpful to the gastrointestinal tract, should be consumed regularly with meals. They include papaya and pineapple juices, and comfrey and chamomile teas.

BALDNESS

Symptoms

Baldness is the thinning of the hair in both sexes between their twenties and thirties. Male pattern baldness comes later on, beginning in the front and gradually proceeding to the back. Little can be done for this type as it is genetic and immutable.

Relief Measures

First thing in the morning upon arising, set on the edge of your bed in a bent over position and vigorously massage your scalp with your fingertips for about five minutes. This brief routine exercise will at least keep further baldness from setting in and provide badly needed stimulation to the hair follicles remaining.

The great French herbalist, Maurice Mességué recommended this to prevent baldness: steep one pinch of stinging nettle flower, one of sage blossom, one pinch of burdock (using the entire plant) and one pinch of bay leaf in a quart of water. Let the mixture stand for 24 hours, then wet your scalp generously with this solution.

Foods and Nutrients

He also suggests drinking a glass of watercress juice at breakfast, as well as rubbing some into the hair itself. But the truth of the matter is this: both of us have experienced baldness in our own lifetimes and have yet to find the ultimate cure for it. Then and if we ever do, we expect to become instant millionaires overnight!

Stress can allow baldness to appear. Hair loss might also be an autoimmune disease sometimes. (Dermatologists will inject small doses of cortisone in the scalp skin: often hair grows in that injected area, suggesting that the problem is autoimmune.)

Low thyroid will also cause the hair follicles to atrophy and hair will then drop out. Many women suffer postpartum (after childbirth) hair loss, but if the mother is provided with the proper nutrients it all comes back in 3 to 6 months.

Kelp or other sources of iodine, plus zinc (50 mg.), vitamin A (50,000 I.U. beta-carotene) and pantothenic acid (75 mg.) will speed hair return.

BEDSORES

Symptoms

Bedsores start as redness over pressure points in bedfast people, and will ulcerate unless promptly treated at this stage of development.

Relief Measures

Dr. K. Bhanganada of Siriraj Hospital of Sri Lanka told one of the authors that he and his staff use white sugar (mixed with a little water) and honey to dress bedsores with. Lesions tend to heal more rapidly this way, since both items draw fluid out of skin cells by osmotic pressure and don't irritate. Even major wounds showed improvement, with the sucrose syrup destroying all major bacteria within 7 days.

Foods and Nutrients

Vitamins A (25, 000 I .U.) and E (400 I. U.) and zinc gluconate (50 mg.) are valuable here. Crush 2 zinc tablets into powder. Cut the end off of a vitamin E capsule and squeeze out the oil into the zinc powder. Mix together with a cotton swab and apply to bedsores directly. This promotes rapid healing. Also a couple of the tablets and capsules of each taken internally helps as well.

BED WETTING

Symptoms

This condition occurs mostly in young children. Fifteen percent of boys and eight percent of girls under age six years wet the bed two to five times a week. Their daytime control is usually good. The elderly may wet because of unawareness, infection or poor control from an enlarged prostate.

Relief Measures

Teas made from different herbs, when admistered while warm stop bedwetting. These include balm, bearberry, botony, cornsilk, fennel, hops, pansy, St. Johns wort, horsetail and yarrow. Bring a pint of water to a boil. Add one teaspoonful of any of the above herbs. If the material is coarse and tough, cover and simmer on low heat 5 minutes; if the material is delicate, cover and remove from heat and steep 30 minutes. Strain, sweeten with honey and drink 2 hours before bedtime.

Foods and Nutrients

Older people should avoid drinking coffee or alcohol several hours before retiring since they may cause urination in the nighttime. Magnesium (500 mg.) at bedtime may help the bladder stretch enough to hold at least 8-10 ounces of fluid, the capacity necessary to retain that night's production of urine. Sixty percent of children will wet because they are eating some food to which they are allergic: dairy, wheat, corn, soy, and citrus are the usual culprits.

A protein snack at bedtime will maintain the blood sugar at a level so that the brain will be able to receive the message of the full bladder and get the owner of the bladder up to seek the toilet. Bedwetting is rarely ever a psychiatric problem.

It is said on good authority that chiropractors find neck or pelvic adjustments control bedwetting in over 507~ of all cases reported.

BEE STING

Symptoms

A bee sting causes sharp jabs of throbbing pain, accompanied by swelling and inflammation. Affected area of skin becomes puffy, itchy and reddened in appearance.

Relief Measures

An attempt should be made to extricate the stinger part from beneath the skin by scraping it away with a blade knife. Don't use tweezers as that may force more venom in the tissue. An ice cube brings immediate relief. So does licking the injury with the tongue for several minutes or else drooling saliva on the surface and rubbing it in with the fingers.

A little water or even some urine mixed with some dirt to form mud and then applied also helps as well. Another method is to put a little water or saliva on top of the sting site and then sprinkle some Adolph's meat tenderizer on top and rub it in with the fingers.

Foods and Nutrients

A slice of cucumber applied on a sting brings quick soothing relief. So does some citrus juice (particularly lemon or lime) rubbed on as well. Or cut the end off of a vitamin E capsule and squeeze out the oil, rubbing it into the skin with the fingers. A crushed zinc tablet mixed with vitaminE oil and applied works, too.

BEHAVIORAL DISORDERS

Symptoms

Behavioral disorders are common in all ages from children to the elderly. In kindergarten-age kids, it is often manifested as pouting, crying, shouting, kicking, hitting, etc. In older children and young adults, it includes rebellion, talking back, leaving home for a while, or the "silent" treatment with parents. In the elderly, it includes grouchiness, selfishness, and shouting.

Males act out, become violent or very aggressive. For them it's sometimes considered macho or part of the manly image. Girls are more likely, though, to run away or engage in sex. However, recent news reports indicate that some inner-city girls, who congregate in gangs, have become just as malicious as their male counterparts, if not more so.

Such erratic behavior patterns of contempt and violence stem mostly from sexual or physical abuse at an early age and hatred for authority figures later on. Negative self-images and virtual worthlessness are at play here. Many Los Angeles-area gang members who've been previously interviewed by authors, social workers, and police, cite loneliness and neglect as two of the major factors which led them into the lives of crime that they now lead.

Relief Measures

Irregardless of what age groups are involved in such disorderly conduct, several common factors are jointly shared. First, they usually *want something*. Determining what it is and if such can be given without much difficulty will obviously alleviate the problem somewhat. Secondly, some wants turn out to be very real and legitimate needs. Love, in the form of lots of attention, usually heads the list and should be freely distributed, whether asked for or not.

A sense of *belonging* to someone or something, was the most common need in those L.A. gang members who've been interviewed by others in the past. They stated that when society no longer wanted them, they turned to a particular gang and there found many of the things their own families and society in general had failed to provide them with.

A different set of attitudes and actions is called for, however, when taking care of Alzheimer's patients, who manifest bizarre behavioral disorders. The first virtue is patience, lots of it as a matter of fact! The second is a real commitment to stay with caring for someone this much out of control especially when the individual has lost nearly all of his or her own reasoning powers. The third is the willingness to give of self, to put up with extreme situations from a person who displays infantile behavior much of the time. And the fourth is an understanding that victims of Alzheimer's disease are really adult "children" in many ways, who desperately require the same nurturing instincts that newborn infants do.

Foods and Nutrients

If a person is a Jekyll-and-Hyde personality, the problem is nutritional more than it is psychological. The food the person loves-or even craves-is usually the one causing the blood sugar fluctuations and the inappropriate behavior. Dairy, corn, soy,

wheat, eggs, chocolate, sugar, and citrus are the common ones. But any food can cause the problem. When the blood sugar plummets, the animal brain kicks in. These types of children and adults need nutritional as well as psychiatric support.

A high-potency B-complex vitamin and a good calcium-magnesium supplement (where the ratio is 2:1) are called for. Additional therapeutic information is given under ALZHEIMER'S DISEASE and HYPO-GLYCEMIA.

BELCHING

Symptoms

Belching is usually due to swallowing a lot of air with food, drinking soft drinks, beer, or wine with the same, or eating too fast or too much at once. It's characterized by loud and strange noises travelling up the gut, through the throat and out of the mouth. Most of the swallowed air is due to talking while eating.

Relief Measures

The late Henry G. Bieler, M.D. had this to say about belching in his book, *Food Is Your Best Medicine* (p. 193): "Most people consider a belch a digestant *faux pas*, but in reality it is the vestigal remains of the infant's 'spitting up.' Learn to heed this little warning of nature!"

Sucking on a piece of licorice root, chewing some parsley and swallowing the green saliva juice, sipping a warm cup of peppermint or chamomile tea, drinking some cool papaya or mango or pineapple juice, and chewing your food more slowly and thoroughly under relaxed conditions provide relief.

Foods and Nutrients

Wrong food combinations should be avoided. Examples include dairy products and tomato items (catsup, soup); beer and baked beans; soda pop and hot dogs; coffee and doughnuts; French fries and hamburgers; tossed salad with dressing; etc.

Also some foods deserve to be consumed alone or not at all. A good rule of thumb to remember relative to all melons is this: "Eat melon alone or leave it alone!" The same thing also applies to nuts and bananas.

BELL'S PALSY

Symptoms

Bell's Palsy is the partial or complete loss of function of the facial nerve, usually on one side. It may be due to a virus and may come on after exposure to cold, or an ear infection may cause an inflammation of the nerve in its passage near the ear canal.

Identifiable characteristics include: stiffness and loss of motor nerve power in the face; an inability to close the eyes or to raise the eyebrows or to pucker up and whistle; a lop-sided smile; slight pain.

Relief Measures

Massage is one of the very best remedies we've found for this particular

malady. The subject should be in a reclined position when this is administered by someone else. The hands of the therapist should be covered with a good oil (olive) or cream to permit them to slide easily over the surface of the skin.

Sitting behind the patient's head, the therapist should begin on the sides of the neck and with fingers spread a part, pull upward towards the ears from the shoulders. Then work across the throat, face and forehead in gentle pulling strokes. Do this procedure about 10 minutes twice daily.

Foods and Nutrients

All the B-complex vitamins help improve nerve function. About 50 mg. of each of the B-s daily is about right for this. Vitamin B-12 shots help; so does folic acid at about the 4 mg. level. Magnesium in about 800 mg. amounts is suggested, too.

BEREAVEMENT

Symptoms

The "bereavement factor" as we prefer to call it, is most common among middle-aged and elderly persons. But moreso with those who've had a happy marriage, a solid bank account and a sense of control over life, than with those who've had lousy marriages, live from paycheck to paycheck and feel dominated by others. This is according to some of the latest research presented by psychologists from the State University of New York at Stony Brook and a sociologist from the University of Michigan in Ann Arbor, at the annual meeting of the

American Psychological Society held in Washington, D.C. during the middle of June, 1991.

Mourning the loss of a friend or companion is quite healthy and normal. But excessive grief that runs into months or even years sometimes isn't that good for the surviving individual. Different studies — *Journal of the American Medical Association* 250:374-77 and the *American Journal of Psychiatry* 144:437-41—have shown that those plagued by continual bereavement, suffer significant drops in their white blood cell counts and are more susceptible to infections than others their own age are. Additionally, such sometimes become more suicide prone and wreckless as well.

Relief Measures

We think that for those plagued by this "bereavement factor" to keep on hand personal momentos (photographs and letters) and souveniers (articles of clothing, gifts) of their dearly departed for very long, isn't always a good idea. Such treasured items can be kept in storage in boxes, but not always displayed out in the open where eye and brain contact can immediately conjure up old memories that bring with them renewed pain and suffering.

A growing body of medical research in the past decade has supported the concept of adopting a pet of some kind to help fill the void. Unless otherwise allergic to such creatures, chronic bereavement victims can find a great deal of love and support from cats and dogs, who like to lick, rub, caress, and curl up next to their new-found masters. This has a way of taking away the hurt and pain that words alone are insufficient to describe.

Becoming involved with the needs of others is an excellent way to overcome personal grief. Or as we prefer to put it, "losing yourself in the service of others" helps you to forget your own problems for a while. Stan Kreutzfeldt, a Jewish rabbi in an East Coast city whom one of the authors knows, lost his dear wife of many years not too long ago.

They were extremely close and loved each other dearly. When she died, his world nearly came apart. Friends and colleagues in the local neighborhood and synagogue who knew him well, became very concerned with his state of mind. Until one day someone suggested to him to become involved in a local organization which helped disadvantaged kids from the ghettos.

Soon Stan became a "grandfather" of sorts to some special needs youngsters in helping them to read and spell better. Those few hours he spent with them every day soon helped him over his terrible slump and he was on the road to complete recovery in no time at all.

Food and Nutrients

Bereavement makes the body lose potassium. When potassium is low, heart arrhythmias and elevated diastolic pressure may cause sudden death. "He died of a broken heart" is an accurate description of the events. One of the authors knew of a specific case in which a middle-aged white woman had just lost her husband through cancer. They had been married for 35 years and she was beside herself as to what she would do without him. She was placed on a special diet of high-potassium foods for 3 months, during which time her state of mourning ended, her depression cleared up, and her attitude significantly improved.

Here is a short list of some of those foods she ate regularly during this mourning period of her life:

Food Item (mg)	Amount	Potassium
Potato, boiled:	1 serving (3/4 cup)	10.50
Banana	1 small 6"	9.50
Carrots, fresh	1 serving (3/4 cup)	8.74
Celery, fresh	1 serving (3/4 cup)	8.70
Tomato, fresh	1 serving (3/4 cup)	6.25
Prune juice	3.5 oz.	6.00
Apricots, canned	3 halves	5.90
Tomato juice	1 oz.	5.82
Orange juice, fresh	3.5 oz.	5.82
Broccoli	1 serving (3/4 cup)	5.64
Orange, fresh	1 small	5.00
Beets	1 serving (3/4 cup)	4.28
Asparagus	1 serving (3/4 cup)	4.25
Strawberries, fresh	10 large	4.20
Cucumber, fresh	1 serving (3/4 cup)	4.10
Grapefruit juice	3.5 oz.	4.10

Dark-leafy greens in the form of salads is also another rich source of potassium. Magnesium (800 mg.) and valerian root (3 capsules) will also help the body to withstand bereavement.

BERI-BERI

Symptoms

This specific form of polyneuritis occurs in endemic form in eastern and southern Asia, but sporadically in other parts of the world without reference to climate. An increasing problem within the United States, mainly in alcoholics and the growing number of homeless people, due mainly from an insufficiency of B-1 or thiamine.

The sensory nerves are more likely to be affected than motor nerves, with symptoms beginning in the feet and working upward with the hands affected late in the course of the disease. Initially, the deep tendon reflexes are increased, but later on they may be absent. The muscles are often tender and may atrophy. Foot and wrist drop occur. Fatigue, decreased attention span and impaired capacity to work are striking.

Relief Measures/Foods and Nutrients

The B-Complex component, thiamine, is the vital key here. Foods rich in B-1 include: blackstrap molasses, brewer's yeast, brown rice, barley broth/soup, other whole grain cereals, fish, meat, nuts (especially pecans and almonds), organ meats (liver), poultry, wheat germ, lobster, sunflower seeds, etc. We think a high-potency B-Complex supplement is important to take (4-6 tablets daily). When B-1 is low, so are all the other Bs.

BIRTH CONTROL MEASURES

Symptoms

Any methods or means used to prevent the development of the fetus within the womb after sexual intercourse is birth control.

Relief Measures

Hundreds of food and medicinal plants worldwide have been evaluated for their contraceptive effects in animals and people. Test animals employed for such purposes have included rabbits, hamsters, gerbils, rats, mice, quail, sheep, and male canines. While it's rather difficult to apply the antifertility results of a particular plant in an animal to a person, those experiments conducted with male dogs can be said to be somewhat relevant to men, "since male dogs are known to have reproductive organs anatomically similar to those of men" (*Indian Journal of Experimental Biology* 18:459, May 1980).

The following list of possible birth control agents from plants in no way suggests that any of them will be 100% effective in people, but at least demonstrates that within the botanical kingdom, there are natural options available besides medical devices and drugs, for those choosing to limit the increase of their offspring.

ALFALFA (Medicago sativa). At certain times of the year, alfalfa is known to generate compounds which suppress hormones necessary for fertility of animal sperm. (*Veterinary Record* 74:1148-50, 1962)

BANJAURI (Vicoa indica). Routinely used by the tribes in Bihar State (India) as a natural contraceptive in women right after childbirth. Clinical testing with it shows remarkable antifertility activity when administered in the postpartum period. (*Indian Journal of Medicinal Research* 78:724-25, November 1983)

BAYBERRY (Myrica cerifera). A flavonoid glycoside, myricitrin, present in the berries is toxic to sperm. (*Journal of Pharmaceutical Sciences* 63:958-59, 1974)

BORAGE FAMILY (Boraginaceae). German scientists isolated lithospermic acid from comfrey, which exhibited strong antigonadotrophic activity. (Gonadotrophins are hormones which stimulate the growth of sex cells within the testes or ovaries of men and women. Thus, something antigonadotrophic in nature would prevent this from happening.) (Journal of Pharmaceutical Sciences 64:546, April, 1975).

CHINA ROSE (Hibiscus rosa sinensis). This is a common ornamental plant widely cultivated throughout India and Bangladesh, where population explosions are a definite problem. Extracts of the flowers were given to pregnant rats in the first several days of their pregnancies, with 50% 70%, and 100% antifertility effects being realized. These effects depend, though, a lot upon the dose, duration of the treatment and the stage of the pregnancy in which it's to be administered. China rose accomplishes this by rapid expulsion of fertilized ova from fallopian tubes and by disturbing or upsetting the delicate estrogen-progesterone balance, resulting in termination of pregnancy. (Planta Medica 29:321-29, 1976) In another study done at Banaras Hindu University in Varanasi, India, effectively inhibited the release of gonadotrophins from the pituitary glands of young male rats, which in turn had a direct inhibitory effect on their testes as well. After frequent sexual engagements with female rats, no evidence of pregnancy was observed. However, the initiation of spermatogenesis in these male rats could be achieved once they stopped taking the China rose extract. (Plant Medica 31:127-35, February 1977) Positive research like this lead at least one scientific journal to pose the question as an article title, "Is Hibiscus rosa sinensis Linn. a Potential Source of Antifertility Agents for Males?" (International Journal of Fertility 28:247-48, 1983)

EUCALYPTUS (Eucalyptus globulus). Zoologist Roger Martin with Monash University in Clayton Victoria, Australia, did some preliminary work with phytoestrogens in eucalyptus and discovered low fertility in some koala bear populations in Victoria, which consumed these leaves in abundance. (Australian Wildlife Research, Vol. 8, no. 21; and personal letter to John Heinerman, dated Feb. 9, 1981)

GARLIC (Allium sativum). Chronic administration of garlic powder resulted in the arrest of sperm production in white albino rats and a shrinkage of their testes as well. (Indian Journal of Experimental Biology 20:534-36,1982)

GINSENG (Panax ginseng and Eleutherococcus sp.) The genetic crossing of Korean ginseng root with Siberian ginseng cells resulted in a new type of hybrid plant, which when made into an extract and exposed to male sperm cells resulted in their heads shriveling and becoming totally inactive. (Münchener Medizinische Wochenschrift 127:60, March 1980).

GUAVA (Psidium gua java). Guava root was boiled in hot water and then the aqueous extract evaporated under pressure. After which the brown amorphous residue was dissolved in distilled water and fed orally to rats and mice. In male rats the testes shrivelled to some extent and sperm production dropped dramatically, while in females a desire to not permit coitus with males resulted. Pretty much the same things were evident in the mice as well. This somewhat substantiates the use of guava root by South Chinese and Japanese monks to suppress their libidos. (The Tohoku Journal of Experimental Medicine 62:287-302, 1955)

JUNIPER (Juniperus species). Twenty plants were studied in India for their antifertility activities. Juniper was one of them and showed a 60% effectiveness. (International Journal of Crude Drug Research 24:19-24, March 1986)

LICORICE (Glycyrrhiza glabra). The root of licorice has been used as an effective Oriental contraceptive in Korea. (Korean Journal of Pharmacognosy 8:81-88, 1977)

MAYTENUS (Maytenus ilicoflia). Employed as a long-term contraceptive in parts of the rural parts of Paraguay. Women drink a decoction of the roots, branches and leaves after giving birth, and they do not conceive again until their children reach the age of walking. (*Economic Botany* 31:303, July-September 1977)

PEAS (Pisum sativum). The antifertility effects of garden peas was discovered quite by accident. An Indian study involving the vitamin contents of different cereals lead to the observation that male and female rats fed on a restricted diet consisting entirely of "matar" or peas didn't produce any offspring like they should have. Another Indian study showed that the litter production in mice was substantially decreased when the animals were fed peas at a level of 20% in their diets; litter production was totally abolished when the level was raised to 30%. Both studies are interesting in light of the fact that the population of Tibet had remained stationary for the past 200 years and, coincidentally enough, that the staple diet there consisted chiefly of barley and peas. (*Journal of Pharmaceutical Sciences* 64:541, April 1975)

PURSLANE (Portulaca oleracea). This food plant occurs in abundance. An alcoholic extract of the seeds was given by subcutaneous injection to male albino mice. The treatment produced tremendous shrinkage of their testes and suppression of sperm production. (*Indian Journal of Medicinial Research* 75:301-10, February 1982)

RED CLOVER (Trifolium pratense). Phytoestrogens (mostly isoflavones) like biochanin A, formononetin, genistein, daidzein and others found in red clover, have manifested definite infertility activity in certain mammals and birds. Some of these effects have been observed in sheep in Western Australia. (*Australian Journal of Experimental Biology and Medical Science* 29:105-13, 1949; and *Canadian Journal of*

Animal Science 60:53-58, March 1980) The presence of large amounts of formononetin and genistein in the red clover and other grasses consumed by California quail, seemed to have a definite inhibiting effect upon their reproduction abilities. (*Science* 191:98-100, Jan. 1976)

STONEWEED (Lithospermum ruderale). In 1941 a treatise by the U.S. Dept. of Agriculture on the medicinal plants of Nevada Indian tribes, contained the following information on this particular plant. "In one settlement...the plant has contraceptive properties, and...a cold water infusion of the roots, taken daily for a period of 6 months, will induce sterility thereafter." (*Contributions Towards a Flora of Nevada,* No. 33, Medicinal Uses of Plants by Indian Tribes of Nevada, Division of Plant Exploration and Introduction, Bureau of Plant Industry, USDA, Washington, D.C., Dec. 1, 1941) Scientific experimentation has shown that alcohol extracts of stoneweed root administered to mice, in their diet, inhibits or abolishes the normal estrus cycle and reduce the incidence of birth. (*Proceedings of the Society for Experimental Biology and Medicine* 73:311-13, February 1950)

WAX MALLOW (Malvaviscus conzattii). This is a common ornamental plant. The flower thereof possesses a resemblance to that of China rose. Similar antifertility effects of an alcoholic extract of the flowers were observed on male albino mice after administration to that reported for China rose. (*Indian Journal of Experimental Biology* 18:561-64, June 1980) Daily administration of this extract of wax mallow flowers orally to adult male dogs for 8 weeks "induced an antifertility state without altering general metabolic activities." (*Indian*

Journal of Experimental Biology 16:245-49, Feb. 1978)

WILD YAM (Dioscorea villosa). A midwife from Bay City, Texas, one Willa Shaffer reported her own experiences with this particular herb in 1986. "I found a source for wild yam in July of 1981, and I lost no time in rounding up the ladies who were interested in testing this herb. Since July of 1981, I have tested this herb, as a contraceptive on approximately 75 women. Out of the original 75 women who began testing this product there are still 56 women who are using it as their *sole* form of contraception. Out of the 19 women who are no longer taking it, three women decided to have a baby and intentionally became pregnant. Six of these women forgot to take it or did not take it as I directed.... The other ten women who are no longer involved in the research dropped out for unrelated reasons and I do not know about them...[This is] a birth control with no known side effects and obviously boasting a terrific success rate.... The ages of the women tested ranged from 17 to 47 years of age. The women involved had zero to six children each. The races of the women tested so far have included Caucasian, Negro and Latin American.... A very important finding is that in the four years I have been testing this contraceptive I have had absolutely no reports of side effects.... My recommended dosage is three capsules in the morning and three capsules at night...four or five weeks in advance [of sexual intercourse].... I believe that the wild yam causes the eggs to become sterile. The woman still ovulates (produces eggs); however, when these eggs unite with sperm they are not productive." (W. Shaffer, *Wild Yam: Birth Control Without Fear*)

YELLOW PINE (Pinus ponderosa). An aqueous extract of yellow pine needles limited the reproductive abilities in female mice in the laboratory. (Canadian Journal of Animal Science 41:1-8, 1961)

Foods and Nutrients

Omission of certain supplements and foods rich in them may also be another means of natural birth control. The primary nutrients here that are necessary for optimal reproductive performance are vitamins C and E, folic acid, and zinc. (*British Journal of Nutrition* 55: 23-35, January- February 1986; and *Indian Journal of Experimental Biology* 18:1411-14, Dec. 1980)

BIRTHMARKS

Symptoms

Birthmarks may be present on the skin of the newborn infant. Some can be seen as reddened patches on the forehead, upper lip, or back of the head and neck. Such "stork bites" as they're nicknamed are common and usually disappear within a few months.

Port wine marks are flat purple stains that may occur any place but mainly in the same areas as stork bites do. They don't disappear, but grow in proportion to the rest of the skin. A famous world leader who bears such a birthmark on the top of his bald head is Mikhail Gorbachev, former leader of the Soviet Union.

Strawberry marks are soft, raised, red and rounded areas, sometimes bluish, appearing in the first few weeks, enlarging for several months and then remaining the same until, in most cases, they gradually disappear altogether.

Moles are quite common, brown or black in color, flat or raised, and sometimes hairy.

Relief Measures

Maria Treben, an Austrian nun and famous European folk healer, claimed that her Swedish Bitter mixture would get rid of just about any birthmark imaginable, including moles, warts, liver spots, corns, etc. She said that these areas of the skin need to be moistened frequently throughout the day with a wad of cotton soaked in her mixture and kept in place for a while until dry.

Here is her formula for Swedish Bitters. Combine ten (10) grams of each of the following powdered herbs: wormwood, myrrh, senna, Chinese or Japanese camphor, rhubarb, zedoary, canine thistle and angelica. Then put into a wide-necked two-litre bottle and pour 1.5 litres of 38% rye whiskey or vodka over the same. The bottle is then left standing in the sun or near the stove for two weeks and shaken twice daily. The liquid is then strained and poured into small bottles, well stoppered and stored in a cool place. This way it can be kept for years! Be sure to shake contents well before using.

Foods and Nutrients

Vitamin A and zinc are the skin support nutrients. They should be used for people who have any skin lesions. Nothing but time works on real birthmarks.

BITES

Symptoms

Bites are the punctures or lacerations that may result from snakes, scorpions, centipedes, spiders, other insects, cats, dogs, and humans. Depending on the nature of the material propelled into the puncture wound of the skin—i.e., venom, saliva, bacteria, viruses—the local reaction will be immediate or delayed, accompanied by varying degrees of pain, itching and burning, and systemic manifestations peculiar to the offending agent.

Those experiencing bites of this type are strongly advised to get immediate medical help wherever possible and not to be satisfied with self-treatment alone!

Relief Measures

The area should first of all be thoroughly cleansed with soap and water. A strong tea made from hot water (1 cup) and some powdered goldenseal root (1 tablespoonful) should be consumed as soon as possible; the mixture will taste horribly bitter and should be taken on an empty stomach. One thing we've observed over the years is that consumption of animal proteins in the form of meat when such bites occur, tends to aggravate things a lot more. So any type of animal flesh shouldn't be consumed during the worst stages of a bite.

Where venomous materials have been introduced into the bloodstream from a bite, especially from poisonous spiders and snakes, the application of heat to the surface of the skin within the first several minutes seems to break down the protein complexes of such toxins and renders them less harmful to the system.

See also under specific entries: SNAKE-BITES and SPIDER BITES as well for additional information.

Food and Nutrients

Vitamin C is a must and most ideally, ought to be given intravenously. Twenty to fifty grams of vitamin C intravenously neuralized with calcium or sodium should be given as soon as possible. If unavailable, this amount or more should be consumed in 12-24 hours. Zinc (100 mg.) and vitamin A (100,000 I.U.) promote healing. Allergic reaction to bites are assuaged with C and pantothenic acid (100 mg.).

BITOT'S SPOTS

Symptoms

These spots are characterized by white, foamy, elevated, and sharply outlined patches on the whites of the eyes, usually caused by a deficiency of vitamin A., rare in Third World countries.

Relief Measures/Food and Nutrients

Dark leafy greens and plenty of vitamins A and D are the keys to clearing this problem up. Lots of leafy spinach or dark Romaine lettuce, plenty of parsley, and similar vegetables rich in beta-carotene should be consumed frequently. Also freshor salt-water fish of different types should, likewise, be included in meals.

A good fish oil vitamin A supplement can be taken as well. About 50,000 I.U. (or two 25,000 I.U. capsules) is recommended each day for 10-20 days. The protein from egg yolks is good for this, too, when mixed in with some vitamin D-enriched milk.

BLACK EYE

Symptoms

Black eye is the accumulation of blood under the loose skin of the lid.

Muscle tissue around the eye becomes baggy and permits leakage of an unusual amount of blood and fluid after a blow. This means that a bruise in this area has a striking appearance, disproportionate with the degree of injury.

Relief Measures

A cold compress is called for here and left on until it becomes warm, and then changed for a fresh one. Or else an ice pack placed directly over the site is recommended.

As the slow healing process takes place, color changes become inevitable, moving from red to deep purple, through green to yellow as the extravasated blood is altered chemically and removed. The entire process takes about two weeks.

Food and Nutrients

A cold, raw beefsteak placed over the eye has been a traditional remedy since at least the turn of the century. The cold slows the swelling. A few minerals and vitamins also are valid for this problem. Calcium (800 mg.), chromium (150 micrograms), iron (35 mg.), pantothenic acid (100 mg.) and vitamin C (3,500) are especially helpful. A good enzyme complex (two tablets daily) will also speed the reduction of the blood and swelling.

BLACKHEADS

Symptoms

Blackheads are properly called comedos by dermatologists. The closed kind are familiarly known as whiteheads, while open comedos or blackheads have a wide opening on the skin surface capped with a blackened mass of skin-surface debris. Comedos are the primary lesions of acne vulgaris.

Relief Measures

Wash the face with pine tar soap (obtained from a veterinary supply house or animal livestock center). Rinse with cold water. Dry thoroughly with a new hand towel by rubbing the face and forehead briskly but not to vigorously. Afterwards splash on a little tincture of witch hazel with the hands and allow to dry.

The famous French herbalist, Maurice Mességué claimed that in the "old country" of his native France, folks would rub the faces of their teenagers "with quarters of fresh tomato or morsels of ripe pumpkin. Gentle massages of this sort can absorb the imperfections," he added. He also made his own anti-blackhead lotion "steeping one pinch of celandine and one pinch of dande-

lion root overnight in a quart of spring water."

Rubbing alcohol on a cotton ball rubbed over the greasy skin will slow the formation of these comedos.

Foods and Nutrients

Some zinc (25mg.) and vitamin A (25,000 I.U.) are useful for this problem. Greasy and sugary foods and things like chocolate should be restricted from the diet as much as possible.

BLACKOUT

Symptoms

This is a temporary loss of consciousness due to decreased blood flow to the brain.

Relief Measures

Joseph Smith III, son of the Mormon Prophet, Joseph Smith, Jr., related this episode in his life's *Memoirs*. In the Summer of 1843, when his folks lived in Nauvoo, Illinois, he and the family took a carriage ride. "Upon getting into my seat...," he recalled, "I thoughtlessly put my hand around one of the carriage posts, and as the driver closed the door, two of my fingers were pretty badly crushed."

His mother, Emma Smith, bound up the bleeding wounds with some clean strips of cloth. But the pain proved to be so intense that young Smith momentarily fainted. To revive him, she took "from her trunk a little bottle of whiskey and wormwood...turned the tips of my fingers upward and poured the liquid upon them, into the dressings..." The jolting effect it had upon his nerves and heart promptly brought him out of his unconsciousness in no time at all!

Also valerian and wormwood in a shot glass of whiskey or some asafetida tied up in piece of muslin, and either of them held beneath the nose will quickly bring someone around from a blackout.

Foods and Nutrients

A piece of fresh gorgonzola or limburger cheese held under the nostrils of someone who has suffered a temporary blackout, is guaranteed to revive the individual just as quickly as smelling salts or ammonia will.

BLADDER PROBLEMS

Symptoms

There can be different types of difficulties associated with this one particular organ. For instance, a nervous bladder is a condition in which there is a neurotic wish to urinate frequently, but sometimes with failure to empty the bladder completely. Bedwetting is another bladder problem.

Then there are infections of the urine itself, usually called cystites. These can be detected by the presence of cloudy or bloody urine, pain on urination, frequency and burning, little or no fever, and occasionally pain in the lower back, and nausea. A specimen of urine under the microscope will show that it is loaded with white blood cells, the usual response to infection. Kidney infections are more serious and will show as chills and fever, backache, but not burning or frequency, but the urine will usually show the pus cells of such an illness.

Relief Measures

Maurice Mességué, a famous French herbalist, prescribed cherry juice or "a cup of cherry stem tea every evening" for those with bladder problems. He also recommended that they eat "a good dish of strawberries every evening during the strawberry season" because it "refreshes the entire body!" He also advised bladder sufferers to take a little onion wine every day as well. Here is his recipe for that: "Take 250 grams of onions and chop them fine. Mix with 100 grams of honey and a pint of white wine. The mixture is curious-tasting," he claimed, "but effective." 3-4 spoonfuls should be taken daily.

Foods and Nutrients

A daily glass of freshly squeezed orange juice is good for the vitamin C content to stop bladder infections. Israeli scientists have recently discovered that both blueberries and cranberries have bacteria-fighting properties that work against bladder infection. Both berries contain a compound that weakens E. coli, the chief cause of bladder infection, by preventing the bacteria from clinging to cells along bladder and digestive tract linings. Frozen or fresh blueberries may be eaten alone and Ocean Spray Cranberry or Cran-Raspberry Juice may be consumed regularly instead of water.

Vitamin C is the key nutrient here as it can control infections as well as acidifying the urine. The usual bacteria that invade and infect the urine will not grow in acid urine. Five to ten grams of C should control the infection. An intravenous dose would do it faster.

BLEEDING

(INTERNAL & EXTERNAL)

Symptoms

Some loss of blood each month in a woman during her menstrual period is normal; an excessive amount, however, isn't and needs prompt attention. A bloody stool may result from bleeding hemorrhoids or a problem inside the colon itself. Blood in the urine will give it a smoky tint or red if the amount is large enough. A bleeding stomach ulcer, an enlarged prostate, a bleeding kidney or a tissue or vessel tear within the colon somewhere, are just a few of the things that may account for bloody stool or urine.

External discharges of blood from the mouth or nose may indicate a ruptured blood vessel somewhere. Surface bleeding on the skin is usually attributed to a cut or wound of some kind. Outward bleeding is easier to treat than internal kinds. We must caution that *any* bleeding from an outward organ must be investigated to rule out cancer or other life-threatening conditions.

Relief Measures

Maurice Mességue, a great European folk healer, called pimpernel a wonderful agent for "controlling all sorts of hemor-rhages, from nosebleeds to blood in the urine and abnormal vaginal bleeding." A decoction is prepared "by boiling a handful of the plant, including a good bit of the root, in a quart of water for about 10 minutes." Then "drink a wine glass of this several times a day." Spotted cranesbill or wild geranium root, sumac, white oak bark, witch hazel, gold-enseal and powdered kelp (a seaweed) are also very effective for this.

Teas can be made from nearly all of them to stop internal hemorrhaging, while powdered goldenseal root or kelp can be dusted on surface bleeding to stop it fairly quickly.

Foods and Nutrients

Strong, day-old black coffee or black tea will also stop internal bleeding. Dusting external cuts or wounds with some white flour is effective when nothing else is avail-able to halt blood flow. So too is some crushed vitamin C tablet powder sprinkled on the skin.

BLINDNESS

(TEMPORARY)

Symptoms

The type of blindness which we speak about here, is that kind which is reversible within a short time with simple care. We don't mean the permanent loss of sight due to caustic chemical injury, eye diseases or the eyeball being penetrated with a sharp object.

The most common forms of temporary blindness usually occur on the water with those who love to sail or on mountain slopes in the wintertime with those who love to ski. Another infrequent form may strike those who spend a lot of time in the desert around white sun. In each of these cases, continuous sun glare off of water, snow or sand tend to produce temporary loss of vision in some.

Relief Measures

Individuals thus afflicted should, first of all, be removed into a dark room or else put on a pair of very dark sunglasses to protect them from further glare. Cool compresses of lavender or hyssop tea can be laid across the eyes or put on top of each closed eyelid for comfort and relief of pain.

Some fresh rose petals should be snipped with scissors into half a pint of distilled water and allowed to set overnight undisturbed. The next morning an eyedropper full of this solution should be put into each eye, and the process repeated several times more each day until not needed any longer. Rose petal water is one of the very best remedies we know for this. And is made even better when fresh rainwater is used to soak the petals in.

Foods and Nutrients

Vitamin A is the first nutrient if there are problems with the eyes. Twenty to thirty thousand units daily for a week or two is the place to begin. Vitamin C (10,000 mg.) and vitamin E (800 I.U.) can be added, if necessary.

BLISTERS

Symptoms

Some blisters may be due to a skin disorder or an eruption of some kind. Shingles, eczema, dermatitis, cold sores, and second-degree burns can all produce blisters.

But here we refer to those that are caused by an injury of some type. They are a collection of serum under the horny layer of the skin. And are caused by friction, such as shoveling, rowing with oars, hiking, marching, and so forth.

Relief Measures

Large water blisters should be opened with a sterilized needle (made red hot in a flame—then dressed with antiseptic cream and a clean but loose-fitting bandage of some kind. The area should be cleansed with a solution of hydrogen peroxide, however, before a suitable cream and bandage are put on. Most authorities feel that it is best to leave the blister intact after the fluid has been evacuated.

If the blister is on the heel or bottom of the foot where sock and shoe agitation can make it worse, then a loose-fitting cotton stocking and a slipper or sandal should be worn until it clears up. A dressing with a hole the size of the blister can be placed on top so pressure will be displaced to the healthy, surrounding skin.

Foods and Nutrients

Rubbing a little vitamin E oil on said blister helps, too. Also crushing single zinc and vitamin C tablets and then mixing the resulting powders with a little oil squeezed out of the snipped off end of a vitamin E capsule, makes a wonderful application to expedite the healing process of a blister.

BLOOD CIRCULATION

(POOR)

Symptoms

Usually evident in the elderly, this problem is commonly characterized by cold hands and feet, a "pins-and-needles" sensation in the lower extremities, blue lips and pale countenance, and fatigue. Some of the symptoms common to anemia may overlap here a little.

Relief Measures

Recently published medical studies within the last decade or so, have amply demonstrated that both gotu kola and ginkgo are ideal for circulatory disorders. The December, 1981 issue of an Italian medical journal called *Clinica Terapeutica* reported that in a double-blind trial carried out in patients experiencing a variety of venous problems, an extract of gotu kola showed definite improvements in all of them. And the September, 1986 conservative French medical magazine, *La Presse Medicale* was entirely devoted to the wonders performed by ginkgo. Several reports from French physicians reported how helpful the extract was in treating patients who suffered circulatory problems in their lower extremities.

Wakunaga of America manufactures a product called Ginkolic, which contains not only ginkgo biloba leaf, but also aged garlic extract and Siberian ginseng and its respective extract. This is available from most health food stores (or see Appendix under Wakunaga).

Dr. Robert Sturgis, a Winnipeg health-care provider, informed one of us (Heinerman) a couple of years ago during a lecture appearance in that city, that he treats his patients suffering from venous disorders with chlorophyll. But not just any kind, mind you. He says that the product called Kyo-Green (see Appendix under Wakunaga) rates tops in his book. This powdered drink of concentrated cereal grass (barley and wheat) juices also includes chlorella, Pacific Ocean kelp, and boiled brown rice. He has each of his patients mix a level tablespoonful in 8 fl. oz. of pineapple or carrot juice or spring water and drink it every morning before breakfast.

Foods and Nutrients

We've discovered that concentrated red beet juice is also helpful as well. An outfit in Laurence, Kansas by the name of Pines, International makes an organic beet powder which can be easily mixed with water and taken for such problems (see Appendix).

Most people with cold hands and feet are not drinking enough fluid. An electrolyte solution with physiologically balanced amounts of sodium, potassium, chloride, carbonate, magnesium, and sulphur, should be drunk a few times each day. Especially so if the person has low electrolytes as shown in the blood test. People with low blood pressure generally have inadequate amounts of sodium in their bodies and have cold extremities and very poor circulation.

BLOOD CLOTS

Symptoms

A blood clot is a soft, coherent, jelly-like red mass which results when fibrinogen is converted to fibrin, thereby trapping the red blood cells (and other formed elements) within the coagulated plasma. Such clots can induce strokes. Warning signs for these would include: unexplained and terrific weakness on one side of the body or in the limbs; slurring of speech; double vision; sudden headaches; unexpected dizziness; and general clumsiness.

Relief Measures

The idea here is to help "thin" the blood, so that clot formation is delayed or even prevented. Powdered ginger root is helpful for this. Daily intake of three capsules with a meal is advised. Drinking tomato or V-8 juice seasoned with a pinch of cayenne pepper is also good.

Foods and Nutrients

A great deal of research has focused on the omega-3 fatty acids in fresh and salt-water fish for their ability to prevent clotting. A lengthy report in a recent issue of the *American Journal of Clinical Nutrition* (54: 438-63, 1991) explains how such omega-3s decrease fibrinogen concentrations and prevent blood platelets from bunching up — factors which contribute to clotting. Rirslane, spinach, buttercrunch and red leaf lettuce, and mustard leaves also contain some omega-3s as well, and should, therefore, be incorporated into the diet more often.

Certain nutrients may, likewise, be useful in preventing the formation of blood clots.

BLOOD POISONING

Symptoms

When dangerous bacteria like bacillus tetani found in cultivated soil or harmful chemical agents, get into the bloodstream through an open cut or wound or directly through the pores of the skin, serious consequences can result within a very short time. Very painful muscle spasms can occur at the back of the neck and around the throat and mouth areas. A red or pink line slowly starting from a sore or cut on the hand or foot travelling up the forearm or leg to the armpit or groin is an indication that infection is in the lymph channels: that is not blood poisoning, but indicates that infection has started to invade the system (a condition known as lymphangitis).

Relief Measures

Imediate medical attention should be sought for at once! In the event that such isn't readily available, a *temporary* antidote can be found until medical services can finally be obtained. Bring a quart of water to a boil. One handful each of elecampane root-stock and turdock root (or yellow dock root). Cover, lower heat and simmer for 5 minutes. Remove from heat and steep half an hour longer. Uncover, strain and add one level tablespoonful of powdered charcoal. Stir thoroughly and refrigerate. A cup of this should be consumed every 45 minutes or so.

An effort should be made to help the immune system. It is not an emergency unless the victim is in shock or there is a raging fever. Lymphangitis is still a localized infection.

Continuous hot wet packs (see ABSCESS) are the cornerstone of treatment. Leave the pack on all night long and the red line is usually gone by morning.

Foods and Nutrients

Vitamin C is the obvious first choice of nutrients. Ten to 20 grams a day until the infection is under control. Intravenous administration would be better. Vitamin A and zinc in large doses for a few days help the skin heal better. A good program with these and vitamin E would go something like this: Vitamin A (75,000 I.U.), zinc (100 mg.) and vitamin E (800 I.U.) daily.

BLOOD PRESSURE (HIGH/LOW)

Symptoms

Most people with hypertension have no visible symptoms. That's why it is called the "silent killer." But the common ones to look for here when they do occur, include headaches, dizziness, ringing in the ears, and fatigue. Bouts of breathlessness, especially at night, chest pain, cough, and misty vision can occur in the more severe cases. One must look to the kidneys as a major cause for this disorder.

Low blood pressure is something to be greatful for in a way, considering that the other, hypertension, is the real culprit because it doesn't produce perceptible symptoms until considerable damage has already been done to the body. Symptoms of low blood pressure include fatigue, inability to do heavy work, light-headedness sometimes, occasional dizziness, and pale countenance due to poor blood circulation.

Relief Measures

Exercise is strongly recommended for hypertension. Get into a regular program whereby you walk at least 20 minutes every day and climb at least three flights of stairs. Also bicycling and swimming helps as well.

Aged garlic extract from Japan called Kyolic is marvelous for treating cases of hypertension. So said different scientists at the First World Congress on Garlic held in Washington, D. C. in August, 1991. About three capsules daily is advised with meals.

Learn to restrict your sodium intake. Stay away from alcohol. Lose weight. Stop smoking. And cut your caffeine intake of colas and coffee beverages.

Drinking several cups each day of black or green tea from the Orient, should help to elevate your blood pressure if you suffer from hypotension. The xanthine alkaloids present in both tend to raise it a little. Also the tarinic acid in some herbs like white oak bark may be useful as well.

Foods and Nutrients

Calcium and magnesium intakes are important. Most calcium can be obtained from low-fat dairy products and some leafy green vegetables like broccoli or spinach. We recommend these sources over the standard calcium pills sold in health-food stores. At the same time we feel that sufficient magnesium should be consumed to offset any disadvantages which excess calcium intake may cause. The best rule of thumb to remember here is that your magnesium intake should be between one-half and two-thirds of whatever your calcium intake is. So, if you're say consuming 1,200 mg. of calcium each day, then your magnesium intake should be between 600-800 mg. Magnesium-rich foods include bran, honey, nuts (especially peanuts and Brazil nuts), seafood, spinach, and kelp. In some cases, however, a magnesium supplement may be necessary to take also.

Potassium is very critical for the function of the kidneys. But your potassium should come from food rather than supplements per se, unless you're under a doctor's care for this. Most fruits and vegetables contain potassium. Figs, blackstrap molasses, tomato and V-8 juices, shrimp, dates, raisins, and organic peanutbutter are high in this mineral.

And when polyunsaturated fats replace the saturated kinds in the diet, there is usually an inmediate drop in blood pressure. But try to restrict your total fat intake to just 30% of your daily calories, with no more than 10% of those calories coming from polyunsaturated fats.

If the blood test shows a sodium level above the mean (more than 140 mg.), it suggests that elevated sodium is partially responsible for the elevated pressure. Acetic acid (in vinegar) is a specific to help the body carry sodium out via the kidneys. One teaspoon of apple cider vinegar in eight fluid ounces of water three or four times a day—as long as it tastes good—is safe and can be carried on for a lifetime, with proper monitoring, of course.

Consumers should become better label readers when shopping in their favorite supermarkets for groceries. Besides the obvious foods to avoid—potato chips, canned nuts, and crackers—there are others in which sodium is less obvious. One example is the new low-fat or fat-free brands of mayonnaise. Very few are aware that such actually have *more* sodium in them than regular mayos to make up for the taste lost by the removal of fats. By carefully monitoring foods, beverages and medications for high sodium, consumers can definitely help to hold the line on their soaring blood pressures.

BLOOD SUGAR IMBALANCES

(See also DIABETES and HYPO-GLYCEMIA)

Symptoms

For specific symptoms of either condition, consult under their respective entries: DIABETES or HYPOGLYCEMIA. The way to distinguish between them, however, is to think of the pancreatic glands as being underproductive with regard to diabetes and overproductive when it comes to hypoglycemia. "Too little" or "too much" is the best way of characterizing each of them.

Relief Measures/Foods and Nutrients

The late Paavo Airola, Ph.D, N.D. was a world-renowned nutritionist who received his early medical training in his native Finland. Until his death in the last decade (1980s) of a ruptured aneurysm, he was a frequent public speaker at many different health conventions. One of the authors knew him personally and had various opportunities to chat with him in private.

Here is what he recommended in a general way for BOTH imbalances. Dr. Airola insisted that a raw foods diet was the primary ingredient in getting well again from either condition. "Emphasis should always *be* on raw foods!" one of us remembers him insisting in his usual forthright way. "Raw foods stimulate the pancreas and normalize their metabolic functions," he said.

His list of raw food therapy included: nuts, whole grains, organic fruits and vegetables (especially cucumbers, string-beans, Jerusalem artichoke and garlic for diabetes), and *fermented* whole milk products (yogurt, kefir, buttermilk). Snacking on 6-8 *small* meals per day instead of eating the 3 big customary meals, was also recommended. And the *most important meal* of the entire day, he stated unequivocally, was BREAKFAST! Pay *strict* attention to that meal if you suffer from blood sugar imbalances of any kind!

BLOOD TRANSFUSION (NATURAL)

Symptoms

When extra blood is needed during a routine operation or to replace blood which has been lost through an accident of some kind, where do you find some that is safe and free of the dreaded AIDS virus? Well, we're not about to give advice on giving yourself a natural transfusion at home by any means. But our research has turned up something rather remarkable, which we pass along by way of interest only!

Relief Measures/Foods and Nutrients

One of us who has specialized in the study of food and medicinal plants worldwide for over two decades now (Heinerman), has discovered something remarkable about the okra pod. Scientists in India made a raicilaginous preparation from it sometime in the mid-fifties and found it made a useful blood plasma-replacement or blood volume expander. Mongrel dogs bled to a state of shock, recovered completely when transfused with this unique preparation, and blood regeneration and recovery were hastened when the preparation was supplemented with a small quantity of the animal's own blood. The preparation caused no reaction to speak of. This study was reported in *The Wealth of India* (5: 86-87, 1959). The Japanese journal, *Chemical & Pharmaceutical Bulletin* (28:2933, 1980) has also explored the mucilage potential of okra as a plasma expander and as a possible intravenous circulation agent. A report on the rich proteins in okra seeds has also been published in the *Journal of Agricultural & Biological chemistry* (23: 1 204-07, 1975).

Science News for January 16, 1988 pointed out that blood hemoglobin has recently been discovered in some plants of the elm family. Based on evidence, it would seem logical to advise patients needing extra blood to consume a lot of gumbo soup and capsules of fenugreek seed and powdered slippery elm (all high in mucilage). And drinking some Kyo-Green every day wouldn't hurt either (see Appendix under Wakunaga)

BODY ODOR

Symptoms

We just can't resist the temptation to quote from Ralph L. Roy's classic study published by Tulane University in New Orleans back in 1931. *In The Ethno-Botany of the Maya*, Dr. Roys translated the ancient Maya descriptions for the most obvious body odors as being "goaty armpits" and "goaty leg areas where village dogs like to stick their noses." We don't think either of these needs any further elucidating from us.

Relief Measures

Roys had access to different manuscripts written by early Jesuit priests who came over with the Spanish conquistadores several centuries ago when the Maya and Aztecs had developed their cultures. These Catholic padres interviewed many different Maya herbalists and healers, and recorded a number of their remedies on paper for the benefit of later generations.

First of all, the ancient Maya believed that you had to clean up the inside in order to get the outside smelling good

again. To accomplish this, enemas and purges were in order. Occasional "mild food" fasting was also encouraged. Green plant food was especially favored for this.

Secondly, the armpits and reproductive organs were to be cleansed frequently with cold water. A strange recommendation of cutting a sour orange or lime in half and then rubbing that half on the skin to reduce perspiration also appeared in this literature.

Foods and Nutrients

Vegetarians can smell the presence of carnivores. But vegetarians themselves, provided they bathe themselves daily, do not emit odors like meat-eating people nor do they need to use a lot of underarm antiperspirants either. When people bathe frequently and thoroughly and still have a disagreeable odor, it suggests they are low in the B-complex vitamin PABA (100 mg.), magnes ium (600 mg.), and zinc (100 mg.).

Various liquid chlorophylls on the market can be used in place of deodorants, if one doesn't mind the skin getting a little green in the process. An even better recommendation comes from Jay Levy of Euless, Texas, who is a sales representative for Wakunaga of America. He told one of the authors in March, 1992, that he makes a combination of chamomile and rosemary tea, which he then strains, puts into a spray bottle, and uses under his arms after showering every morning. He claims it's the best thing he's ever tried, and doesn't have to expose his skin any more to potentially harmful chemical deodorants.

BOILS

Symptoms

A boil is an infected nodule on the skin with a central core of pus surrounded by inflamed and swollen tissue. A boil usually occurs when the skin tissue is weakened by chafing, lowered resistance due to disease, or inadequate nutrition. Boils reveal themselves as swollen, red, hot, and tender.

After receiving a series of tragic news reports concerning the loss of all his livestock and personal fortune and the sudden and untimely death of all his sons and daughters, the Old Testament patriarch Job, was probably overcome with so much grief and stress that he promptly broke out in boils all over his body.

Relief Measures

Boils should be washed several times each day with a strong solution of white oak bark tea and then swabbed with tincture of witch hazel and fanned until dry for relief. Hot compresses can also relief pain and promote healing. They should be wet, hot, and continuous. (See ABSCESS)

Foods and Nutrients

We read about the prophet Isaiah advising King Hezekiah to make a poultice from some figs and then apply it directly to his boil, which he did and was able to draw out the pus therefrom.

Snip the ends off of several vitamin E capsules and squeeze out the oily contents into a small dish. Then crush two vitamin C tablets and mix in with it. Apply this mixture

to a lanced and drained boil to expedite the healing process nicely.

BONE INJURIES

(BROKEN/DISLOCATED/FRAC-TURED)

Symptoms

Fractures and breaks are synonymous with each other. When a bone snaps but the skin remains intact, the fracture is described as being "closed" or "simple. " But if the break penetrates the skin allowing for invasion by bacteria, then it becomes an "open" or "compound" fracture. Fractures can occur as a result of an accident, tumor, osteoporosis, or even a vitamin-mineral deficiency.

Fracture symptoms include limb deformities, limited limb functioning, shortening of the limb in fractures of long bones, pain, a grating sensation if the broken bone ends rub against each other, and swelling and skin discoloration overlying the immediate fracture area.

A dislocation is a disarrangement of the normal relation of the bones entering into the formation of a joint. Usually pain and inflammation accompany such, followed by an obvious difficulty in mobility, such as in lifting or walking, for instance.

Relief Measures

Properly splinting the broken bone part in the same position it was found, until regular medical help can be obtained is the right thing to do in emergency situations. In the early frontier days of America, some pioneers went about setting their own fractures but we don't recommend that this be done unless an individual has some knowledge of the anatomy and general bone structure.

Alfalfa tablets (ten per day) and yarrow capsules (6 daily) are recommended for quicker recovery. The first contains significant amounts of calcium and vitamin D and the latter contains an interesting protein complex, both of which are necessary for knitting bones together again and reducing the inflammation in muscle tissue.

Dislocations can be treated several different ways. One is to soak the injured limb in solutions of hot and cold water for about a minute each, and keep repeating this procedure for 30 minutes or more at a time. This reduces swelling and lessens the pain somewhat.

Another is to consult a good chiropractor, who with some simple adjustments can usually manipulate such dislocated bones back into their proper sockets again. Heat pad and ice pack treatments are advised for areas of the body which can't be easily soaked in hot or cold water for very long.

Food and Nutrients

Agnes M. (who wishes to have her last name remain anonymous) contacted one of the authors several years ago in the hopes of finding something that would make her fractured femur (thigh bone) heal more speedily. She was placed on the following foods and nutrients, which brought about the desired results some six weeks later:

Calcium, 1,000 mg.
Vitamin D, 600 I.U.

Magnesium, 500 mg.
Vitamin C, 5,000 mg.

Goat milk and cheese, yogurt, almonds, dark leafy greens, bone meal, granulated kelp (to be used as a seasoning), broccoli, green bell peppers, and fresh orange juice. An additional recommendation was that she spend as much time as she could in the sunlight.

BOTTLE FEEDING/BREAST FEEDING PROBLEMS

Symptoms

The most evident sign is that the infant refuses to take to his or her bottle or nurse properly when hungry for nourishment.

Relief Measures

The old adage that "honey draws but vinegar repels" applies here. Infants are more inclined to suck on that which is sweet instead of bitter. Nature intended for breast milk to be sweet, whereas the contents of a bottle may require a little honey to make them more pleasant to such sensitive taste buds. In England the old nannies used to give babies what was called a "sugar teat" before they were bottle-fed. It consisted of a small lump of sugar wrapped tightly in a clean muslin cloth, tied with some thread, dipped into a little warm water and then inserted into the baby's mouth for a couple of minutes before the bottle was given.

The position of the baby's face to the breast is important because it is difficult to swallow if the head is turned to the right or left. The cheek reflex—the nipple only needs to touch the baby's cheek and the baby will open his mouth—starts the successful nursing. When the mouth is open, the mother jams as much of the nipple and the surrounding areola into the mouth. The gums have to get a hold of the areola area and not just on the nipple itself.

Foods and Nutrients

If the breast milk doesn't seem to flow, as if it is caked up inside the breast, the mother may find that the calcium in her milk isn't soluble enough, and it needs acidification. One teaspoon of apple cider vinegar in a cup of warm water drunk every 3-4 hours might just allow the milk to flow more easily.

In the event a particularly fussy baby won't feed routinely as expected, several sweet inducements can be offered to it in the forms of apple sauce or pureed pears or figs or carrot juice. One of the authors recalls his father recomending to a woman in Provo, Utah many years ago to feed her infant son, Jesse Kevin Young, carrot juice instead of bottle or breast milk. This author, who temporarily lived with this family and helped to care for their older children, remembers how readily the youngster took to this form of nourishment, in spite of the awful looking and hard-to-wash diapers! Some years later, this author happened to see this kid when he was in high school and playing football. He was the most powerfully built lineman on the team, suffered no allergies at all, and had rosy red cheeks. This contrasted sharply with the other milk-fed kids, many of whom were anemic-looking and suffering often from sinus and throat problems. Jesse was the epitome of health and a walking testimony to the advantages of carrot juice over breast or cow's milk.

BREAST CANCER

Symptoms

Here's what to look for when doing a self-exam of your breasts.

Begin by standing in front of a mirror with your arms at your sides. Become familiar with the general appearance of your breasts and nipples, including their shape, texture, and any normal asymmetry. Lean over to see breast contour in that position. After finding out what is typical for you, look for any of these signs: bulging or flattening in one breast but not in both; redness on the surface; unusual toughness or inversion of the nipples.

Next raise your arms over your head and check for the same signs. Inspect your breasts while keeping your palms together above your head, and then again with your hands on your hips. Both of these positions tend to contract chest muscles and could make it easier to spot any changes in your breasts.

Then, proceed to gently squeeze each nipple in order to check for any blood-tinged discharge.

After this, stand in the shower and soap the upper part of your torso good. Using a little baby shampoo for this purpose will help your fingers to slide a lot easier over both breasts. But to do the lower part of them, you'll need to shower, dry off, and then lay down on your bedroom or front room rug with a small pillow beneath your shoulder blades to help flatten your breast against your chest better. Now use the flat part of your left fingers and commence pressing the right breast lightly against the rib cage. Begin at the outside edge of the breast, and rotate in a spiral toward the nipple, without lifting your fingers, until you've covered the entire area of the breast.

Next, move your arm down by your side and start to feel the upper and inner part of your armpit, the area between your armpit and your nipple, and finally between the outer lower part of your breast and the nipple. Repeat these steps for your other breast, using the opposite hand.

Relief Measures

A growing trend among many people today who've decided to take health-care matters into their own hands, is self-treatment for cancer. While neither of us advocates this as the ideal solution to a very complex problem, we can mention several herbs which have had proven track records for rnany but not all cases of cancer.

The herbs of which we speak are red clover blossoms and chaparral twigs and stem. The first is a common meadow and pasture grass, while the second grows in the semi-arid regions of the American West and Southwest. They work best in tea form.

Bring a quart of distilled water to a boil. Add 3 tablespoonfuls of chaparral; cover, reduce heat and simmer 10 minutes. Remove from stove, uncover and stir in 2 tablespoonfuls of red clover flowers. Cover again and steep for *ten hours*! Strain and drink 4-5 cups per day in between meals. Save the crude plant materials for making a second batch of tea before discarding. But we issue a warning to your taste buds: this is gosh-awful stuff and a vivid imagination of vanilla ice cream together with a little honey mixed into the tea is going to be needed in order to get the stuff down! But it seems to work for those who've used it in times past.

Foods and Nutrients

Animal protein in the form of red meat and chicken and turkey ought to be eliminated from the diet. Better stick with fish and other seafoods. And stay away from margarine and other hydrogenated fats, including anything that is fried or deep-fried. Skip pizza and other fast foods. Stop drinking coffee, colas and soft drinks. And, more importantly, *do not fret* about your problem even if it happens to be cancer. Anxiety can spread cancer faster than a crummy diet will, believe it or not! Learn to relax and calmly decide how you intend to lick this problem.

A handful of nutritionally-minded doctors that we know of, employ Kyolic Aged Garlic Extract and the wonderful chlorophyll mix called Kyo-Green (both made by Waku-naga of America) for treating cases of breast cancer in many of their female patients. Benjamin Lau, Ph.D., M.D. of Lama Linda School of Medicine in California is one of these who not only believes in the efficacy of aged garlic extract, but has done considerable research on the same and has presented and written numerous scientific papers on it in medical conventions and journals. We advise taking the liquid Kyolic extract, which can be put into gelatin capsules and swallowed that way. Or else a tablespoonful of the same mixed into an 8 fluid ounce glass of Kyo-Green and taken in that manner twice daily. If taking the capsules, we recommend about 6-8 per day. (See Appendix under Wakunaga if neither of these products is readily available at your local health food store.)

Recent clinical evidence strongly suggests that women who are vegetarians and consume very little animal flesh and fat and more plant fiber, face far less risk of contracting breast cancer than their counterparts who consume a lot of fat and meat. (American Journal of Clinical Nutrition 53:798, January-March, 1991)

Other nutritional supplements are of definite advantage here as well. Because of the enormous publicity which vitamin C has received in the popular press in the last decade or so, we should all by now be aware of its tremendous benefits for recovering from cancer. At least ten grams a day will slow the progress of this dreaded disease.

And foods containing this important vitamin should be included in the diet often. Fresh citrus juices, dark leafy green vegetables in the form of various salads, and certain fruits play a therapeutic role for the average cancer patient.

Vitamin A holds great significance as well. Fifty thousand of the suggested 100,000 I.U.s taken daily should be betacarotene, while the other half is from fish oils of some kind. There are several relatively new products in the health food market place these

days that are derived from shark oil and quite good for a sound cancer nutrition program.

Additionally, foods high in this important vitamin should also be consumed regularly. Besides fresh and salt-water fish, there are also a wide variety of green and yellowish-orange fruits and vegetables to choose from: bell peppers, carrots, zucchini and banana squashes, pumpkin, and cantaloupe are a few of these. Dairy products and certain organic meats devoid of growth hormones are high in vitamin A, too.

We should point out that surgery to remove cancerous growths from the breast is prudent. But the extensive and radical surgery down to the ribs, promoted so heavily by doctors in the past, isn't preferable any more and may, in fact, be detrimental in the long run. The authors think that a total nutritional and herbal program should be the first choice of every woman before considering chemotherapy or radiation.

BREATHING DIFFICULTIES

Symptoms

An inability to breathe properly can be due to a number of different factors. Some of those are highlighted in greater detail under such entries as ASTHMA, BRONCHITIS, EMPHYSEMA and HAY FEVER. Generally speaking, though, either an accumulation of excess mucus or else a constriction of the muscles within the lungs themselves, can impair normal breathing.

Relief Measures

One of the very best remedies we've discovered a number of doctors using throughout North America, is advising their patients to drink hot black coffee without cream or sugar. The caffeine in a heated form seems to do wonders in relaxing tightened lung muscles and clearing up the breathing passages of excess mucus. Hot black tea also works well.

Foods and Nutrients

Foods to be avoided by those experiencing such breathing difficulties include all sweets and items with sugar in them, all dairy products, eggs, pork, and some white flour products.

Calcium (600 mg.), magnesium (400 mg.), vitamin C (1,500 mg.) and vitamin A (20,000 I.U.) will be helpful in such situations.

BRIGHT'S DISEASE

Symptoms

Also called nephritis and involves a dysfunction of kidneys marked by discharge of considerable protein into the urine (albuminuria). Ordinarily, while waste products are present in the urine, valuable constituents of the blood such as sugar and protein aren't.

Acute nephritis occurs about 10 days after a streptococcal infection. Generalized edema, most prominently in the face and abdomen make the child look bloated. There may be scanty and bloody urine.

Subacute nephritis occurs more gradually. The patient has a pale countenance, face is puffy, a general laziness is manifested, and headaches are common.

In chronic nephritis, an increased quantity of urine discharge becomes evident, usually at night. Headaches occur upon awakening in the morning, the vision is somewhat blurred, fatigue is common, and vomiting may also happen.

Relief Measures

A lot of bed rest is advocated. Up to six capsules daily of Wakunaga's Goldenseal Root and six capsules of Kyolic aged garlic extract (see Appendix under Wakunaga) are recommended. NOTE: If you suffer from hypoglycemia, then switch to wild Oregon grape root capsules or juniper berry tea instead of the goldenseal; however, the Kyolic garlic can still be used without any problems.

Foods and Nutrients

The diet should include a lot of plant protein in the form of tofu, soy milk, okra, and so forth. Cranberry juice is also very helpful to drink during this period instead of water. Avoid salty foods and high-sodium items such as kelp and some seafoods.

BRONCHITIS

Symptoms

This malady is an inflammation of the tissues lining the air passageways leading to the lungs. Symptoms include mild fever, muscle and back pain, sore throat and even a dry cough followed by the hacking up of mucus as the inflammation becomes more severe.

Relief Measures

The patient should obtain a lot of rest in a stress-free environment. Some decades ago, a female writer of children's books was stricken with bronchitis, but doctors could do very little for her in the late thirties when she became ill. However, she cured herself of this ailment by renting a cottage by the ocean where she spent an entire year relaxing and writing. Her daily walks and deep-breathing exercises along the beach proved to be the best therapy of all.

A tea made from equal parts of coltsfoot leaves, wild cherry bark and horehound herb, sipped in half cupful amounts while still warm, is a real treat for injured lungs. Some mullein can also be added for good measure and the brew sweetened with a little pure maple syrup or blackstrap molasses. Simply bring a quart of distilled water to a boil, and add the cherry bark and horehound. Cover and simmer 5 minutes, then remove from heat, uncover and add the coltsfoot and mullein before covering again and allow to steep 45 minutes. Strain while still quite warm, sweeten to taste and slowly sip.

Foods and Nutrients

Vitamins A, C, D, and E are all good for this condition. Suggested intake is 25,000 I.U., 3,500 mg., lots of sunshine, and 800 I.U. respectively. Salmon, cod-liver oil, dark leafy greens, and wheat germ are foods loaded with these same nutrients, too.

BRUISES

Symptoms

Usually characterized by a discoloration of the skin, which can turn blue, black-blue or even a deep purple in more serious injuries.

Relief Measures

The following herbs are all wonderful for treating bruises but in different forms. Aloe vera gel, arnica tincture, calendula salve or expressed juice, comfrey leaf poultice or comfrey tea compress, stewed fig poultice, hyssop ointment or tea, lobelia tincture or fluid extract, cooked and cooled mashed okra poultice, olive oil, evening primrose tea or ointment, wintergreen oil, witch hazel tincture, and wormwood tea compress.

Foods and Nutrients

Several B-complex vitamins are useful here. These include folic acid, pantothenic acid and PABA (paraaminobenzoic acid). Also vitamins C, D, K, and the bioflavonoids are helpful. Of the minerals, iron and zinc seem to be especially good for bruises. Some of these work better topically in ointment form, but others like a complete

B-complex, C, bioflavonoids, and zinc can be taken internally.

Digestive enzymes are helpful in dissolving the blood that has leaked from the capillaries. Most notable are papain and bromelain, which are derived from ripe papayas and papaya juice, and fresh pineapples and pineapple juice.

BUBONIC PLAGUE

Symptoms

Bubonic plague or Black Death—why even its two common names sound terribly ominous to the average person unacquainted with this most destructive of all diseases. When it swept Europe from 1348-1350 A.D., it claimed over 20% of the population, especially in the British Isles, reported *The New England Journal of Medicine* for Sept. 5, 1985.

The plague is acutally two diseases working simultaneously: bubonic plague, transmitted by fleas that have bitten infected animals and pneumonia plague (also known as pulmonary anthrax), a lung infection.

The most likely symptoms include fever, prostration, delirium, and swelling of the lymph gland, especially in the armpit or groin. These swellings become hard and are called buboes; sometimes black blotches appear with them, too.

Right now, in the Western Hemisphere, serious outbreaks of bubonic plague have been reported in dozens of rural villages in northeastern Brazil, in portions of Bolivia, and in the western part of the United States, particularly New Mexico, Colorado, and Arizona, where it has become somewhat prevalent on certain Native American Indian reservations.

Dr. Allan Barnes, formerly with the Centers for Disease Control in Atlanta, Georgia, warned health officials that "the plague is all over the West" right now, and that "it could take only a spark to get the country on an epidemic course" again. Some think that with the outbreak of AIDS in the last decade and the resurgence of old diseases such as cholera and leprosy, that it's very likely the Black Death will come back again to haunt mankind in modern times with devastating effects.

Relief Measures

The late herbalist, John Ray Christopher recited a historical incident concerning one remedial possibility employed by some thieves in the Middle Ages. When the plague hit the city of Marseilles, France quite hard, there were four thieves who went around plundering the bodies of dead plague victims without ever getting the disease themselves. While when they were captured by authorities and arraigned for their heinous crimes, they were asked by the magistrate how it was they never became sick. Only after extracting a promise from the court that they wouldn't be prosecuted for their previous crimes, did they reveal their curious secret. It was this: they chopped up a bunch of peeled garlic cloves and soaked them in a gallon of fermented apple vinegar. Whenever they went out to rob the dead, they would drink some of this stuff and take it along to wash their hands, faces, and mouths with it, as well as to inhale some of the aromatic vapors after completing their sinister work. Their remedy has since become known as the "Four Thieves Vinegar."

History seems to bear this tale out. We think, however, that daily intake of *liquid* Kyolic aged-garlic extract with some apple cider vinegar is just as good. Add one level teaspoonful of the liquid aged-garlic extract with 4 tablespoonfuls of apple cider vinegar, and take first thing in the morning on an empty stomach.

Foods and Nutrients

Any infection calls, irregardless of being major or minor, calls for vitamin C. It must be taken orally and intravenously to do any lasting good, even up to 50 to 1,000 grams per day. Also, for epidemics such as this, 100,000 I.U. of vitamin A per day is advisable.

BULIMIA

Symptoms

This is a chronic morbid disorder involving repeated and secret episodes of eating, marked by uncontrolled rapid ingestion of large quantities of food over a short period of time, followed by self-induced vomiting or purging. Typically accompanied by feelings of guilt, depression, or self-disgust.

In Roman times, the nobility would often hold all-night orgies in which an abundance of food accompanied their sexual extravaganzas. Guests would consume to their hearts'content, then repair themselves

to an inner chamber where there was a large receptacle known as a vomitorium, where they could throw up the entire contents of their recent meals before romping off to nearby bedrooms for more lascivious and licentious fun.

Relief Measures

Psychological counselling is obviously in order here for those who suffer from this problem. In some instances, it can be due to an imbalance of some kind, such as hormonal or nutritional. We believe that a good blood workup of the individual, together with a thorough examination of the physical body as well as the inside of the head is fitting in such cases. Therapists treating such cases should look for "hidden" stresses in the patient's life—early negative childhood memories locked away for years, stifled repression towards authority, poor self-image, and so forth.

Something as relaxing as warm catnip tea or peppermint tea or fluid extract of valerian or skillcap may be appropriate here.

Foods and Nutrients

These people, usually women, are subject to rises and falls of their blood sugar. When it falls, they will eat 5,000 calories or more of cookies, pasta, chocolate milk, and mashed potatoes—the sweeter and the softer, the better it is. When the blood sugar rises and the judgment part of the brain becomes operative, they realize what they have done and put their fingers down their throats or take a laxative to purge themselves. It is the ultimate in control. Most of these women have never felt they had any autonomy over their lives until now.

A high-potency B-complex (4 tablets daily) and magnesium (1,200 mg.) comes to mind here.

BUMPS

Symptoms

Similar to bruises in some ways, but not always discolored. Hard lumps beneath the flesh can be due to a sustained injury of some kind. Or can be more serious in the form of developing tumors. Certainly any bumps that refuse to go away with simple remedies should be looked at by a competent doctor of your choice.

Relief Measures

One of the authors had a rather unpleasant experience back in the beginning of 1980. He was in the back lot of a large food wholesale discount warehouse putting some wooden pallets on the back of his pickup truck, which had been given to him free of charge by store management. In the process of doing so, he accidentally hopped up on the tailgate and without looking behind him, hit his back pretty hard against a circular metal flange sticking out of one end of the store garbage dumpster. He paid no mind to the incident, but endured the pain quite well for several days thereafter.

Until one morning, upon getting out of bed, and, looking in the mirror, he noticed a terrific lump on the lower right side of his back just above the kidneys, which looked an awful black-and-blue. He promptly called this to the attention of his father, who resided with him at the time. His father remembered an old family remedy from his own Hungarian mother, and immediately applied it to his son's injury with excellent results. Which was simply this: he had his son lay face down on the bed with his shirt and pants removed and proceeded to put hot and cold packs on the injured site every couple of minutes. This routine was kept up for 30 minutes four times in two days. The bump went away and the author resumed his normally busy schedule of activities.

Food and Nutrients

Some vitamin C (3,500 mg.), PABA (100 mg.), rutin (500 mg.) and zinc (50 mg.) are in order here.

BURNS & SCALDS

Symptoms

Burns or scalds are tissue injuries caused by heat, electricity, radiation or chemicals. There are three degrees of burn severity. The first-degree kind is reddened in appearance (sunburns can fall into this category); a second-degree burn includes blister formation, while a third-degree type involves destruction of the entire thickness of skin and possibly of the underlying muscle as well.

Because of tissue destruction, massive losses of body fluids, proteins, sodium, potassium, and nitrogen can occur. Because large amounts of fluids are lost in extensive burns, the possibility of shock exists. Infection is a definite reality to burn victims.

Relief Measures

There is a wide variety of home remedies for the successful treatment of burns. The Jehovah's Witnesses' publication, *Awake* magazine contained an account in their July 22nd, 1966 issue of ice cold water being the very best thing to submerge a burned limb into for immediate relief. One of the authors discovered just how true this was for himself when he lived in southcentral Utah 30 years ago. He accidentally scalded his arm with hot boiling honey and rushed outside and plunged his injured limb into a snowbank, where he stayed covered with a quilt until he could no longer endure the freezing chill. Afterwards, his father applied a mixture of olive oil and baking soda on the injury and loosely covered it with a light gauze dressing. In several days, healing became very evident with little or no scarring to speak of.

This same author has spent considerable time in the Yucatan, studying the Maya Indians as part of his work in medical anthropology. There he has witnessed first-hand the successful treatment and quick recovery of very serious burns with nothing more than a dressing of egg yolk and lime juice. An old Aztec remedy calls for mashed ripe guava fruit or guava juice to lessen the severity of the intense pain accompanying such serious burns.

In Australia, the Aborigines have used tea tree oil or eucalyptus leaf tea for reducing the chances of infection on open wounds and burns. Tea tree oil is available in most health food stores nationwide, but should *only be used externally!*

Newsweek magazine for May 7, 1990 and Michael Resnick, M.D. on the H.O. M. E. show on ABC on Friday, August 10, 1990, both recounted the amazing ointment developed by Dr. Nu Rongxiang of mainland China. This herbal salve which can be applied to burn victims like a popsicle stick, leaves virtually NO scarring in the wake of major burns. "In the past doctors have treated the complications of burns instead of curing the burned tissue," he observed. "But we use nutrition in the body to repair the skin." American physicians who've carefully investigated his remarkable salve, have declared that his remedy is nothing short of amazing. While most of the ingredients still remain a secret, Dr. Xu has admitted that two of the chief components are whipped honey and fresh sesame seed oil. Another researcher thought possibly that Dr. Nu's formula also included zinc gluconate powder and vitamin E oil as well.

Some medical journals over the years have reported on novel methods for treating burns. Take, for instance, the July, 1926 issue of *Annals of Surgery*. The lengthy article mentioned that gas and kerosene lamp burns, and burns from "lighted Christmas trees, exploding stills, boiling water, automobile and industrial injuries" could all be successfully treated with tannic acid solution. Now certain herbs are high in tannic acid content. Chief among them is white oak bark and acorns. If these items are boiled in water for awhile and the resulting liquid applied to burns when cool in compress form, healing should be evident fairly soon.

The May 1982 issue of the medical journal, *Plastic and Reconstructive Surgery*, contained a lengthy article by a physician reciting numerous Native American remedies for burns. Boiled pine needles (probably for the rich vitamin C content to stave off infection), fresh crushed leaves of yellow dock or cinquefoil, boiled sage tea, burned cedar ashes, fresh dog or horse or buffalo excretement (probably for the ammonia to resist infection), yarrow tea, egg white applied with turkey feather, crushed plantain leaves, and boiled wormwood tea, were some of the effective things mentioned.

In a related incident found in Melvin R. Gilmore's *Uses of Plants by the Indians of the Missouri River Region* (p. 79), a Winnebago medicine man boasted of chewing plenty of fresh echinacea herb in order to make his mouth insensitive to pain so that he could take a live hot coal from the fire and insert it, much to the amazement of fellow tribe members. Equally astonishing is the fact that other Native American shamans would "bathe their hands and arms in the juice of this plant so that they could take out a piece of meat from a boiling kettle with the bare hand without suffering pain, to the wonderment of onlookers."

Foods and Nutrients

The *Bulletin of The History of Medicine* carried a report in its February, 1944 issue about a remarkable French cure for burns involving common onions. The famous French surgeon Ambroise Pare (1510-1590) employed expressed onion juice to dress all of his bern injuries with. The article also reported that fluid extracts of belladonna, plantain, henbane, prickly lettuce, poplar leaves and rose petals were excellent for washing such injuries with. The latter (rose) seems especially useful for this.

In addition to these things, the article also cited some other vegetables employed by Russian doctors in treating war victims who suffered serious burns from invading German artillery units. These included garlic, radish, and mustard. We think that Kyolic aged-garlic extract (liquid) would be very helpful in such injuries, both internally as well as to be used topically (see Appendix under Wakunaga).

Certain minerals and vitamins appear to have a purpose here as well. Intravenous and oral vitamin C of up to 20-30 grams a day will speed the healing process nicely. Vitamin C can be used in an ointment form and will help to control local infection.

BURSITIS

Symptoms

Bursitis is an inflamation of the liquid-filled sac, called a bursa, found near the joints, muscles, tendons, and bones, which helps to promote muscular movement and reduce friction. Usually found in the shoulder, elbows, hip, knee or feet, the malady known familiarly as "Tennis elbow" is nothing more than bursitis. Symptoms include swelling, tenderness, and stabbing pains in the afflicted area which frequently limits muscle-and-nerve motions to some extent.

Relief Measures

Rubbing on a few drops of oil of pepperment, followed by some fluid extract of lobelia and eucalyptus, and then covered briefly with a heating pad, is one way of finding relief.

Foods and Nutrients

Vitamins A, B-12m, C, and E are helpful here. While some of these can be taken orally, an intramuscular injection of B-12 will help better and faster.

CAFFEINISM

Symptoms

Caffeinism is the addiction to caffeine. Excess consumption of coffee or colas can produce trembling, nervousness, chronic muscle tension, irritability, throbbing headaches, disorientation, sluggishness, depression and insomnia, otherwise known as "coffee nerves." The clue that one is hooked is the onset of withdrawal symptoms occurring about 12-24 hours after the last intake. The symptoms noted above would all be exaggerated.

Relief Measures

The most obvious thing to do is to limit one's daily intake of coffee or cola to just a single cup or can or bottle, if total abstinence is impossible. Even then, such junk should only be sipped sparingly to satisfy the body's cravings for it. Better to find healthier substitutes in the form of roasted whole grain and herb root powders that mimic coffee and ginseng-based soft drinks that resemble colas.

Anything else that may contain caffeine should be watched very closely. This ranges from some over-the counter medications to herbal energy stimulants that have kola nut or guarana in them. Switching to mint teas like catnip or peppermint or herbal sedatives such as chamomile, skullcap and valerian should help ease a person off of caffeine for good.

Foods and Nutrients

Those attempting to kick the caffeine habit should probably avoid consuming too many spicy foods for awhile. These tend to excite the central nervous system more and also seem to increase the desire for more caffeine as well.

Extra water should be consumed. The drinking of at least eight fluid ounces of water 6 times each day will minimize the effects of this substance within the body. And the B-complex vitamins should allow one to get off caffeine more quickly. Between 2-4 tablets of a high-potency brand is suggested here.

Helping to keep the blood sugar at a safe, constant level will prevent the ups and downs of mood. About 500 mg. of magnesium and 750 mg. of calcium will help control stress.

CAKED BREAST

Symptoms

Caked breast describes the full, heavy, painful breast that will not allow the milk to flow.

Relief Measures

Rubbing a little olive oil after each feeding on the sore nipple should help. And keeping the breast nipple dry after each infant feeding is recommended, too.

Foods and Nutrients

Linda Ann, a Registered Nurse with an open mind to holistic health alternatives, decided to have a child, her first one as a matter of fact. Everything went well as expected. She decided to breastfeed her infant daughter. She discovered that drinking alfalfa and stinging nettle teas twice daily, helped enormously in producing more than enough milk for her hungry child, as well as a richer quality. She told one of the authors that she drank a cup of alfalfa in the morning and a cup of nettle in the mid afternoon for this.

The consumption of certain oily foods such as avocados, pecans, bananas and olive oil dressing is of benefit. Taking some vitamin E oil internally and mixing a little with a crushed zinc tablet and applying this simple paste to sore nipples helped.

CALLUSES

Symptoms

Calluses generally show up on the bottoms of the feet and on the palms of the hands due to excessive wear of the skin. The epidermal layer becomes quite thick and tough, almost like stiff cow leather left out in the wind, rain and sun for awhile.

Relief Measures

Wearing the right kind of shoes and gloves is the best way to solve this problem. Sanding them down with an emory board used for nail cuticles is one method for getting rid of them. Another is to carefully snip the hardened ends away with a small pair of curved sewing scissors. The application of some lecithin helps to keep them soft.

Foods and Nutrients

The intake of vitamin A (25,000 I.U.) and zinc (100 mg.) will help reduce calluses. Using vitamin E internally (800 mg.) and externally on the skin, is of definite benefit. Just cut open the end of a capsule and squeeze its contents into the palm of one hand and then lightly rub it into the callus. Repeated applications should clear it up in no time.

CANCER

Symptoms

Readers should be alerted to the fact that cancer is a very serious disease which requires multiple therapies. First and foremost should be competent medical care by skilled surgeons. In addition to this, a growing number of orthodox physicians believe that various alternative care programs involving the mind, herbs, exercise, diet, and nutritional supplements can be used in conjunction *with* surgery, chemotherapy and radiation but never by themselves.

Next to coronary heart disease, cancer is now the number two cause of death in North America. It claims 500,000 victims each year. Broken down, this averages out to about 1,400 every day, 60 per hour, and 1 per minute.

The big "C"— cancer to common folks and carcinoma to medical people—is a large collection of many different malignant tumors, most of which invade surrounding health tissues, and can spread to several sites at once, and are apt to recur after surgery or drug treatment.

Cancer is a complex disease, usually involving multiple factors such as diet (35%), alcohol and tobacco (35%), sexual activities (10%), occupational and industrial hazards (5%), environmental pollution (5%), geophysical things like solar radiation (4%), modern medical practices and prescribed drugs (3%), and other unknown factors (3%).

But in the most simplistic explanation we know of to describe its probable origins, this much can be said about it. Mental, emotional and environmental stresses assault the biochemical functions of the body on a cellular level, inducing electrical "shorts" in the body's own energy production system. Such temporary "brownouts" or "blackouts" cause cell production to become out of sync with its regular programmed activities. The result is an abnormal multiplication of new cells, which produce the growths or tumors we fundamentally recognize as cancer.

External growths and internal lumps that become evident, unusual changes in routine bowel habits, loss of weight and appetite, unexplained fatigue, and remark-

able discharges of fluid for no reason at all, are some of the more common manifestations of this disease. Still, when suspecting cancer, it's always a good idea to get two or three opinions from not only medical doctors, but also an alternative healer of your choice—i.e., Chinese herbalist, naturopathic physician, chiropractor, nutritionist, and so forth. Physicians can ably diagnose the disease on a biological level, but the others can do so on dietary and spiritual as well as physical levels.

Relief Measures

One of us (Heinerman) has written several major books on the subject of cancer. They are: The Treatment of Cancer with Herbs and East/West Remedies for Wellness & Recovery (co-authored with Henry Yun, Ph.D., N.D.). (This three-volume set is available for $175 from John Heinerman, FOB 11471, Salt Lake City, UT 84147. This is mentioned if readers wish to have more data on the subject than space allows.)

While a number of medicinal plants have been previously screened by the National Cancer Institute for possible anti-tumor properties, there are only a few that seem to work. It should be pointed out that their ultimate efficacy over this disease is largely determined by how early the treatments begin and just how far the cancer has already advanced. While herbs are certainly no magic bullets for cancer, they can prove to be effective in many cases.

The following short list explains how some of them work inside the body to promote tumor regressions:

BLACK WALNUT. The juglone in the bark and roots deny the growth of moss and other vegetation on or immediately around the tree. Suggested intake of capsules is four daily.

CHAPARRAL. Grows in the West and Southwest. Nothing—not even other chaparral or weeds of any kind—will ever grow within several feet of its perimeter. The root system secretes a potent anti-growth substance called NDGA. Both the *Rocky Mountain Medical Journal* (Nov. 1970) and *Cancer Chemotherapy Reports* (April, 1969) have favorably discussed its value in cancer therapy. Best taken as a tea, one cupful every four hours on an empty stomach until bedtime. Be sure to steep the tea for at least *ten hours* before drinking it!

GOLDENSEAL. The yellow-colored berberine in the root has destroyed live cancer cell cultures in lab petri dishes. About six capsules daily is advised, unless you're hypoglycemic. (Wakunaga is the best brand to look for in health food stores for this.)

GARLIC. Benjamin Lau, M.D., Ph.D. of the Dept. of Microbiology at California's Loma Linda School of Medicine, has carefully researched aged garlic extract supplied to him by the Wakunaga Pharmaceutical Co. of Japan on different kinds of tumors. And has found, as he states in his recent book, *Garlic For Health*, that Kyolic aged-garlic extract suppresses tumor growth by enhancing the body's own immune defenses. About 8 capsules of the liquid Kyolic each day with meals is advised. (See Appendix under Walkunaga for both.)

RED CLOVER. One of us (Heinerman) discovered an amazing account of how this tea cured a very stubborn case of facial melanoma in the December, 1867 issue of *Phrenological Journal*. While it's too long to relate here, suffice it to say an 80-year-old fellow named Truman Woodford failed to find relief for his problem from some of the best physicians whom he consulted in his time. Only after drinking red clover tea in large quantities instead of water, did his cancer finally clear up after a decade of persistent growth. Four glasses daily with meals is suggested.

SPIRULINA AND WHEAT GRASS. Both are rich in chlorophyll, though one is an algae and the other a land-based crop. They contain a wealth of minerals, vitamins and trace elements which stimulate the immune system to stronger action against such malignancies. Wakunaga of America makes an excellent powdered green drink mixture containing these items and barley grass and boiled brown rice. A level tablespoonful in an 8 fluid ounce glass of water or juice, twice daily, is advised.

In treating cancer, a multi-faceted approach must be used. Besides drugs or surgeries, or herbal therapies, diet, and nutrition, there must also be other considerations as well. In Chapter 176 of the *Comprehensive Textbook of Oncology* (2nd Ed.), some contributing authors discuss the emotional and psychological ramifications of the management of this disease. They point out that grief, fear, covert hostility ("Why me of all people?"), hopelessness, loneliness, helplessness, a sense of isolation, and utter depression must all be adequately dealt with by the practitioner or else all other treatments will inevitably fail. They emphasize that caregivers need to be very understanding, extremely patient, full of love, and willing to listen and offer encouragement wherever appropriate.

Foods and Nutrients

This same massive reference work (published in 1991 by Williams & Wilkins) estimates that about 35%, of cancers may be attributable to dietary factors. A growing number of epidemiologic studies indicate that too much fat, not enough fiber, and inadequate consumption of vitamins, minerals and trace elements could be associated with cancers of the esophagus, stomach, colon, rectum, pancreas, and liver, as well as some hormone-specific locations like breast, prostate, ovaries, and endometrium. It is worth noting that the increased incidence of cancer can be correlated with the increased use of margarine and the depletion of our top soil (admitted by the USDA in 1935.)

Some interesting things have emerged from specific cultural groups which have been extensively studied by scientists of late. Doctors who've monitored the Seventh-Day Adventists (who are mostly vegetarians) and the Mormons (who are heavy meat eaters) have noticed that both groups have less breast and colon cancers than comparable U.S. white populations of similar socioeconomic status. Neither group smokes and alcohol, coffee, colas, and black/green tea are either held to an absolute minimum (Adventist) or else not used at all (Mormons).

But where it really becomes amazing is in the diets of the Navajo Indians. Dr. De Lamar Gibbons and other Adventist physicians, who've labored many years in religious hospitals located on or near the Navajo Reservation, have noticed a virtual absence

of cancer, period! This isn't to say that the Navajos are healthy by any means. They have more than their share of obesity, diabetes, hypertension, infant mortality, Bubonic plague and so forth. But, as Dr. Gibbons observed in his article "Indians Hold Key to Cancer" in the November 29th, 1987 *Salt Lake Tribune*, "None of us have ever seen a breast cancer or a lung cancer in a Navajo" despite the fact that a lot of fat is consumed and many of the men smoke like chimneys! The answer to this riddle is two-fold: First of all, the Navajos never eat chicken or turkey (believing them to be birds of evil omen); and secondly, they thoroughly boil most of the red meat (mutton and beef) they do consume. Dr. Gibbons noted that "most of these people avoid animal-source foods that may contain the viruses known to cause cancer" in man and beast alike.

But the most comprehensive and ambitious task ever undertaken in the 20th century was carried out in 65 different counties in mainland China from 1976 to 1989. During that time some 20 million deaths were investigated and some 6,500 living men and women surveyed as to their diets. Both deaths and diets of the living were studied for their relationship to cancer. The final results were tallied and jointly published by Oxford and Cornell University Presses in 1990, a massive, nearly one thousand-page volume appropriately entitled: *Diet, Lifestyle, and Mortality in China.*

One statement prominently featured in the book (p. 56) is this: "The lowest risk of cancer is generated by the consumption of a variety of fresh plant products." Particularly, sulphur-bearing vegetables. The following sulphur foods are routinely consumed in those mainland Chinese counties with the lowest cancer mortality rates: apricots, broccoli, brussel sprouts, cabbage, cauliflower, collard greens, garlic, horseradish, kale, kohlrabi, mustard greens, onion, radishes, spinach, and sunflower seeds.

There are, of course, many other foods which offer a certain amount of protection against cancer. Some of them include bran, Brazil nuts, brown rice, butternut squash, cantaloupe, carrots, chard, figs, grapefruit, great northern beans and kidney beans, kiwis, mangoes, cooked oatmeal, oranges, papaya, peas, popcorn, potatoes, prunes, pumpkin, raisins, salmon, sardines, strawberries, sweet bell peppers, swordfish, tofu, tuna, turnips and rutabagas, wheat germ and whole wheat, and yogurt. But the evidence from China clearly speaks in favor of sulphur-rich foods to afford the best protection against cancer.

A variety of different vitamins, minerals and amino acids, likewise, help to prevent as well as treat this dreaded disease. A brief discussion of them follows below. Vitamin C is the keystone of therapy in cancer. At least 10 grams to be taken daily. Most patients will increase the dose by one gram per day until the bowel movements become sloppy. That is called titrating the dose by bowel tolerance. When one has found this saturation dose, one moves back to a sub-diarrhea dose. Vitamin A is added if the cancer involves the eyes, the skin, the bowels, or the lungs. 100,000 International Units (lUs) would not be toxic in such cases. Beta-carotene may be taken simultaneously in 50,000 I.U. amounts.

Certain key trace elements are absolutely essential in cancer nutrition. The first of these is sulphur, and is to be principally obtained from those foods highest in

this odorific mineral: cabbage, kale, kohlrabi, brussel sprouts, broccoli, cauliflower, garlic, onion, mustard greens, spinach, watercress, and blackstrap molasses.

Next come selenium and germanium. About 200 micrograms of the first and 25 mg. of the second are suggested each day. They seem to work best with Korean ginseng (2 capsules) and should be taken simultaneously with that herb.

For some cancer patients, folic acid (1,000 mcg.) therapy seems to help as well. A vegetarian, low-fat diet with plenty of fresh fruit and vegetable juices and cooked whole grains will stress the body functions less and expedite recovery more quickly.

CANDIDIASIS

Symptoms

This particular fungal infection affects the intestines, the genitalia of both men and women, and the mouth and throat. Under healthy conditions, Candida albicans exists in harmony with other types of bacteria and yeasts within the system; but when the immune system becomes weakened by physical, mental and especially emotional stresses, then it rapidly multiplies and becomes candidiasis.

In the mouth it appears as thrush, forming white sores many times on the tongue, inside cheeks and tooth gums. In the vagina area of a woman's body, it's known as vaginitis and usually results in a large discharge of white, cheesey stuff and accompanied always by uncontrollable itching. It's thought that other skin problems like athlete's foot, ringworm, jock itch and diaper rash may be caused by a combination of food allergies and candidiasis.

Symptoms vary considerably depending on wherever Candida decides to set up shop. In the G.I. tract they can include constipation, diarrhea, colitis, gut pain, and heart burn. In muscle tissue, it can sometimes mimic the painful inflammation common to rheumatoid arthritis. Mental and emotional imbalances also are likely to occur as well—hyperactivity, anger, and depression.

It is also important to point out that such symptoms may often occur with hypoglycemia and chronic fatigue syndrome as well. In fact, there are related crossovers to all three of these conditions, which makes it even more difficult for doctors to correctly diagnose.

Relief Measures

Two of the very best antibiotic herbs to use in controlling candidiasis are aged-garlic extract and goldenseal root, both from Wakunaga of America (see Appendix). The first can be taken with meals (1 capsule) three times a day, while the latter works best on an empty stomach (2 capsules).

Practicing a so-called "rotation diet" helps to limit the spread of candidiasis. Both authors have discussed aspects of this diet in their own books. But their collective wisdom on just how well this diet works is given in the synopsis below:

First Three Weeks

1. Whole grain cereals (hot or cold), breadstuffs, pastas, tortillas, and popcorn are permitted. But breadstuffs made with baker's yeast should be avoided!

2. Organic (unsprayed) vegetables (except iceberg lettuce may be eaten raw, lightly cooked or baked.)

3. A variety of cooked legumes is highly recommended.

4. Unprocessed nuts and seeds are good to eat (except peanuts and peanut products).

5. The judicious use of some spices with antibacterial activities to them is advised: bay, cinnamon, cloves, garlic, lemon grass, mustard, onion, rosemary, sage, and thyme.

6. Butter and cold-pressed vegetable oils may be used.

7. Fish (with fins and scales only) and lean red meat (veal, lamb and rabbit) except pork ought to be used more often than poultry.

8. Avoid regular milk and eggs and just use goat's milk.

Second Three Weeks

1. Gradually work back in small amounts of dark grain yeast breads.

2. Slowly add back one fresh fruit or fruit juice at a time. Overripe and canned fruits should continue to be eliminated.

3. Natural sweeteners may be put back, but restricted to blackstrap molasses and pure maple syrup only. All honey and white sugar foods should still be avoided!

4. Certain types of cheese can be added back into the diet, but mold-derived kinds (Roquefort) should be avoided.

5. Other foods can be steadily worked back into the diet so long as they do not evoke serious reactions in the person with candidiasis. All forms of alcohol and deep-fried/fried foods, however, should continue to be eliminated from the diet.

Foods and Nutrients

We recommend the consumption of *live* (not pasteurized) cultured yogurt or its application inside the vagina because it seems to help inhibit the spread of candidiasis. KyoDophilus capsules (2-3 daily) from Wakunaga (see Appendix) can assist in restoring normal balance to the colon and vagina.

Caprylic acid (2 tablets daily), high potency vitamin B-complex (3 tablets daily), germanium (50 mg. daily), and an omega 3-6 fatty acid combination are recommended. Vitamin A (50,000 I .U. daily), vitamin C (3,500 mg. daily), selenium (200 mgg. daily)

and L-Cysteine (500 mg.) daily should be taken, too.

CANKER SORES

Symptoms

Cankers sore s have white centers and surrounding red borders to them that occur on the inside of the mouth and lips. Their sizes range from pinhead to half-dollar in some cases.

Relief Measures

Here's what we've found to be the most effective treatment for getting rid of them. Crush a small zinc tablet. Then snip off the end of a vitamin E oil capsule and squeeze out the contents and mix in with this powdered zinc to make a paste. Spread on to a small postage-stamp size piece of adhesive tape and apply directly to lips or corners of the mouth where such sores frequently occur. If inside the mouth, just spread a very thin layer of peanut butter on to half a slice of white bread. Then apply this zinc-oil paste to an inch square section of the bread center with a cotton swab, cut it out with a knife and then insert into the mouth and firmly affix to the sore itself. Repeat as often as needed in both cases.

Also frequently gargling with goldenseal or chaparral tea helps get rid of them as well.

Foods and Nutrients

Eat fresh salad made with shredded cabbage, chopped cauliflower and onions, and minced garlic. Sulphur helps sores to disappear. Avoid eating sugary foods and citrus juices and soft drinks.

CARBUNCLE

Symptoms

A carbuncle is a painful, localized infection beneath the surface of the skin which usually produces pus. It often appears as a group of boils, but is more painful, deeper and slower-healing than a boil is.

Relief Measures

Proper hygiene is one way to get rid of a carbuncle. The area around the site should be frequently scrubbed with a strong soap and plenty of hot water. A good pine-tar soap from a local veterinary supply house is recommended for this. Or something with rough granules in it like Lava to penetrate the skin is advised.

Hot compresses can relieve and promote healing, too. Lemon grass or hyssop are recommended for this. Adequate sleep is helpful and so is a healthy diet.

Foods and Nutrients

Vitamins A (25,000 I .U.), C (1,500 mg.), and E (800 I.U.) are recommended on daily basis. Also, some vitamin E oil from an opened capsule can be applied externally to the carbuncle after it has been thoroughly cleansed and dried. The application of some tincture of witch hazel following this may further help it to disappear.

CATARACTS

Symptoms

This is a condition in which the lens of the eye becomes clouded or opaque. (This is the part which enables us to focus and see objects close up or distant with greater clarity.) Symptoms of cataracts include painless, but gradual blurring of the vision, hypersensitivity to bright lights, and the appearance of halos around lights.

Relief Measures

Washing the eyes with a solution of eyebright tea may help to diminish their progress in the early stages. Using antioxidant spices such as rosemary, thyme, sage and garlic in cooking helps to destroy the free radicals which cause cataracts.

Foods and Nutrients

Calcium-rich, dark leafy green vegetables and B-l (75 mg.), B-2 (100 mg.), C (1,500 mg.) sod E (600 I.U.), along with pantothenic acid (250 mg.) are suggested on a routine basis.

CARPAL TUNNEL SYNDROME

Symptoms

Long hours spent at repetitive hand-intensive tasks can lead to carpel tunnel syndrome. Assembly-line work such as boning chickens in a processing plant, typing or computer keyboarding, or even hobbies like knitting or playing the piano, are all capable of causing this. Symptoms begin with pins and needles effect and numbness in the hand. In time, they worsen, extending to wasted thumb muscles, a weakened grip, and severe hand pain that sometimes radiates to the forearm or shoulder.

Relief Measures

While working with your hands, keep your wrists straight. Flexing, extending, or twisting them stresses your carpal tunnel. Use your entire hand and fingers when you grip an object. Cut down on repetitive gestures as much as possible, and take a break from handwork every half hour or so.

Also rubbing the surface of the skin with some eucalpytus ointment or a few drops of peppermint oil, and then gently massaging the hand for a few minutes will help to reduce pain and inflammation.

Foods and Nutrients

Daily intake of pantothenic acid (75 mg.) and zinc (50 mg.) should help to bring some relief also.

CAVITIES

Symptoms

This is the lay term for the loss of tooth structure due to dental caries. Caries is a localized, progressively destructive disease of the teeth which starts with the enamel, then graduates to the protein matrix and dentin, and finally destroys the organic matrix of the tooth itself.

Throbbing pain (see TOOTHACHE), bad breath and rotten teeth are the most prolific evidence of cavities by far.

Relief Measures

Brushing the teeth after every meal with a wet medium-soft toothbrush and a little common table salt instead of the customary toothpaste is recommended. Flossing is also important to help prevent plaque buildup as well. And rinsing the mouth after every meal or snack is a very important thing to do. One of the authors (and we won't say which of us) is in the habit of doing this quite frequently, even in public restaurants, with a glass of water—sometimes to the embarrassment of others including himself. But the fact of the matter remains, it does help to curtail cavities quite a bit!

Foods and Nutrients

Certain foods seem to rot teeth faster than other foods do. All soft drinks and colas tend to increase the demineralization of tooth structure more rapidly than other fluids do. And also sticky foods like jams, jellies, peanut butter, raisins, dates and so forth, tend to produce decay more quickly unless the teeth are immediately brushed after eating such things, which isn't always possible.

CELIAC DISEASE

Symptoms

Some people can't tolerate a protein called gluten found in wheat, rye and barley. It tends to irritate their intestinal lining terribly, causing diarrhea, gut pains, nausea, bad smelling bowel movements that float instead of sink like they should, loss of weight, skin outbreaks, and joint/bone pain.

Relief Measures

Powdered cardamom, an aromatic kitchen spice, seems to allay most of these symptoms. This can be mixed in with cooked grain cereals or taken in capsules (4) or spoonfuls (.5 tsp.) in some liquid.

Foods and Nutrients

Kyo-dophilus (3 capsules) from Wakunaga (see Appendix), papain (3 tablets), magnesium (750 mg.) and vitamin B-6 (300 mg.) should be taken daily as needed.

CELLULITIS

Symptoms

In simple terms, cellulitis is that digusting form of fat which accumulates on the buttocks, thighs, hips and arms, mostly in women. It's a combination of fat globules, waste material, and water captured in muscle tissue. It's most evident by the skin being pulled inward because of fibrous strands of tissue, and, in the process, plumping the fat cells outward.

Relief Measures

Exercise, massage and sweating are three of the best ways to get rid of this stuff. Wrapping portions of the body in air-permeable plastic (such as Saran Wrap), while

pedaling on a stationary bike for up to 20 minutes at one time, helps to break up some of this cellulite.

Rubbing into the skin essential oils of sandalwood or juniper is still another way to go about this. Follow it up with a vigorous massage of these areas, before entering a spa for 15 minutes. Also dry-brushing the skin with a natural bristle brush helps to improve circulation and remove cellulite.

Foods and Nutrients

People with cellulite usually have poor bowel movements. Eating some bran or taking 4 capsules of psyllium seed hulls will overcome this for sure. Drinking at least 6 glasses of mineral or spring water every day helps, too. Some vegetable juices, like 1/4 carrot and 3/4 mixed greens (celery, parsley, Romaine lettuce) should be added to the regimen as well.

CEREBRAL PALSY

Symptoms

When the brain becomes injured due to a fall or blow to the head of some kind or because of a viral infection, there is a substantial loss of motor nerve power and muscular coordination. Partial paralysis or extremely awkward muscular efforts are the most noticeable. This best describes cerebral palsy.

Relief Measures

There isn't much that can be done in such cases without competent medical assistance. However, one European doctor in Prague, Czechkoslovakia whom one of the authors interviewed awhile back, seems to think that massage and St. Johnswort tincture may help to some extent. The massage he emphasizes is more of a vigorous rubbing, slapping and pinching along the spinal column and neck using a tiny amount of peppermint oil. The St. Johnswort is given beneath the tongue (15 drops) three times daily.

Foods and Nutrients

Those foods high in copper (nuts, oysters, and avocados), magnesium (dark leafy greens, kelp, spinach), and phosphorus (organ meats, yellow cheese, egg yolks), as well as individual amounts of each of these nutrients themselves appears to be helpful, some European doctors declare.

CHAPPED LIPS & SKIN

Symptoms

A condition like this is brought on by excessive exposure to wind and sun. Afflicted areas become sore, red, and tend to peel as a result.

Relief Measures

Some type of lip balm or protectant is very helpful under such adverse weather conditions. Besides Chap Stick, there are also several creamy lipsticks made by Revlon and Max Factor, which can prove useful at times when the former isn't readily available. And rugged men shouldn't hesitate to use these things; it's a lot better than having your lips so cracked and inflamed that they feel like the parched Mojave Desert floor. Only don't be seen in public wearing the same, we advise the guys, or you're bound to draw a few stares from startled passers-by.

One of the best things for protecting your skin against too much wind and sun, besides the usual sunscreen agents, can only be found in a farm supply house or veterinary supply center. It's called Bag Balm and is petroleum-based. Dairy farmers use it all the time on their cows' udders when they become cracked and sore. Just rub some of the stuff on your hands, arms, neck and face, and you'll be surprised at just how well it works. One of us (Heinerman) has used it in times past when working on his family cattle ranch in the southern Utah wilderness.

Foods and Nutrients

A nifty remedy one of the authors has devised for chapped lips and cracked skin, consists of mixing a little vitamin E oil, the powders from two crushed zinc and PABA tablets and some melted beeswax together, then allowing the mixture to harden just a trifle before rubbing on injured skin surfaces. Avocado oil is also very good for this. And taking a teaspoonful of olive oil internally doesn't hurt either.

CHEMICAL POISONING

Symptoms

Prolonged exposure to harmful chemicals can lead to excess toxicities within the body. Symptoms for such aren't always easy to detect, as they often take years before they become readily apparent. However, some general signs can be traced to this type of problem: the appearance of sudden and unexplained rashes; extreme allergies to ordinary things; the development of mysterious lesions and boils that refuse to go away; continual bouts of low-to-moderate grade infections; etc.

Relief Measures

An effective cleansing and detoxification program of the entire body must be commenced at once. Liquids in the form of red clover and burdock root tea are useful for the blood stream, while dandelion root tea and tomato juice are important for the liver. Additionally, powdered chlorophyll such as Wakunaga's Kyo-Green (see Appendix), which has been re-constituted with water according to label directions, is essential to take.

Foods and Nutrients

The consuiption of water-containing fresh fruits and vegetables is to be strongly encouraged. Berries of every description, peaches, pears, and melons (when in season), tomatoes, cucumbers, and so forth are excellent cleansers for the body in this respect.

Protein in the form of a good free-form amino acid supplement (3 capsules or tablets daily) is useful. So is a high-potency B-complex (4 tablets daily) supplement, too. And about 7,500 mg. of vitamin C with bioflavonoids wouldn't hurt either.

CHICKENPOX

Symptoms

Chicken Pox is a highly contagious childhood disease, which sometimes manifests itself again in late adulthood in the form of shingles. Both are caused by the herpes virus. Symptoms include skin eruptions, headache, fever, weakness, and itching.

Relief Measures

Bathe the afflicted parts often with rose petal water or lavender tea. To expedite the healing of the blisters, bathe the skin with a strong solution of white oak bark tea or tincture of witch hazel.

Foods and Nutrients

Internally, vitamin A (25, 000 I .U.) and vitamin C (1, 500 mg.) should be given to the child each day with a cup of warm mullein tea. Externally, a paste made out of small amounts of powdered goldenseal root and vitamin E oil should be applied topically, often. The sick child should be given some warm catnip tea to drink every few hours, to bring the fever down.

CHILD ABUSE

Symptoms

Child abuse is very common at present. Physical abuse of children can include hitting, slapping, and kicking by mean and aggressive adults. Obvious symptoms would be bruises, welts, and bone fractures.

But a more sinister kind, which is quite pervasive, is sexual child abuse. While there is little or no physical evidence for this, the mental and emotional scarring which transpires can remain for years and require an entire lifetime to get over.

Children suffering from this latter abuse become withdrawn, sullen, antisocial, fearful, despondent, full of low self-esteem, and occasionally suicidal.

Relief Measures

While we would like to think that psychological counseling could and should help in such instances, the sad fact of the matter is that it doesn't always do this. Both of us in our respective professions of pediatrics and anthropology have been aware of many such cases like this through the years. And have discovered for ourselves that words alone can't suffice.

The well-intentioned parent or adult care-giver responsible for such a suffering child, needs to understand that extreme patience, much love, and a good deal of hope are needed to make sunshine out of real darkness. And when love is to be expressed, it ought to be done so in words and deeds, but not necessarily with physical touching, such as hugging. For the child thus abused, is apt to recoil from the mere suggestion of touch in many instances, recalling to mind the sickening touches of his or her abuser.

Giving a child a pet such as a puppy, kitten or bunny rabbit, to take care of and adore may be helpful. Both the adult and the child can share in petting and handling such a creature with minimal difficulty and virtually no embarrassment or discomfort between them. While both are petting such an animal, the adult can frequently remind the child through verbal encouragement, that there are positive benefits to be derived from *proper* touching.

Foods and Nutrients

It has been the experience of some European therapists, where child abuse occurs less frequently, that spicy and sugary foods tend to upset the abused youngster. Therefore, they should be ruled out of the diet for awhile. Also, an abused child might do well to be given a high-potency B-complex vitamin (2 tablets) and a magnesium supplement (600 mg.) each day with meals. Warm catnip tea is also good on occasions.

CHILDBIRTH

Symptoms

Childbirth is that very special moment when a woman is delivered of the life which she has carried inside of her for some nine months, more or less. And while the final event itself is obviously quite joyful by the healthy youngster just delivered, there is much pain and trauma accompanying it beforehand.

Relief Measures

However, there are certain things which can be done to reduce some of these unpleasant aspects and to make the entire process more enjoyable for everyone concerned, including the mother herself.

For one thing, the nausea and vomiting experienced during the first trimester of pregnancy can be greatly alleviated by the woman drinking some warm ginger tea every few hours. (See also under MORNING SICKNESS for additional things to be done.)

And the risk of possible miscarriages can be greatly reduced if an expectant mother will just take a couple of capsules of Wakunaga's Premium Kyolic-EPA (see Appendix) every day. The rich marine lipids provide lots of vitamin A and the aged garlic extract supplies the body with sufficient sulphur amino acids to fight viral infections that may cause spontaneous abortions or premature deliveries.

A pregnant woman should never wear high heels, should never smoke, should never drink coffee or alcohol, should watch her intake of sweet things, and should get plenty of rest. All of these factors will guarantee a healthier and happier baby.

And to make birth less complicated, the expectant mother should drink 3-5 cups of hot raspberry leaf tea every day in the last several days just prior to her actual delivery. Smuggling hot herbal tea into her hospital room in a thermos by her husband or friends,

is a good way to get around a doctor's objections to this.

Foods and Nutrients

Whole grain cereals and breads, dark leafy greens (cooked side dishes or else in salads), some dairy products (yogurt and cottage cheese especially), eggs occasionally, and certain organ meats (liver) will give an expectant mom the essential minerals her body requires for a safe and happy delivery.

The intake of vitamin E (800 mg.), lecithin (1 teaspoon of the liquid), and a high-potency B-complex (4 tablets), along with ample magnesium (800-1, 200 mg.) will strengthen the nerves during this period.

CHILLS

Symptoms

Such can occur for several different reasons, one being lack of adequate circulation throughout the body. Secondly, lack of proper clothing during cold weather. Yet a third reason might be consumption of very cold liquids, such as icy drinks, which plunge body temperature dramatically.

Typical sensations would include shivering and pallor, and an elevated internal temperature. The onset of an infectious illness of some kind is usually preceded by the chills.

Relief Measures

Warm red clover tea or slightly heated tomato or V-8 juice to which has been added a pinch of cayenne pepper will improve blood circulation. Full cotton, woolen or flannel clothing are great for insulating body heat and keeping a person warmer in cold weather. The hands, head and feet should always be properly covered, as these are the main exits for heat from the body.

Foods and Nutrients

If chills are due to viral infection, the diet ought to consist of mostly liquid nourishment. Including plenty of sleep and *night-time* supplementation with kyolic aged-garlic extract (four capsules), vitamin A (50,000 I.U.) and vitamin C (3,500 mg.), washed down with a glass of reconstituted Kyo-green (1 level tbsp. to 8 fi. oz. of water) (see Appendix under Wakunaga). In such instances, dairy products, eggs, soft drinks, and solid foods should be avoided.

CHOLERA

Symptoms

Throughout most of the 19th and even into the early part of this century, doctors referred to a variety of gastrointestinal disturbances of unkown etiologies as cholera. But in reality this is a serious epidemic infection caused by Vibrio cholerae. While occurring primarily in Asia, it has made terrible comebacks in some South American countries of late.

Customary symptoms include profuse watery diarrhea, an extreme loss of fluid and electrolytes, and a state of dehydration and collapse. Between the constant

vomiting and continual diarrhea, the victim becomes very weak, suffers loss of energy, and can be reduced to a state of near or actual death, unless immiediately attended to.

Relief Measures

Early medical reference works, published in the 19th century, suggested that using one of various types of enemas was the most effective way to treat cholera and bring immediate relief. A strong base solution of warm black coffee (1 pint) and a little bicarbonate of soda (1 tsp.) mixed in with it, is made first of all. After this can be added 1/2 cup of strong white oak bark tea to which has been added either .5 teaspoonful of powdered echinacea or gun Arabic. Also swallowing 3-4 capsules of kola nut with some white wine appears to be helpful.

Food and Nutrients

Liquid nourishment is to be preferred here in place of solids. Barley soup and chicken or fish broth are heartily recommended. Tonics consisting of small parts of brandy or Burgundy or port wines and white oak bark tea are excellent as well. About 1,200 mg. of potassium may also be necesary.

CHOLESTEROL (ELEVATED)

Symptoms

Hypercholesterolemia is brought about because of our preference for fatty and greasy foods that taste good, but in reality, do a lot of damage to the body. Poor blood circulation, difficulty in breathing, gallstones, obesity, colon cancer and polyps, and hypertension are some of the more obvious symptoms. Mere recent evidence suggests that it may now be triglyceride elevations with which we should be more concerned, however.

Relief Measures/Foods & Nutrients

The frequent consumption of garlic, onion, leek and scallion with meals that contain meat or fried foods, will subtantially cut down your elevated cholesterol and triglyceride levels. The consumption of cereal grains once or twice daily, such as cooked oatmeal for breakfast and granola for an evening snack, help too.

The following supplements should also be taken on a daily basis as well: choline and inositol (250 mg. each); Coenzyme Q-10 (60 mg.); Kyolic aged-garlic extract (4 capsules); liquid lecithin (1 tbsp.); niacin (250 mg.); vitamin C (3,500 mg) and emulsified vitamin E (800 I.U.).

CHRONIC FATIGUE SYNDROME

Symptoms

By its very name, the most suggested and obvious symptom appears to be a chronic and continual lack of energy for great lengths of time. Believed to be caused by a member of the herpes family (Epstein Barr virus or EBV), this traumatic disorder also elicits other symptoms which are common to influenza and hypoglycemia as well—appetite loss, mood swings, intestinal tract problems,

unexplained aches and pains in bone joints and muscle tissue, sensitivity to light, insomnia, and so forth. In fact, trying to separate the three is real tricky for inexperienced physicians unfamiliar with chronic fatigue syndrome.

Relief Measures

Goldenseal and garlic and onions are all good for controlling the herpes virus causing this, provided the victim isn't also suffering from low blood sugar as well. These three items tend to be very hypoglycemic in nature and those with this blood sugar imbalance may want to substitute wild Oregon grape root and Kyolic aged-garlic extract instead. About four capsules daily of each is suggested on an empty stomach.

Foods and Nutrients

Dietary considerations are more vital here than one may realize. At least 65% of consumed foods should be raw and alive: some fruits, root and leafy vegetables, nuts, seeds, and freshly made juices. Cooked whole grains in the form of breads, cereals and pastas as well as poached or baked fresh or salt-water fish and limited amounts of veal, lamb and certain hormone-free organ meats (particularly liver) do well in promoting energy. Likewise, so do cooked beans, lentils and chickpeas.

An arsenal of supplements is definitely needed in order to fortify the system against further havoc by this malicious little virus. Buffered vitamin C (7, 500 mg.), Kyodophilus (3 capsules), vitamins A & E (50,000 and 800 I .U .'s respectively), any high-potency vitamin B-complex (4 tablets), and an all-around mineral supplement (4 tablets). Additionally, daily intakes of powdered Kyo-Green (1 level tbsp.) in 8 fl. oz. of tomato juice will provide more fuel for the body to run on. (See Appendix under Wakunaga for the various products listed here.)

Since about two-thirds of all chronic fatigue syndrome sufferers also are infected with Candida albicans, it may be worthwhile checking under CANDIDIASIS for further information.

CIRRHOSIS OF THE LIVER

Symptoms

Cirrhosis of the liver is a degenerative, inflammatory disease induced by consumption of too much alcohol and greasy foods, as well as by infectious hepatitis. Obvious symptoms in the early stages are yellow skin, indigestion, and poor colon functions. Later symptoms include bruising, gout, and anemia.

Relief Measures

Dandelion or chicory root teas (2 cups daily) with meals is recommended. Or 3 capsules of either when eating. Peach bark tea (1/2 cup twice daily) on an empty stomach is useful. Four goldenseal root capsules is also helpful if the subject isn't hypoglycemic. Alfalfa tea (1 cup or 4 capsules) with a meal works wonders for the liver. So does a liquid chlorophyll preparation like Wakunaga's Kyo-Green.

Food and Nutrients

A nice vegetable "cocktail" for revitalizing weak livers calls for an 8 fl. oz. glass of tomato or low-sodium V-8 juice into which a pinch of cayenne pepper and .5 teaspoon of lime juice have been added.

Useful supplements include liquid lecithin (1 tbsp.), brewer's yeast powder (1 tsp.) mixed in with some juice, powdered vitamin C (2 tsps. which is the equivalent of 3,500 mg.), and some soybean protein (1 tsp.). These can be mixed in with the above-mentioned juices. Also dessicated liver tablets (2) from your local health food store is advised.

COLD SORES

Symptoms

Cold sores are known as fever blisters, and are caused by the herpes simplex I virus. They originate mainly because of mental, emotional, physical or environmental stresses upon the body and turn into highly contagious sores.

Relief Measures

Localize the infection first by washing the area with a strong solution of white oak bark tea. Then apply a paste made of powdered goldenseal root and honey to the skin.

Foods and Nutrients

L-lysine applied as a cream is helpful. A zinc gluconate (25 mg.) tablet dissolved in the mouth is good. A chewable vitamin C tablet is suggested, too. A high-potency B-complex (3 tablets) is advised, along with magnesium (1,200 mg.).

COLIC AND COLITIS

Symptoms

Colic and colitis are disturbances in different parts of the gastrointestinal tract. Colic is characterized by sharp, agonizing bouts of pain which cause writhing agony. Sometimes a cold feeling and vomiting occur. Pains can be similar to those associated with appendicitis, gall stones and kidney stones.

Colitis occurs when the mucosal lining deep inside the colon becomes severely inflamed. Small pouches of purulent matter form. Symptoms include cramps similar to those for colic, watery stools and continuous trips to the bathroom.

Relief Measures

Remedies for both conditions are similar and work equally well. Warm catnip or ginger tea, and cool marshmallow or slippery elm teas (1 cup with each meal) are recommended. Capsules (2 per meal) may be substituted, but the tea is preferred.

Foods and Nutrients

Barley broth soup, cooked oatmeal (the instant kind), cooked Cream o' Wheat cereal, yogurt, cottage cheese, melons, cucumbers, and carrot juice are good to eat. But avoid very starchy, sweet, acidic, fatty foods for awhile.

COLOR AND NIGHT BLINDNESS

Symptoms

Color blindness makes it very difficult to distinguish red and green; usually they appear as gray. Specific types of color blindness are protanopia, deuteranopia, and tritanopia.

Night blindness is a decreased ability to see in reduced illumination (nighttime), but without any apparent organic disease involved. The lack of adequate amounts of visual purple in the retina is believed to be responsible for this.

Relief Measures/Foods and Nutrients

Both conditions require the expert care of a qualified opthalmologist. But a German eye doctor, S. Niedermeir, M.D., mentioned in the medical periodical *Deutsche medizinische Wochenschrift* (76:210, Feb. 16, 1951), that he used a lique-fied blend of dandelion flowers and vitamins A and B-2 on his patients suffering from either of these, with apparently good results. The addition of the herb eyebright may bring additional improvement to some.

COMA

Symptoms

Coma is a condition brought about by a traumatic blow to the head, by a stroke or brain tumor, by drug or chemical poisoning, by diabetes mellitus sometimes when there is a lack of adequate sugar in the blood, by an epileptic seizure, by meningitis and other acute fevers, by severe hemorrhaging, by extreme temperatures such as sunstroke, and very rarely by ordinary hysteria and grief.

The usual symptoms are loss of consciousness, with a gradual deepening of the same. Such passing out is often accompanied by slow, stertorous breathing, which is more prolonged in its effect than would be for ordinary fainting spells.

Relief Measures

Maria Treben, one of Europe's greatest living herbalists, currently resides with members of her family in Grieskirchen, in northern Austria. Her first book, *Heilkrauter aus dem Garten Gottes* was published in 1980 by Wilhelm Ennsthaler of Steyr. It became an instant best-seller overnight with sales now totalling close to 4.5 million copies with editions in 7 different languages.

One of the authors contacted her a few years ago relative to comas. She recommended that tiny pinches of tragacanth gum (Astragalus gumifer) and valerian root be mixed together and the powders placed under the nostrils of said victim or else put into a forded piece of paper and blown directly up the nose with the aid of a straw. The natural occuring stink from both should arouse the person, she thought.

Another more involved remedy for serious comas calls for lifting the patient's head, opening his or her mouth, and pouring some of her special Swedish Bitters blend down the throat very slowly. While Swedish Bitters can be bought at most health food stores, she prefers that people take the time to make their own. Combine 1/2 ounces of powdered wormwood, hops, angelica, myrrh, camphor, rhubarb, and senne in a large fruit jar and add 2 1/2 pints (1.5 litres) of vodka. Seal the bottle with a tight lid and let it stand in a warm place for about three weeks. Only be sure to shake the contents vigoroustly each day. A tip she says, is that the potency of this mixture becomes greater the longer it's permitted to stand. 2-3 tablespoonfuls should be administered each time until recovery to normal senses becomes apparent.

She also insists that the vital points on the hands, wrists, feet, and neck be vigorously rubbed with Mentholatum, too.

Food and Nutrients

Under these difficult circumstances, we really don't see how such would apply. However, we think the administration of some hot clear chicken broth, heavily spiked with crushed jalepeno peppers and lime juice, should get the brain's attention in no time at all. One of us (Heinerman) witnessed this being used by a Mexican curandero on a comatose young man in the Yucatan several years ago with amazingly good results!

COMMON COLD

Symptoms

Typical symptoms include the usual pounding headache and accompanying congestion, wheezing, coughing, fever, irritability and nervousness, runny nose, watery eyes, and general aches and pains. Yet how can something so simple, be so darned hard to cure? Probably because the virus keeps on changing in size and shape and into a multitude of different forms every few hours as it were. And also, because people refuse to *go to bed* when they should in order to sleep it off, among other things.

Relief Measures

One of the authors gave a lecture before 150 health food retailers, manufacturers, and distributors at the Sheraton Hotel in Hasbrouk Heights, New Jersey in mid-January, 1992. He was astonished to see so many of his audience present, coughing and sneezing and clearing their throats. When he asked some of them sitting at tables near his podium, how much sleep each of them had been getting, the answer was typically "between four to five hours." And when he persisted in further questioning as to why they didn't get more, the standard reply was this: "Because I (or we) simply don't have enough time to do it right now!" *That* right there is proof enough to show just how many of us ignore the first fundamental rule of getting over a common cold: *get lots of sleep!*

In fact, so widespread is this health problem, that one of us (Heinerman again) included it in the opening chapter of his recent best-seller, *Double the Power of Your Immune System* (Prentice-Hall, 1991). Here are some quick guidelines for knocking your next cold:

(1). Stay away from antibiotics. Instead take Kyolic aged-garlic extract and goldenseal root capsules (4 of each daily)!

(2). Aoid eating in public restaurants!

(3).Keep your nerves steady. The nervous and immune systems are more closely linked together than you may think. Drink lots of warm catnip tea for this!

(4).Wash your hands frequently and avoid large crowds.

(5). Inhale cool air and avoid extremely warm air.

Foods and Nutrients

(6). Eliminate eggs, milk, cheese, red meat, and sugary and fried/deep-fried foods from the diet until fully recovered. They tend to produce a lot of unnecessary mucus.

(7). Fortify the body with these simple supplements: vitamins A (100,000 I.U.) and C (up to 15,000 mgs.), zinc gluconate (1lozenge sucked on about every 2 hours), Kyolic aged garlic extract (6 capsules), Nature's Way cayenne pepper (4 capsules), and Wakunaga goldenseal root (2 capsules). All of these should be taken on a daily basis. (See appendix.)

COMPLEXION PROBLEMS

See under individual headings such as ACNE VULGARIS, BLACKHEADS, CHAPPED LIPS/SKIN, etc.

CONCUSSION

See under **BLOOD CIRCULATION (POOR) and COMA** for further information on this.

CONJUNCTIVITIS

Symptoms

Conjunctivitis is brought about by an inflammation of the mucous membrane that lines the eyelids and covers the scleras (white portions) of both eyes. Likely symptoms to be seen are itching, redness, some swelling, and purulent matter exuding from said membrane. Often caused by rubbing or picking around the eyes with dirty fingers or hands, contact with cigarette or cigar smoke or automobile/truck/bus exhaust fumes, contact with certain weed/tree pollens, and various chemical irritants.

Relief Measures

Washing the affected eye out with a solution of powdered boric acid (1/2 tsp.) and some red eyebright tea (1/2 cup, strained) seems to work well in such cases. Or heating one tea bag of chamomile in some potato water and then placing the moist bag over the eyelid, may help, too.

Foods and Nutrients

Children under the age of twelve who are afflicted with this problem, should be given some vitamin A (10, 000 I.U.) and C (1, 000 mg.) each day. Figure on triple this amount for adults who have it.

CONSTIPATION

Symptoms

Infrequency of bowel movements can stem from a variety of causes. Insufficient peristalsis action of the colon muscles due to lack of exercise is one. Another is the repeated failure to answer nature's call to go to the bathroom when needed. And nervousness, anxiety, traumatic stress, and general excitement can also prevent normal elimination, as well as a diet lacking adequate fluids or sufficient roughage.

The most evident signs of constipation are in the stools themselves. Small, rock-like nuggets or difficulty in elimination or the occurrence of a bowel movement every couple of days, are some of these.

Relief Measures

Warm herbal enemas made from senna or buckthorn or even coffee grounds for that matter, should evoke a bowel movement very quickly. Herbal laxatives such as cascara sagrada can be taken internally as well, in capsules (4 at a time) or tea (1 1/2 cups on an empty stomach).

Foods and Nutrients

But it has come under our observation of late that those cultures (Chinese, Indian, Mexican, Korean, etc.) which eat a lot of spicy foods, seem to have more frequent bowel movements than the rest of us do. And foods such as pulpy prune juice, orange juice, and guacamole with vinegar, also inspire regularity without necessarily becoming habit-forming.

CONVULSIONS

Symptoms

Convulsions are extraordinary muscular contractions, characteristically marked by involuntary jerks, twitches, or spasms of tightening. They can be either generalized or else in just one particular area of the body.

Generalized convulsions would include the following:

CHILLS: Bouts of shivering cold and teeth-chattering wretchedness. Marked by very cold or very hot hands and feet and excessive thirst. May be due to pneumonia, flu, tetanus, tonsillitis, polio, mononucleosis, abscess formation, malaria, and so forth.

CHILDHOOD CONVULSIONS: Child's eyes become fixed or else roll upward; the arms, legs, or entire body twitch convulsively. Often due to a high fever at the onset of an infection. Same factors in chills may be responsible for this as well. Epileptic seizures in children, however, will evoke similar symptoms as for adults: unconscious, falling, body rigidity, extreme twitching, recovery and inclination to sleep awhile.

ADULT CONVULSION: Usually come quickly and unexpectedly. Marked by falling down, jaw clenching, noisy and belabored breathing, considerable muscle jerking and rigidity, uncontrollable urination and bowel activity inside of clothing, bubbling up of saliva at corners of mouth, and temporary unconsciousness.

Localized convulsions would include the following:

FATIGUE: Involuntary twitching after someone has gone to sleep. In nervous or highly excitable people, such spasms can occur frequently, often in the face, following a surprise of some kind.

LOCKJAW: Stiffness or twitching may first occur around the wound where infection has gained entry. Due to blood poisoning.

BRAIN IRRITATION: Often a result of a tumor, internal hemorrhaging, an infection, or an injury. Mostly confined to just one spot.

TICS: Automatic movements begun with purposeful actions to them that usually get out of control, however. An example would be the innocent shrugging of a shoulder because it itches.

Relief Measures/Foods and Nutrients

A toddy made with heated rum (.5 cup) and distilled hot water (.5 cup), some lime juice (1 tsp.), and pinches of cinnamon and cayenne pepper can be given in very small amounts to victims of convulsion. Also rubbing some tincture of capsicum and oil of peppermint on their wrists, hands, feet, and neck works well, too. Some fresh, grated horseradish or horse-radish sauce or Tobasco sauce placed on the tongue or in the nostrils should revive a person, too.

CORNS

Symptoms

Corns are a localized thickening of the horny layer of the skin, as a response to pressure on the soles of the feet. A cone of hard material, pointing inward, presses on the sensitive deeper layers, causing pain.

Relief Measures

One of the authors had the fat pads on his feet completely wear out as a result of excessive standing on wooden slats during his earlier years in the restaurant business as a chef and on cold, concrete floors during his several years in the funeral business as an apprentice mortician. As a result of this, he incurred frequent corns and calluses which made walking somewhat difficult and rather painful for him.

The first thing he did was to see a competent podiatrist (foot doctor), who removed them and promptly fitted him with the proper shoe supports. This made walking a pleasure and jogging no longer an impossibility. But still the corns would recur every so often, though not with as much frequency as before.

In such instances, he has resorted to soaking his feet in a warm solution of Epsom salts and then carefully removing the top horny portions with a sterile, sharp knife. As well as buffing them down when totally dry with an emery board such as what manicurists would use in nail care.

Foods and Nutrients

Vinegar seems to be particularly useful for removing them, as does zinc. Crush a single zinc tablet into powder, before mixing with a few drops of vinegar to make a stiff paste. Then spread on a small circular bandage the size of a coin and apply directly over the corn to hold in place. You'll be surprised just how much this helps. A little bit of vitamin E oil can also be added to this mixture.

CORONARY BY-PASS RECOVERY

Symptoms

General fatigue and weak immunity following open-heart surgery.

Relief Measures

Kola nut (4 capsules daily), guarana (4 capsules), and yerba maté tea (1 cup daily) are recommended for quick energy boosters.

Foods and Nutrients

An 8 fl. oz. glass of tomato juice with a pinch of cayenne pepper and 1 tsp. of lime juice in it each day, is great for the heart ! So is barley broth, Kyo-Green drink (see Appendix under Wakunaga), iron (ferrous gluconate) supplement (15 mg. prescribed by your doctor), folic acid (800 mcg.), and vitamin B-12 injections from your physician.

CORONARY HEART DISEASE

Symptoms

The symptoms for coronary heart disease are very similar to those for arteriosclerosis. Look under this particular entry for more details regarding the likely signs of CHD.

Relief Measures

Fluid extracts of hawthorn berry, arnica, broom, aixi mistletoe are all highly recommended. Any of these ought to be taken on an empty stomach, sublingually (beneath the tongue) in 10-15 drops once or twice daily. A well tried infusion suggested by France's greatest herbalist, Maurice Mességué, calls for pinches of aniseed, savory, mint, chervil, aix! fennel seed, steeped in 1.5 cups of boiling hot water for 15 minutes, covered, before straining to drink.

Foods and Nutrients

Diet should include frequent soups or broths heavily spiced with paprika, horseradish, sage, and thyme. Also, sufferer should consume 1 tablespoon of olive oil or black currant oil every day.

A chelated calcium-magnesium supplement with about a 2:1 ratio should be taken (4 tablets) every day, too. Equal parts of wheat germ oil and liquid lecithin (one tablespoonful each) are to be taken simultaneously, usually in the morning.

Potassium (1, 200 mg.) and selenium (100 mcg.) ought to be included. S.O.D. (superoxide disnutase) can be taken in small amounts. The amino acid, L-taurine and vitamin B-6 work nicely together when taken with carrot juice or a glass of reconstituted Kyo-Green (see Appendix under Wakunaga).

COUGHING

Symptoms

The action is so common that just about everyone is familiar with what constitutes a cough. But there are different kinds: short dry (cold, sore throat, smoking); night cough (throat congestion or snoring); nervous type (habit-forming spasm); long, barking, and showy (due to hysteria); short and suppressed (pleurisy); brassy sounding (possible pressure on the bronchi from undetected swelling in the chest); and a silent, ineffectual kind (probable paralysis of the vocal cord; something for a doctor to look at right away).

Other coughs may yield very little expectoration, as in the case of whooping cough or emphysema. Spasmodic coughs can be attributed to asthma, emphysema, and heart trouble. In recurrent, wheezy coughs, such as that associated with bronchitis, raicus is often brought up.

Relief Measures

Adult coughs are treated a little differently in some ways than those in children would be, although there is some overlapping between them both.

Dry coughs can be treated with something as simple as a warm glass of water, or the use of a humidifier to create a warm steamy atmosphere in a room. If a humidifier isn't readily available, then an alternative solution can be resorted to. Fill a large roast pan half full of hot water; throw a bath towel over your head to form a tent of sorts, and then inhale the steam for about 7 minutes every 3 hours or so. Or just turn on the shower in your bathroom, close the door and breath in the warm mist from the hot water that steams up.

Gargling with and slowly sipping warm horehound herb tea is something which adults and kids can both safely do. For finicky tastes, a little honey or pure maple syrup can be added to sweeten things up a bit. Warm catnip tea, flavored with a little blackstrap molasses also works well for children's coughs. Sucking on a piece of eucalyptus or horehound candy or cough drop, lets small measures of medicated saliva trickle down the throat to soothe irritated mucosal linings.

Foods and Nutrients

Hot chicken or beef consommé flavored with minced white onion and squeezed lime juice and a pinch of cayenne

or ginger, makes a wonderful and soothing nourishment to stop an incessant cough with.

CRACKED NIPPLES

See under CAKED BREAST for more information on this.

CRADLE CAP

Symptoms

Cradle cap is common on infants, especially over the fontanel located in the middle and towards the back of the head, where parents sometimes forget to wash their babies' scalps. Characterized by scaly patches on the skin of the newborn.

Relief Measures

*Daily washing wi*th a good shampoo containing some salicylic acid is suggested. Make a strong solution of white willow bark tea, using the coarsely dried and cut materials instead of the powder. Add a teaspoonful of this to 1/2 tsp. of Johnson & Johnson baby shampoo. Rubbing a little olive oil on to the baby's scalp at night also helps.

Food and Nutrients

Nursing moms should take vitamin A (50,000 I .U.), vitamin E (800 I .U.), vitamin C (3, 500) and a high-potency B-complex every day. When these nutrients wind up in the infant's body, they may assist in clearing the problem up.

CRAMPS

Symptoms

Cramps are an involuntary tightening of a single muscle or several muscles, either all at once or at spaced intervals of time. Sharp stabbing pain accompanying them and often a temporary inability to move. They occur more frequently in the feet, legs, and calves.

There are also occupational cramps, which are somewhat different in nature than the aforementioned general kind. Typical of these would be the common writers' cramp suffered by authors like us who may write our drafts in long-hand first of all, before committing them to a word processor (another kink of cramp by the way). Also cramps are common to concert pianists or violinists and Olympic swimmers, where anxiety and intense concentration contribute to them.

Relief Measures

The best we've ever found is to massage the painful muscle in a rotating fashion, as well as to stretch and pull it back and forth. You'd be surprised just how well such simple techniques work. Putting a hot or cold pack on the cramp could also give some measure of relief.

Foods and Nutrients

Three minerals seem to work well here in combination with each other—calcium (1,600 mg.), magnesium (800 mg.) and silicon (3 capsules of shavegrass/horsetail herb). Lecithin (1 tbsp. daily), and

vitamins D (400 I.U. daily) and E (800 I.U.) also are beneficial.

CROHN'S DISEASE

Symptoms

Crohns disease is autoimmune and marked by chronic and long-term inflammation of a part of the gut. Said inflammation extends through all layers of the stomach lining even to include the lymph nodes. Usual symptoms include but are not limited to watery stools, abdominal cramping on the lower right side (similar to what appendicitis may evoke), lack of energy, loss of desire to eat, and decrease in weight.

Relief Measures

One of the very best concoctions we've discovered came from an old Hawaiian folk healer on the island of Molokai. With some slight modifications, it calls for combining equal parts (1 cup each) of liquid aloe vera and concentrated papaya juice and then drinking it with 4 capsules of Kyo-Dophilus (see under Appendix for Wakunaga).

Foods and Nutrients

A study published in the November-December 1984 *Human Nutrition & Applied Nutrition* magazine indicated that many of the offending foods which aggravate Crohn's victims, can be slowly worked back into their diets in about 3 time after avoiding them for this long.

Helpful foods include those high in sulphur content: cabbage, kale, kohlrabi, Brussel sprouts, cauliflower, spinach, mustard greens, and turnips. Spicy, greasy and sugary foods as well as coffee, alcohol, milk, soft drinks and colas, red meat, and chocolate should be avoided during an attack. But fresh or salt-w ater fish, preferably steamed or baked, is acceptable. Manganese (5 mg.), chromium (2 m g.) and zinc (25 m g.) work well together here.

CROUP

Symptoms

Croup encompasses a variety of conditions in which there is a high-pitched cough and difficulty in breathing, often caused by a viral infection. In turn, the larynx or trachea narrow down in size, resulting in the unlucky victim gasping for air. A raspy cough, laryngitis, muscle tension in the lungs, and a general feeling of suffocation are the most evident symptoms.

Relief Measures

Warm coltsfoot tea (1 cup for adults, .5 cup for children) can be slowly sipped for relief. Some goldenseal root capsules (2 for adults, 1 for children) can be swallowed with some water to help fight the infection.

Foods and Nutrients

Cod liver oil (1 tbsp.) and wheat germ oil (1 tsp.) each morning gives the immune system and nerves a definite boost. Sucking on a zinc lozenge several times throughout the day is important to promote

healing. Citrus juices (preferably fresh) or Wakunaga's Kyo-Green (1 tbsp. to 8 fl. oz. water) provide all of the vitamin C needed for this.

CUSHING'S DISEASE

Symptoms

Cushing's disease results from an increased secretion of a steroid hormone (hydrocortisone) from the adrenal cortex. An over-abundance of it produces excessive obesity in the hips, moon-shaped face, acne vulgaris, high blood pressure, decreased carbohydrate tolerance, rapid breakdown of absorbed proteins, and psychiatric problems, among others. When this disorder becomes associated with a benign pituitary tumor of a particular type, then it's referred to as Cushing's disease.

Relief Measures

A combination of goldenseal root (3 capsules daily) and licorice rootbark (6 capsules daily) would be of some usefulness. Additional intake of Kyolic aged-garlic extract (4 capsules daily) might provide some help, too.

Foods and Nutrients

Potassium-rich foods (blackstrap molasses, figs, sunflower seeds), a homemade chlorophyll drink in which a lot of parsley and celery are utilized, and frequent consumption of chamomile tea with meals is highly recommended. While none of these things will correct the problem entirely, they should offer some nutritional benefits to a malady that requires medical and pharmaco-logical assistance as well.

CUTS

Symptoms

Any slicing of skin tissue by a sharp object, whether accidental or intentional, may be defined as a cut. An instant result is bleeding, accompanied moments later by throbbing pain.

Relief Measures/Foods & Nutrients

There are several easy methods for staunching the flow of blood from a cut. One is to sprinkle generous amounts of cayenne pepper or paprika over the injured surface. Powdered kelp (a seaweed) is also good for this.

Afterwards, a tiny mixture of aloe vera gel and one crushed zinc tablet can be applied to expedite healing. Or an emptied capsule of vitamin E oil and a crushed zinc tablet will suffice for the same purpose. If none of the former are readily available, resort to simply licking the injury with your tongue, if possible, since saliva contains some very potent healing agents, including epidermal growth factor.

CYSTIC FIBROSIS

Symptoms

Cystic fibrosis is a hereditary disorder affecting different glands of the body. Chief among those disturbed are the gallbladder, the pancreas, the sweat glands, the lungs, and male reproductive organs. Respiratory mucus membranes generate an unusually thick mucus that blocks breathing passages and breeds unfriendly bacteria. Symptoms start early in life for those afflicted.

Malnutrition ranks as one of the foremost dangers here because of an under-production of gastric juices inside the stomach. As a result, ingested foods, espe-cially fats, are poorly digested and absorbed. This leads to an evident deficiency in all major nutrients, especially the fat-soluble vitamins such as A, D, E, F, and K.

Relief Measures/Foods & Nutrients

Papaya or mango juice should be taken with every meal. A good enzyme supplement is recommended, along with Wakunaga's Kyo-Dophilus (2 capsules per meal or as needed; see Appendix). And obvi-ously vitamin A (25, 000 I .U. fish oil /25, 000 I .U. beta-carotene), D (400 I .U.), E (400 I .U .), F (1 tsp. wheat germ oil), and K (1 tsp. blackstrap molasses) should be taken regularly each day. Some practitioners prescribe raw animal glandulars, but unless such can be obtained from organically-raised livestock, we think they should be avoided. Manganese and copper (each 5 mgs.), along with chelated zinc (50 mg.) wouldn't hurt either. Or foods rich in them: egg yolks, nuts, brewer's yeast, clams, mushrooms, sunflower seeds.

CYSTITIS

Symptoms

Synonymous with bladder infection. See under **BLADDER PROBLEMS** and below for additional information.

Relief Measures/Foods & Nutrients

A good combination which some doctors have discovered for this is Kyolic aged garlic extract (4 capsules daily) and the amino acid, L-cysteine (800 mg. daily). These should be taken in between meals with some cranberry juice for best results.

Another equally good blend is some powdered or liquid vitamin C (about 1 tbsp.) and a little apple cider vinegar (1 tsp.) stirred into some Ocean Spray Cran-Raspberry juice (8 fl. oz.) and taken in conjunction with 2 Kyo-Dophilus capsules from Wakunaga (see Appendix).

CYST

See under BOILS for further information on this.

DANDRUFF

Symptoms

Dandruff can be recognized by loose flakes falling from the scalp when the hair is brushed or combed. It will then lay on the shoulders like some type of coarse powder.

There are two basic types of dandruff. One is called seborrhea and appears in yellowish greasy-looking scales, while the other is just dry scales. The chief cause is an excess production of discarded particles of the horny layer of the skin on top of the scalp, induced by stress, certain vitamin and mineral deficiences and improper hair care.

Relief Measures

Regular and frequent shampooing with pine tar soap or something just as strong, is an absolute must. Scrupulous hygiene of brush and comb should also be practiced; this means no lending or borrowing of the same to others.

Rinse the hair good after an initial shampooing, then pour on a second rinse of equal parts of apple cider vinegar and any comercial beer (1/2 cup of each). Don't rinse again with water! This somehow manages to curtail about 50% of the dandruff, especially if this solution is massaged into the scalp good.

Foods & Nutrients

Vitamins A (25, 000 I.U. fish oil), D (400 I .U.), E (400 I.U.), and F (1 tsp. wheat germ oil), lecithin (1 tbsp. of the liquid), and zinc (50-75 mg.) each day are recommended.

DEAFNESS

Symptoms

Any condition which impairs the ability to hear sounds clearly, can be classified as temporary or permanent deafness. Sometimes, it's just as simple as long-term accumulation of old wax plugging the ears. In which case, a good cleansing should rectify that. Again, the intrusion of sound may be obstructed by a boil or possible eardrum damage caused by an infection or injury.

But, more often than not, it's perceptive rather than conductive deafness. In which case, certain high frequency and letters like G, D, K, P, and T aren't heard, while the rest of the words are. Such victims can't stand loud sounds, and will usually complain, "You don't have to shout! What do you think I am, deaf?" This perceptive deafness is common with old age, following measles or mumps infections, and may also be inherited from birth as well.

Relief Measures

Over the last few years, the great advancements made in hearing aid technology have been nothing short of phenomenal. Today's hearing impaired folks can wear devices small enough inside their ears with minimal detection and discomfort, but remarkably quite strong to still capture the full depth and range of all sounds.

Scientists have now established that constant exposure to loud and irritating noises, can induce permanent ear damage over a period of years. This includes rock music, airplane engines, jack-hammers, diesel trucks, car and ship horns, gun

reports, etc. Such noises should be avoided as much as possible. Also, the continuous wearing of earphones plugged into clip-on cassette tape recorders may inflict injury as well, and should be kept to a minimum.

In mainland China, the expressed juice of crushed onion has been judiciously used in the Shanghai Second Medical College by some physicians for treating temporary deafness. But whether this might work in every case, remains to be seen.

Foods and Nutrients

Vitamin E (800-1, 200 mg.) and liquid lecithin (1 tbsp.) taken every morning together, seem to offer some benefit in early cases of nerve deafness. Also the addition of copper and iron to the diet in such foods as blackstrap molasses (1 tbsp. daily), liver, fish, and avocado, may be helpful.

DEBILITY

See under CHRONIC FATIGUE SYNDROME and HYPOGLYCEMIA.

DEHYDRATION

Symptoms

Dehydration is basically a water deficit within the body at which time adequate amounts of fluid are lacking for proper physiological functions. Characterized the most by an incredible thirst, often due to rapid sweating, profuse urination or continous diarrhea.

Relief Measures

The most helpful thing here, of course, is to drink plenty of water, especially spring, mineral or distilled kinds which are devoid of chlorine or fluoride. Doctors estimate that the average human body needs about half-a-dozen 8 fl. oz. of water daily.

Foods and Nutrients

A health myth has been perpetuated among college and professional athletes for many years now. And it is the false assumption that by consuming lots of soft drinks such as Gatorade, for instance, a person's body will be protected against dehydration. In fact, just the opposite is true because of the high amounts of sugar in them! Water is still the best thirst quencher by far, bar none!

Calcium (600 mg.), magnesium (800 mg.) and potassium (1, 200 mg.) are useful minerals to take for preventing rapid loss of fluids from the body through means such as sweating and urination.

DELIRIUM

Symptoms

Delirium is a clouded state of consciousness or confusion, characterized by difficulty in sustaining attention to surrounding stimuli. Other common symptoms include disordered thinking, defective perception (illusions and hallucinations),

disordered sleep-wakefulness cycles, and motor nerve disturbances.

Relief Measures

Several cups of hot ginseng tea spiked with a little rum (1 tbsp.) and a pinch of cloves will definitely increase mental awareness. So, too, will hot black or green tea spiked with some brandy (1 tbsp.) and a pinch of nutmeg. Also, one cup of hot, black coffee has been known to work at times for such things.

Foods and Nutrients

A high-potency B-complex (3 tablets) and some blackstrap molasses (1 tbsp.) for its copper, iron and phosphorus contents restores equilibrium to a confused mind.

DENTAL PROBLEMS

See under CAVITIES, GINGIVITIS, and TOOTHACHE for more information.

DEPRESSION

Symptoms

Depression is a state of mind and heart in which a sinking of one's own spirit is experienced, often accompanied by a certain sense of hopelessness and individual worthlessness. A more severe form of this is melancholia.

Both are marked by an absence of pleasure, insomnia, changes in brain wave and nerve transmission patterns, guilt, lack of appetite (or just the opposite in binge eating), headaches, backaches, mild diarrhea or constipation, and sometimes an antisocial attitude.

Relief Measures

One of us who happens to be an anthropologist by profession, has observed a curious fact in many different societies and cultures which he has studied worldwide. And it is this: those groups who only use alcohol in moderation and enjoy a rich variety of spicy foods, seem to be a lot happier and considerably less depressed than those with blander diets and heavier booze consumption. He has never quite been able to correlate the two together, except that to his way of thinking, excessive intake of alcohol doesn't cloud the mind, while spices appear to stimulate the pleasure centers within the brain more.

In their fascinating little book, The Pleasure Connection, authors D. Beck, R. N. and J. Beck, R. N. discuss the role of very unique opium-like peptides generated from within the brain that make the rest of the body feel good. Deep within the brain is located its middle layer, known as the limbic brain. Here may be found more receptor sites or keyholes for these wonderful narcotic substances than anywhere else in the system. People who are depressed have very low levels of such materials, but folks who are happy and contented with life have an abundance of them. Certain substances like spices can stimulate an increased production of such "feel good" agents.

Foods and Nutrients

A high-potency B-complex supplement (4 tablets), brewer's yeast (1 tsp. in 8 fl. oz. juice or milk), liquid lecithin (1 tbsp.) and vitamin E (400 I.U.) together, L-tyrosine (800 mg.), niacin (2 00 mg.), B-6 (1 00 mg.), magnesium (800 mg.), and bee pollen granules (1 tbsp.) should all be taken every day during periods of mild or severe depression. Alcohol, coffee, tea, tobacco, and most over-the-counter drugs should be avoided. However, we definitely recommend lithium by prescription only.

DERMATITIS

Symptoms

Dermatitis is an allergy which produces scaling, flaking, thickening, changing of pigment, and itching upon contact with the skin. It can be due to contact with metallic jewelry such as gold necklaces or rings, perfumes, cosmetics, rubber gloves, medicated creams and ointments, and plants like poison ivy.

Relief Measures

Combine equal parts (1/8 tsp. each) of powdered goldenseal root and myrrh gum with some wheat germ oil (just enough to slightly thicken) in order to make a loose paste. Then apply it to the skin with the back of a wooden spoon. The afflicted area can also be frequently bathed in a strong solution of pau d'arco tea.

Foods and Nutrients

A high-potency B-complex (3 tablets daily), Wakunaga's Premium Kyolic-EPA (2 capsules daily), zinc (50 mg. twice daily), and emulsified vitamin A (75,000 I.U. daily).

DIABETES

Symptoms

There are two kinds of diabetes—insipidus and mellitus. The latter is the more common, being segregated into two separate categories: type I, known as insulin-dependent or juvenile, and type II in which the onset of the disease occurs during adulthood.

Symptoms include crankiness, frequent urination, insatiable thirst, inclination to throw up, physical weakness, lack of energy and a ravenous appetite. These manifestations are seen the most often in children and teenagers. The adult variety includes some of these, plus blurred vision, itchy skin, pins-and-needles feeling in lower extremities, and wounds that are slow to heal. Almost six million Americans currently are under doctors' care for diabetes.

Relief Measures

A LOT of physical activity is important here, besides severe dietary adjustments. Intense exercise in the open air is highly recommended. Jogging, power walking (fast walking), swimming, and playing tennis are just a few of the ways by which to actually diminish the need for so much insulin.

A dry brush massage is absolutely essential to get health in such instances. Get a natural bristle brush with a long handle to it, so you can reach all parts of your body. If you can't find such an item, then settle for a coarse wash rag or a loofah sponge instead. Don't use nylon or synthetic fiber brushes of any kind; they can really damage your skin.

Beginning with the soles of your feet, brush vigorously in rotary motions upwards over the entire body, ending at the top of your head. Follow this general pattern: feet and legs first, thighs and calves next, then abdomen and chest, followed by hands and arms, ending up the neck and to the scalp. Best times for brushing are when you get up in the morning and before retiring to bed at night.

Diabetics should avoid drinking soft water. And settle for mineral or spring or tonic water instead. Soft water can be somewhat injurious to the pancreas and spleen.

Foods and Nutrients

While there are many different kinds of edible foods and medicinal herbs which obviously benefit diabetics, there is a small handful that really works wonders! They are goldenseal root (4 capsules of Wakunaga goldenseal root); aged garlic extract (4 capsules of Kyolic); and one 8 fl. oz. glass of liquid chlorophyll (1 tbsp. Kyo-Green in water). These three items, constituting a medicinal herb, a culinary spice, and some powdered cereal grasses from one of Japan's leading food and drug companies, Wakunaga (see Appendix), form a perfect nutritional program for diabetics in general.

Then there is also onions, cayenne pepper and pau d'arco, which exhibit hypoglycemic properties and can bring elevated blood sugar levels down nicely. Diabetics should think about investing in a good juicer. Two of the very best fresh vegetable juices for them to drink would be raw stringbean and parsley juice mixed together. Cucumbers are good for the pancreas, too.

Mineral supplements would include: chromium (150 micrograms daily); manganese (75 mg. daily); and copper (5 mg. daily). A teaspoonful of brewer's yeast in some juice or water every morning is highly recommended.

Bear this in mind with regard to diabetes: a high-carbohydrate, high-fiber diet reduces the need for insulin and also lowers the fat levels in blood.

DIAPER RASH

Symptoms

Portions of an infant's skin become very red and irritated. Sometimes infection can set in if the problem is left unattended for very long.

Relief Measures

Leave buttocks and genitals exposed whenever possible. Don't use plastic underpants, which tend to make the skin perspire more often. Apply Johnson & Johnson baby lotion or talcum powder liberally. Or try some tincture of witch hazel. Crush a zinc tablet (50 mg. strength) and mix it in with a little vaseline and rub on the affected area.

Foods and Nutrients

Don't feed baby foods that are very acidic, like citrus juices, for instance.

DIARRHEA

Symptoms

Diarrhea is commonly characterized by loose, watery stools. Occasionally it may even be accompanied by nausea or vomiting, especially when travelling in Third World countries where hygienic conditions and the food and water supplies leave a lot to be desired. Sometimes there can be a fever as well, but not that often.

Diarrhea is NO laughing matter, however. Its persistence for very long can lead to severe dehydration and definite loss of important minerals like potassium and calcium from the body.

Relief Measures

There is a two-fold approach to this problem. One is to take items that will initially stop the "runs." While the second is to take those things which will help to form more substantial stools.

The first regimen ought to include: 4 charcoal tablets, 2 kelp capsules, 3 capsules of Kyolic garlic, and 2 capsules of Kyo-Dophilus every couple of hours until the diarrhea subsides. (See Appendix under Wakunaga.)

The second involves 4 capsules of white oak bark, 4 capsules of myrrh gum, and 2 capsules of guar gum every 4 hours or on an "as need" basis until discharged stools become firmer.

Foods and Nutrients

Calcium (1,000 mg.), magnesium (1,600 mg.) and potassium (2,000 mg.) are three essential minerals you want to be taking under such conditions.

DIPTHERIA

Symptoms

Diptheria was once a common health problem in American and Canadian schools many decades ago. But because of routine immunization programs, it virtually became extinct. That is, until now. News reports of isolated pockets of this disease recurring in young children living in inner city ghettos, have been surfacing from time to time with disturbing consequences.

Not only is malnourishment and poverty partly responsible for this, but also the belief systems of some parents, who have elected to withhold their children from receiving free immunizations, because they deem them more dangerous than the problem itself. Also the widespread AIDS epidemic of late, may also have contributed to its rise as well.

Symptoms include pains in the limbs and joints, lack of appetite, a foul breath, putrid, sore throat, swollen neck glands, and sometimes the signs of fever.

Relief Measures

Goldenseal root tea and fluid extract are of immense benefit here. The child's throat should be swabbed with the fluid extract (10-12 drops). And he or she should be persuaded to gargle with some of the warm tea (1/4 cup). But it may have to be flavored with a little maple syrup or honey before the kid will do this, owing to its bitter taste. A warm garlic enema is also helpful to evacuate the bowels.

Foods and Nutrients

The child should be given plenty of citrus, tomato, and carrot juices. And fed warm beef-barley broth every few hours. Liquid nourishment is the key here to recovery. Liquid or chewable forms of vitamin C and cod-liver oil (1 tsp.) are suggested as well until recovery is imminent.

DIVERTICULITIS

Symptoms

Diverticulitis is when the mucous membrane tissue of the small or large intestine (colon) becomes inflamed. These small pouches or sacs (known as diverticula) cause no problems in and of themselves, unless they happen to get digested food particles trapped in them. Which can then lead to stagnation and the formation of pus. In time, if left unchecked, the infection can spread out of the sacs to the rest of the colon and to other organs of the abdomen.

Symptoms of this disease include cramps and pain in the lower abdomen accompanying bowel movements, extreme tenderness on the left side of the abdomen, bloating, difficult or loose stools, nausea, and occasionally fever.

Relief Measures/Foods and Nutrients

An American-born Japanese fellow from Hawaii by the name of George Izawaya was diagnosed by a Honolulu physician as having diverticulitis. His alternative-minded doctor put him on a strict diet of grain fibers to begin with: cooked oatmeal in the morning, barley broth soup for lunch, buckwheat pancakes for dinner, and millet/wheat bran muffins for snacks. Next, the doctor had George drink two large glasses of Kyo-Green chlorophyll mix with meals (see Appendix under Wakunaga).

Every morning George had to mix one level teaspoonful of brewer's yeast powder into a glass of pineapple or papaya juice and drink that separate from his regular meals. This restored B vitamins to the intestinal tract again. He also took alfalfa capsules (four) and Wakunaga's Kyo-Dophilus (2 capsules) with every meal. In less than four days, George was pronounced in good health once again.

DIZZINESS

Symptoms

Dizziness is any momentary or prolonged state of feeling faint or unsteady. Disorientation of space or a sensation of rotatory movement of self or surrounding objects, may occur. In more severe cases, the person may swag, stagger or even fall down.

It is usually a disturbance of the balancing mechanism, either direct or through a temporarily inadequate supply of blood to the brain.

It sometimes can be due to eating the wrong type of food. Or climbing to lofty elevations and experiencing sudden vertigo (fear of heights). Or coming on after lying down or prolonged stooping, especially in those over the age of 50, or in convalescents. There is a delayed readjustment of circulatory arrangements for the upright position, so that the brain is temporarily short of blood. In some cases, an illness (Ménière's Disease) may cause dizziness.

Relief Measures

The subject should sit down and bend forward, or lie flat on the floor if possible. Getting up should be done very slowly. If such episodes are severe or frequent, by all means, see a doctor to have your blood vessels, heart, brain, blood pressure and circulation, etc. thoroughly checked.

Rubbing the palms of the hands, the soles of the feet, the back of the neck, and the sides of the forehead in a gentle circular motion often helps. Drinking some lukewarm chamomile or peppermint tea soothes an unsettled stomach.

Foods and Nutrients

Drinking a cup of cold, undiluted papaya juice and taking 1-2 capsules of Wakunaga's Kyo-Dophilus helps overcome giddy feelings (see Appendix).

DROWNING

Symptoms

A drowning is usually accidental in nature and results when an individual suffocates by submersion in water. Within moments the lugs become filled with liquid, cutting off the usual supply air. And without oxygen, the body soon turns blue and the brain starts deteriorating.

Because this is a medical emergency, only paramedics, doctors or nurses, who are trained for this type of thing, should be administering first-aid measures!

In the unlikely event that none of them are readily available, the following items may prove of benefit if done quick enough.

Relief Measures

The following remarkable account happened on March 29th, 1864 just off the Hawaiian island of Maui, and was later included in the published biography of the man to whom it happened.

Three Apostles of The Church of Jesus Christ of Latter-Day Saints—Elders Joseph F. Smith, E. T. Benson and Lorenzo Snow—were about to leave their big mother ship anchored a mile from shore and conclude the rest of the journey inside a small dinghy. Elder Smith believing this to be an unwise course to pursue while a typhoon was raging at sea, decided not to go with his companion but remain on board the larger vessel.

Elder Snow, however, went along in the rowboat with three other Mormon Elders, the ship's captain, an unnamed Caucasian fellow, several native Hawaiians, and some of the boat's crew.

It wasn't too long before a huge swell struck the boat and carried it forward several yards, landing it in a trough between two enormous waves. A second swell immediately raised the stern of the boat so high that the steerman's oar was out of the water and control of the rowboat was lost. Without further warning, it capsized, spilling all of its human cargo into the water.

Everyone except Elder Snow managed to save themselves by swimming to shore. A frantic search by the natives turned up his rigid and apparently lifeless body about ten minutes later. As one of that number later recounted: "On reaching the shore, we carried him a little way to some large empty barrels that were lying on the sandy beach. We laid him face downwards on one of them, and rolled him back and forth until we succeeded in getting the water he had swallowed out of him.

"...All were willing to do what they could. We washed Brother Snow's face with camphor...We did not only what was customary in such cases, but also what the spirit seemed to whisper to us. After working over him for some time, without any indication of returning life, the by-standers said that nothing more could be done for him. But we did not feel like giving him up, and still prayed and worked over him, with an assurance that the Lord would hear and answer our prayers. Finally, we were impressed to place our mouth over his and make an effort to inflate his lungs, alternately blowing in and drawing out the air, imitating, as far as possible, the natural process of breathing. This we persevered in until we succeeded in inflating his lungs. After a little, we perceived very faint indications of returning life. A slight wink of the eye, which, until then, had been open and death-like, and a very faint rattle in the throat, were the first symptoms of returning vitality. These grew more and more distinct, until consciousness was fully restored."

Foods and Nutrients

A doctor who routinely treats such accidents in one large California city hospital Emergency Room, told one of the authors that he prescribes "spicy foods with lots of pepper." The idea, he said, is to promote quicker circulation throughout the body. Also the idea of having a revived drowning victim drink some hot peppermint tea to increase oxygen intake in the body is good to implement.

Intramuscular injections of vitamin B-12 and C (10 grams) also are beneficial to new blood cell formation, blood vessels, and blood circulation in cases of recovery from accidental drowning.

DYSENTERY

Symptoms

Dysentery is an acute infection of the intestines through the consumption of milk, food or contaminated water, or indirectly through dust or flies. This is a common cause of epidemics in schools and other institutions of some Third World countries.

Symptoms resemble food poisoning in some ways—abdominal pain, diarrhea, nausea, vomiting, and headache—but they are more acute and severe.

Relief Measures

Strong herbal antibiotics are called for here: Kyolic garlic from Wakunaga (see Appendix) (4 capsules every 6 hours); Wakunaga's goldenseal root (2 capsules every 6 hours); chaparral tea (1 cup every 3 hours); black walnut bark (4 capsules every 6 hours). Also plenty of rest is highly advised.

Foods and Nutrients

Oral intake of liquid or powdered vitamin C, enough to equal 5,000 mg. every 5 hours is recommended. And fresh citrus juices also helps.

DYPEPSIA

See under INDIGESTION for further information.

EAR DISORDERS

Symptoms /Relief Measures

Second only to the eye in its marvelous complexity is the ear! Not only does it serve as a channel for one of our five senses (hearing), but it also is essential to maintaining our upright balance so that we don't suddenly fall over due to the constant, downward pull of gravity upon our bodies.

There are a small variety of problems which can occur with this important organ. In most cases they are easily treated if caught in time.

Otis externa is an inflammation of the lining of the ear canal. Identified by irritation, worse if the jaw is moved, scanty discharge, tenderness on pressure over the tragus (the flap in front of the ear hole). Immediate treatment at the doctor's office is the most preferred. A gentle and complete clearing out of the ear passage is necessary. And after washing, always dry the ears gently with a clean, soft towel. Avoid swimming or allowing water into the ears. Don't scratch them, no matter how much they may irritate you.

A boil within the ear passage produces a pain that is on par with a horrible toothache. A hot water bottle or other local heat placed over the ear directly, acts as an effective analgesic to reduce the pain. Some of the cleansing herbs and foods mentioned under ADDICTIONS are recommended here to clean the body out in hopes the boil will eventually go away.

Acute otis media is an acute inflammation of the middle ear. This is a common, important, painful condition, frequently occurring in children who may scream with the pain. It usually starts with a simple head cold, tonsillitis, the flu, or an infectious fever such as measles, whooping cough, or scarlet fever. **Infection of the middle ear must never be taken lightly and the skill of a qualified medical specialist needs to be sought at once!**

Besides the terrible pain, a high fever, temporary deafness and ringing in the ears may occur, especially in adults. Vomiting may occur in children. The mastoid bone behind the ear will feel tender. A discharge of purulent may occur, at first mucoid, but later turns to a thick yellow.

While a doctor's services are obviously needed here, at least one aspect of the treatment can be self-generated. This has to do with the selection of appropriate antibiotics with which to stop the infection. Kyolic garlic (2 capsules), Wakunaga's goldenseal root (2 capsules), vitamins A (50,000 I.U.) and C (10,000 mg.), twice a day for adults, can replace the standard prescription antibiotics usually ordered up by the doctor. (About half this amount for children.)

Tinnitus is any strange noises detected inside the ear, other than what a person may be used to hearing. These can include the traditional ringing, buzzing, or even hissing. Leota Lane of Eugene, Oregon told one of the authors back in August, 1981 what she did to clear this condition up in her own ears:

"I put about 2.5 full soup spoons of fenugreek seeds in 3/4 quart of cold water and let it stand overnight. Next morning I stirred it and poured off a cup of cold tea and drank it. I then added another cup of water to the remaining seeds. That evening I drank another cup of tea. I followed that routine for 2-3 days until the seeds lost most of their strength. I then discarded the seeds and started over....The tea eliminated the cricket noises if I drank it daily. It is the only relief I've had from ear ringing in several years." A professional reflexologist from

Canmore, Alberta, Canada, by the name of Mary Underhill, informed one of the authors of what she advised one patient to do for his tinnitus:

"A middle-aged gentleman came to me for a reflexology treatment after having been told by two medical specialists that there was nothing wrong with him, and that he would simply have to live with the ringing in his ears. He had reached the point of intense irritability and weight loss, to say nothing of the negative attitude toward the entire medical profession. After the treatment I suggested that he might have a zinc deficiency, since the prostate area on his feet had been particularly painful. It turned out that he had stopped taking the zinc prescribed by his general practitioner, since no reason had been given for its need. Within two weeks after resuming the zinc intake, the tinnitus had completely disappeared, his good humor and appetite had returned, and the prostate area was much less painful. [The fellow took 100 mg. of zinc daily.] Another case: after using various acupressure points around the ear and TMJ area, I suggested that a client go to her dentist for a possible TMJ problem. The resulting action from her dentist completely eliminated her tinnitus. It seems that the main thing to remember when one has tinnitus is that it is a symptom of a great many disorders, and is not a cause in itself."

Cerumen buildup is nothing more than an excess accumulation of earwax. This material is produced by glands near the outer part of the canal and keeps water, dust, and dirt away from the eardrum. The amount of wax varies from person to person. Wax buildup isn't a problem for most people, since the ear canal is basically self-cleaning. Wax accumulates, dries up, and falls out of the ear; or it migrates to the outer ear, where it is washed off. It's okay to use your well-washed little finger to wipe off wax near the outer part of the canal.

If wax does build up in your ear canal, however, you can try an over-the-counter wax softener twice daily for a few days. After inserting the drops, wait a few minutes, then flush your ear gently but thoroughly with warm water, either in the shower or using the rubber syringe that comes with some wax softeners. Don't use any medication that causes fizzing in your ear, since this can cause pressure to build up and may perforate your eardrum. One old-fashioned way to soften wax buildup may work just as well as commercial preparations: insert a drop or two of warm (not hot) mineral oil or olive oil into each ear periodically, using an eyedropper and then flush with warm water. Remember, never put any liquid into your ear if you have a perforated drum. If your ear continuous to be remain blocked because of hardened wax buildup, then check with your physician about this.

Primary otalgia is an earache originating from the external, middle, or inner ear, or from other sites in the head, neck, or, less frequently, other locations in the body (secondary otalgia). As many as half of all complaints concerning earaches can be traced to secondary sources. Symptoms of such pain have been described by patients as "aching, burning, throbbing, stabbing," or "like an electric shock." It may also be dull or sharp and constant or intermittent.

An earache can be due to any number of considerations. Within the ear canal there may be a possible furuncle, abscess, or sebaceous cyst forming. If a dull ache progresses gradually to severe pain over several days and the ear canal is red, swollen, and very tender, the problem is most likely to be otitis externa, or swimmer's ear, the most common source of earaches. An infection in the canal, like an infected cyst, may produce similar symptoms. Sometimes cleaning the ear canal with a cotton swab or inserting objects into the canal itself, can cause a type of dermatitis which produces an aching sensation.

Herpes zoster oticus may sometimes produce an earache similar to that of otitis externa. It's harder to detect, however, until tiny vesicles appear on the concha, in the ear canal, or sometimes on the face on the third or fourth day.

Antibiotic drugs prescribed by the drug can take care of such cysts and infections as these. Natural alternatives might include powdered goldenseal root mixed with some vitamin E oil or a few drops of liquid Kyolic aged-garlic extract. (See under Wakunaga in the Appendix.)

Once in a while insects like cockroaches, earwigs, or ants can enter the ear canal in sleeping adults and children. These can definitely cause excruciating pain as they move around inside of the ear. Putting a small amount of warm mineral or olive oil or lidocaine hcl into each canal will help to remove them easily.

According to the September, 1986 *Journal of Laryngology and Otology*, a heated onion is the best thing to clear up an earache with. Just "warm an onion [in the oven] and then either put the core of the onion in the aching ear, or [just] squeeze some of the drops from the onion into the ear canal or cut the onion in half, wrap it in a piece of muslin and hold it against the ear." This medical journal article claims "relief from pain [is] obtained in this way."

In a few instances, certain medical problems unrelated to the ear, may, in fact, be traced to the ear itself. The Monday, November 7, 1983 edition of the *Philadelphia Inquirer* (p. C-8) reported that dyslexia, a learning disability in some children—was due to inner ear disorders. Psychiatrists treated such youngsters with a combination of motion-sickness drugs. A safer alternative would be ginger root (2-3 capsules daily), which works in a similar fashion to many of these over-the-counter medications.

A short time ago, two prestigious medical journals—*Modern Medicine* (57(lo):l26) and the *British Heart Journal* (6ll(4):36l)—reported that an ear crease might indicate the sign for an impending fatal heart attack. According to them, a diagonal crease across your earlobe at a 45-degree downward angle toward your shoulder may be an early warning sign of a potentially deadly heart attack. So, you may want to check your ear lobes the next time you stand in front of the bathroom mirror.

Meniere's Disease afflicts a small percentage of the population. Common symptoms include dizziness, tinnitus, fluctuating hearing loss, and a feeling of fullness and pressure in the ears. According to

Indiana Medicine (79:961) for 1986, various remedies have been tried for it, including weight loss, low-sodium diet, herbal diuretics, antiemetics, and sedatives, but usually to little or no avail. The only reliable treatment for it, says this medical journal, is surgery. One type of operation decompresses the inflamed structures of the inner ear, while another divides the nerves that connect the inner ear to the brain. By these operations, the symptoms of Meniere's Disease can usually be abolished in over 90% of the cases, but lost hearing ability cannot be restored as a rule. And while the general contents of this book offer numerous alternatives to surgery and drugs, in a few instances such as this, both authors concur with the suggestion of *Indiana Medicine.*

Foods and Nutrients

We suggest that vitamin A in 100,000 I.U.'s be taken each day. This should by divided up between fish oil (50%) and vegetable-derived beta-carotene (50%). Also 800 I.U. of vitamin E is recommended. It can also be obtained by taking 1 tsp. of wheat germ oil every morning before breakfast. Intramuscular injections of vitamin C (10 grams) are helpful, too. A high-potency B-complex (two tablets daily) is called for here. An additional 75 mg. of vitamin B-6 is usually included. A zinc gluconate lozenge (25mg.) should be slowly sucked on a couple of times a day to boost immunity. High garlic enemas are good for cleaning the colon out. A little warm garlic oil dropped in the ear, followed by some fluid extract of lobelia will relieve pain. Smokers tend to have more ear problems as a rule.

ECZEMA

Symptoms

Eczema is a particularly bothersome skin condition often marked by inflammatory itching and the formation of scales. Sometimes (but not always) eczema can be connected to an allergic response of some kind.

Relief Measures

One of the easiest ways to avoid localized eczema in a particular part of the body, is to discover what one is *wearing* that might be the cause of it. And then to remove this offensive material at once. Such things can include perfume, deodorants, jewelry, and some fabrics.

The medical journal *Cutis* (49:43, 1992) mentioned that costume jewelry, watches, zippers, buttons and nail-polish can produce eczema-like dermatitis at their contact points with the body. Also toiletries and some synthetic fabrics (including natural fabrics dry-cleaned with solvents) can produce eczema, too. The underlying culprits here are the many different chemical agents found in each of these items to which the body may have a negative reaction. Avoiding them will obviously solve the problem for many individuals thus afflicted.

An ideal topical application is aloe vera straight from the plant or aloe vera gel or lotion. Also herbal salves that contain chickweed or comfrey or calendula or chamomile are equally helpful. The area intended for application should first of all be cleansed before anything is put on it. Repeated applications may be necessary.

Foods and Nutrients

Certain types of foods are prone to incite eczema in some people. A different issue of Cutis (48: 363, 1991) told the interesting story of a 76-year-old woman who had suffered for 30 years with attacks of severe hand eczema, which made her skin suddenly redden, swell and break out in blisters. Ultimately, it was discovered, the skin of her hands was reacting to an ingredient of barbecue sauce. However, this was thought to be an allergic reaction that occurred on her hands even when she had not touched the food. In some people, it appears that the skin of the hands may be the only part of the body to react when one consumes, but does not otherwise touch, a food to which one is allergic. Pork and eggs are the most frequent offenders. Another issue of Cutis (49:19, 1992) told of a similar case, a small boy with frequent rashes on his cheeks, who turned out to be reacting to tomato sauce.

One of the authors' elderly father has eczema-like flare-ups whenever he eats strawberries or tomatoes. So figuring out what foods are the culprits and removing them from the diet, will help considerably in this regard.

Nutritional supplements include: Vitamin A, 50,000 units of which equal parts should be fish oil and vegetable-derived (beta-carotene); vitamin B-6, 50 mg.; pantothenic acid, 50 mg.; PABA (para-aminobenzoic acid), 50 mg. as well as applied externally in a cream solution; vitamin C, 2,000 mg.; vitamin D, 800 units; unsaturated fatty acids like olive oil, 1 tsp. daily; magnesium gluconate, 800 mg.; zinc gluconate, 50 mg. and a zinc ointment applied externally as well. Also oil of evening primrose (2 capsules) when combined with vitamin E oil (400 I.U.) is an effective measure.

EDEMA

Symptoms

Edema is a disorder in which excess fluid is retained by the body, either localized in one area or else generalized throughout the system. This retention of fluids appears as swelling. In former times it was called dropsy. It's most persistent in the feet and ankles or around the eyes. Obese subjects tend to have it more often than lean people do. Problems relating to the kidneys, bladder, heart, or liver may often be the underlying causes for this disorder.

Relief Measures

An herbal detoxifier and diuretic are called for here. One of the very best herbs for getting rid of poisons within the system that may be causing fluid retention is aged garlic extract. It is sold through health food stores under the name of Kyolic. We recommend the Kyo-Chrome with chromium piconinate and niacin (3 capsules daily) or the Kyolic with some B vitamins (3 capsules daily). (See Appendix under Wakunaga.) An excellent diuretic is buchu leaves (3 capsules daily on an empty stomach). Look for this herb under the Nature's Way label at a health food store in your area.

Another herb which qualifies both as a detoxifier and diuretic is alfalfa tea. A warm cup with a meal once or twice daily will help to flush out impurities and reduce swelling.

Another good diuretic herb is horsetail. Being high in silicon it can readily remove excess fluids from the body in no time at all. Two capsules a day is suggested.

Foods and Nutrients

A lumberjack from Vancouver, B.C. by the name of Michael O'Faraday didn't know what to do for his edema problem. The prescription drugs he took only made him sicker than he really was. So he decided to visit a naturopathic doctor in the city, who put him on vitamin B-6 (50 mg. 3 times daily), potassium (500 mg. four times daily) and potassium-rich foods (dates, figs, peaches, raisins, seafood, blackstrap molasses, bananas, baked potato, sunflower seeds), and a glandular supplement (raw kidney extract).

Within just five days, Michael reported that he began to experience more freedom from his usual muscle aches and pains. He was able to move around a lot better and noticed a drop in his weight (5 pounds) after being on this nutritional program for one week.

EMPHYSEMA

Symptoms

Emphysema is a lung disorder marked most often by a definite shortness of breath which occurs during any type of physical exertion. This is due to a loss of elasticity and the dilatation of the lung tissue itself. Exhaling becomes a difficult chore. Stale air remains trapped in the lungs, preventing the needed exchange of oxygen and carbon dioxide. The most common symptoms are breathlessness followed by coughing, no matter how slight the exertion may be.

Relief Measures

There is no known cure for emphysema, but the situation can be remedied somewhat with a few simple measures. Avoiding air pollution is the first major concern. This includes city smog, second-hand smoking, room air filled with animal odors or fried grease, perfumes and body deodorants, air fresheners, and so forth.

Frequent trips to the mountains, lakes, rivers, or more preferably, the seashore or a waterfall will help immensely. The negative air ions generated at such sights are of tremendous value within the body and replace harmful positive air ions, which can make a person feel tired and lousy much of the time. The air from such places is also oxygen-rich as a rule and can be quite exhilirating, as is the air following a good thunderstorm in which there has been a considerable display of lightning.

Certain herbs of the mint family, notably peppermint and spearmint, have the ability to help the body take in more oxygen. A warm cup of mint tea twice daily in between meals, taken in a relaxed setting, is ideal for emphysema.

Foods and Nutrients

Junk foods should be minimized, if not entirely avoided. Occasional cleansing fasts using carrot, pineapple and dark leafy greens juices is advised. Stay away from gas-forming, deep-fried and fried, and sugary foods, as well as those foods that include thick sauces or gravies. Instead choose hot, clear liquids to eliminate mucus better. Dairy products and eggs should likewise be avoided, including ice cream!

Wakunaga products (see Appendix) like Kyolic with B-1 and B-12 (3 capsules daily), and Kyo-Green are all good to take for this and related respiratory problems.

ENDOMETRIOSIS

Symptoms

Endometriosis is a condition in which the cells lining the inside of the uterus, or the endometrium, also grow elsewhere. The growth of endometrial tissue outside of the uterine body occurs most often in or on the ovaries, the fallopian tubes, the urinary bladder, the bowel, the pelvic floor, the peritoneum, and within the uterine musculature. According to a recent Stanford University report, the most frequent site of this problem is the deep pelvic peritoneal cavity, or the culdesac.

What exactly causes it still eludes physicians. But this much is known, that the majority of sufferers (an estimated 10-12 million American women) have *never been pregnant* in their lives! In overpopulated countries such as Indonesia, Mexico, and India, which one of the authors has visited in times past, endometriosis is virtually unheard of. It is more often a disorder of middle-and-upper income career women by and large. Not too many Hispanic or Afro-American women with large families ever have this.

Symptoms are many and varied: uterine pain, lower backache, pelvic pain, painful menstruation, painful intercourse, excessive bleeding, passing of large clots and shreds of tissue during the menses, nausea, vomiting, constipation, and even infertility at times. Endometriosis produces adhesions, which are formed when endometrial tissue is not fully discharged. Adhesions attach to various pelvic organs, causing them to bind together. This produces the characteristic severe abdominal pain and "chocolate" cysts on the ovaries.

Relief Measures

Simple walking or leisure strolling can help to ease the pain induced by these adhesions and scar tissue. Randi Fletcher of Phoenix, Arizona told one of the authors that she is in the habit of walking up to 3 miles a day and runs about 4 miles, three times a week. She discovered that this type of exercise has been of great assistance in alleviating her symptoms.

Dr. Allison Kramer of Southern California recommends that women avoid drinking soft drinks, cola beverages and coffee. Because, she thinks, the sugar and caffeine in them can aggravate the pain some women with endometriosis may be feeling.

Dr. Kim Woo, a Chinese doctor, uses moxibustion and acupressure to help treat his endometriosis sufferers. He uses moxa sticks, which are sticklike cigars of the herb mugwort rolled up tightly. One end is lit until the stick glows. Then he holds the burning white leaf-stick close enough to the acupressure points that correspond to painful areas, until the skin turns pink and feels very hot but is not burned. This relief lasts for hours, he declares. Sometimes he will alternate this heat treatment with cold packs, which works successfully for some patients better than just moxibustion alone.

Dr. Woo showed one of the authors a spot on the inside of a woman's leg, just about 2 inches above her ankle bone, which can be pressed for relief. Another pressure point is at the base where the bones of her thumb and index finger meet. Press as hard as possible on this for several minutes.

Foods and Nutrients

Judy L., of Los Angeles, shared with one of the authors the program she employed back towards the end of 1981, when major surgery was required to remove her polyps.

"Two days before my surgery commenced, I started taking a high-potency B-complex vitamin (Schiff, 4 tablets daily). I also followed this up with magnesium (1,000 mg.) and calcium (500 mg.). I took an additional amount of B-6 (50 mg.) and pantothenic acid (50 mg.), along with some vitamin C (2,000 mg.). I took these with each meal and at bedtime, too. "I ate high-protein meals consisting mostly of fish and legumes. I used a lot of raw garlic when preparing such foods, and took heavy amounts of Kyolic EPA (garlic and marine lipids)—4-6 capsules a day, or 2 per meal. I took 4 ginger root capsules every night at bedtime to control any nausea and vomiting.

"My surgery came off without a hitch and was pronounced very successful by my doctors. My postoperative regimen 24 hours later included, carrot, tomato and apple juices, canned pears and peaches, yogurt, a banana milkshake, papaya juice and ripe melons. Forty-eight hours after surgery, I started taking Kyo-Dophilus (6 capsules daily, two with each meal) and drinking a glassful of Kyo-Green in the morning and again in the evening. (See Appendix under Wakunaga for these fine products.)

"I can truly testify to the benefits of my nutritional program. I had a much higher tolerance for pain, normal blood pressure, no fever, no kidney or bladder dysfunction, no constipation, no abdominal swelling or pain, no nausea, and an overall feeling of well-being that even amazed my doctors !"

ENTERITIS

Symptoms

Enteritis is an inflammation of the intestine, particularly that of the small intestine, characterized by patchy deep ulcers that may produce abnormal passages, and narrowing and thickening of the bowel by fibrous tissue. Symptoms can include fever, diarrhea, and abdominal cramps and pain.

Relief Measures

In his book, Foods is Your Best Medicine, physician Henry C. Bieler, M.D., strongly recommended the neutralizing of trapped toxins by diet in order to relieve an overworked and upset liver by rest from junk food, and the elimination of such poisons from the body through natural channels like the kidneys, liver, lungs, skin and bowels.

Dandelion root, aged garlic extract, goldenseal root, cascara sagrada, buchu leaves, burdock root, yellow dock root, sarsaparilla root, and horsetail are just a few of the herbs which can help to accomplish this very nicely. They are mostly recommended to be taken in capsules (3 per day).

Foods and Nutrients

Whole grain cereals and breads, legumes, and raw vegetables are very good. Also investing in some type of automatic juicer whereby fresh fruit and vegetable juices become readily available, is a worthy action to take.

Wakunaga's Kyo-Dophilus (3 capsules daily), Kyo-Green (1 glass every morning), and Kyolic 101 (3 capsules daily) form part of this nutritive therapy (see Appendix).

EPILEPSY

Symptoms

One of the authors (Heinerman) recalls going to his local public library a couple of years ago to read some back issues of a newspaper at the microfilm machine. Next to him sat another fellow also reading microfilm. Within minutes this other individual suddenly fell over on to the floor to everyone's amazement.

In his unconscious state, his body became very rigid and manifested occasional but terrific muscle jerks. His breathing was very shallow and his skin started turning blue. It was also evident that he had just wet his pants as well. By the time paramedics arrived five minutes later, he had come out of his seizure but was quite confused, exhausted and unable to remember anything of what had just happened. What this author had just witnessed was someone having a grand mal or epileptic seizure.

Relief Measures

What this author did was the following:

First of all, he removed from the other fellow's clenched fist a pen he had been taking notes with, so that he wouldn't injure himself while thrashing around.

Secondly, he loosened the fellow's tie and belt.

Thirdly, he rolled him over on to his right side with great difficulty.

Fourthly, he himself remained calm and reassured others around that the person experiencing the seizure was feeling nothing.

Finally, this author gently massaged the pressure points located on other fellow's wrists and ankles after he had come out of his seizure. This was done in a slow, rotating motion and seemed to help relax him considerably.

There is also a very important pressure point located on the inside upper portion of the thigh near the groin which could have easily been pushed and held for a few minutes, that would have brought him out of his fit more quickly. But because of public prejudice and ignorance about such things, it was left unattended.

Foods and Nutrients

An epileptic should include in his or her diet plenty of fresh yogurt and kefir, as well as cultured buttermilk and Kyo-Dophilus (3 capsules daily). Fresh juices made from pears, pineapples, papaya, string-beans, carrots, beets, and red grapes should be consumed. Snacking on raw nuts and sunflower seeds, carrot and celery sticks, and unprocessed cheese is good, too. A table-spoonful of olive oil every morning before breakfast is advised. Alcohol, coffee, soft drinks, colas, cigarettes, candy, and anything sweetened with aspartame (NutraSweet) should be avoided at all costs.

Plenty of vitamin D from lots of sunshine and oxygen-rich air found in the warmer, drier climates of the American West and Southwest seems to be very beneficial for epileptics. Put another way, they appear to have *less* seizures in such environments than they would in cold, humid climates.

ERYSIPELAS

Symptoms

Erysipelas is a specific, acute, inflammatory disease of the outer skin caused by streptococcus bacteria infection of the red blood cells. It is characterized by hot, red, edematous, brawny, and sharply defined eruptions. Such is often accompanied by severe constitutional symptoms as well.

Relief Measures

Maria Treben, a renowned Austrian herbalist who resides in Grieskirchen, recom-mends the following herbs be used for treating this condition. Fresh coltsfoot leaves are washed and crushed to a pulp with a wooden rolling pin and applied to the inflamed areas. A decoction can also be made from the dried leaves. A pint of boiling water is poured over two tablespoonfuls of them and infused for a short time. Then when this decoction is sufficiently cool, it can be applied as compress.

Fresh cabbage leaves, washed, crushed and soaked in ice water for awhile, can be used as effective poultices. And, believe it or not, grated and squeezed Bermuda onion from which the juice has been extracted, can be rubbed on the surface of the skin with remarkable results. Also boiled black figs, left to cool and the juice thereof soaked into strips of clean gauze and applied to the face is great.

Stinging nettle tea, made ahead and left in the refrigerator overnight, is wonder-fully soothing as well. Refrigerated aloe vera gel or lotion is good to use in some instances.

Foods and Nutrients

Hot, spicy and vinegary foods should be avoided. As well as condiments like catsup, mustard, pickles and mayonnaise. The intake of red meat and poultry ought to be restricted to some extent; instead one should choose more fish to eat. Soft drinks, colas, coffee and alcohol should not be consumed either until the condition has cleared up.

EYE DISORDERS

(See also BLINDNESS, CATARACTS, CONJUNCTIVITIS, GLAUCOMA, and NIGHT BLINDNESS)

Symptoms

A large number of eye problems can be traced back to lousy eating habits. Many of them, in fact, could have been prevented with good nutrition.

While some eye problems have been covered elsewhere in this book under their respective sections (see the above sub-entries), there are others which we have included here.

Bitot's spots are distinct, elevated, white patches on the white part of the eye known as the cornea.

Bloodshot eyes can be due to excessive eyestrain, lack of sleep, alcoholism, illicit drug use, or allergies.

Blurred vision is fortunately only temporary as a general rule and results when objects appear hazy and unclear at times.

Color blindness is the inability to distinguish colors.

Dry tear ducts result when the eyes fail to produce enough fluid to keep them moist.

"Floaters" are bits of debris floating around within the eye. Because they cast shadows over the retina, a person will see small specks, but most of them eventually float out of view and aren't considered too serious of a problem.

Farsightedness is a condition marked by burning, itchy, scaly, and tired eyes, and by red-rimmed eyelids. Since the eyeball is abnormally short, light rays fall behind the retina. Those who are farsighted can see objects in the distance very clearly, but can't make out those things close by.

Itchy eyes can be due to an inherent allergy and various environmental factors like pollen, dust, and smoke.

Mucus-filled eyes is often attributed to an excessive consumption of dairy products, particularly cheese and ice cream. Junk food is also a deciding factor as well.

Nearsightedness often results from stress. Tension can appear when there is an undersupply or poor absorption of calcium. Adolescents are especially susceptible to this eye disorder due to the stress of growth, allergies, and often an inadequate diet. Symptoms include squinting, dizziness, fatigue, headaches, and low blood pressure sometimes.

Pain behind the eye may be traced to eyestrain or an eye muscle problem. It may or may not need medical attention.

Photophobia occurs in people who simply can't stand light, even when it's turned down low.

Retinitis pigmentosa is a gradual degeneration of the retina, resulting in blindness. The early stages are marked by night blindness and other vitamin A-deficient disorders.

Shingles or painful blisters can sometimes develop very close to the eyes. When this happens, damage to the cornea may result that could eventually lead to blindness.

Styes form from an infection within the oil glands of the eyelid. Since the tissues of the eye become inflamed from the infection, the styes will appear as pimples.

An ulcerated eye occurs when the normal coverings of the eye itself become damaged and inflammation results. Such an ulceration usually occurs because of a viral infection of some kind.

Xeropthalmia is an inflammation of the covering of the eye in which the eye is marked by dryness.

Relief Measures/Foods and Nutrients

Bitot's Spots. Avoid eyestrain and smoke-filled rooms. Supplement your diet with fish, wheat germ oil (1 tsp. daily), and 75,000 units of vitamin A (50% fish oil and 50% beta-carotene derived).

Bloodshot Eyes. Make some chamomile tea. When cool, soak a clean washcloth in the solution, gently wring out and apply over the eyes for relief.

Blurred Vision. Avoid salty foods. Take 1,500 mg. of potassium gluconate and 50,000 units of vitamin A daily. The A should be equally divided between marine lipids and vegetable beta-carotene.

Color Blindness. 100,000 units of vitamin A every other day, equally divided between fish oil and vegetable beta-carotene.

Take in conjunction with dandelion (3 capsules) and alfalfa (6 capsules).

Dry Tear Ducts. Oil of evening primrose (3 capsules), cod liver oil (1 table-spoonful), zinc (50 mg.), Kyolic EPA (3 capsules), and vitamin E oil (1 tsp.) daily are recommeded.

"Floaters." Flood the eyes with distilled water several times. Blink hard for a minute or two. If a large number of them persist for very long, consult an ophthalmologist.

Farsightedness. A high-potency B-complex vitamin (3 tablets daily) is encouraged. Extra B-2 (10 mg.) and thiamine-rich foods like blackstrap molasses, figs, liver, almonds, granola cereal, and kiwi fruit should be consumed. Consult an optometrist, tco.

Itchy Eyes. Same nutritional and dietary recommendations for farsightedness apply here as well. Flood the eyes with distilled water. Then dry them in front of a low-running fan, holding your top and bottom lids down for as long as possible with your fingers.

Mucus-Filled Eyes. Avoid dairy products, white flour products, and fried and sugary foods. Rinse the eyes often with a mild boric acid solution made from cold spring or distilled water and boric acid powder purchased from a local drugstore.

Nearsightedness. Vitamin B-2 (10 mg.), pantothenic acid (50 mg.), C (1,500 mg.), D (400 I.U.), wheat germ oil (1 tsp.), calcium (400 mg.), magnesium (800 mg.), and olive oil (1 tsp.) each day will help in this condition. Consult an optometrist as well for possible prescription eyewear.

Pain Behind The Eye. Gently massage with the fingertips the area immediately around the eye, above, below and on other side of it for a few minutes while in a reclined position. Take a high-potency B-complex (2 tablets) daily.

Photophobia. 50,000 units of vitamin A, equally divided between marine lipids (25,000 IU) and vegetable beta-carotene (25,000 IU) is suggested.

Retinitis Pigmentosa. One of the authors flew to the airport in Oakland, California from his home state to attend a health convention in downtown San Francisco in April, 1992. He took the B.A.R.T. (Bay Area Rapid Transport) subway into that city. In the seat next to him sat a man in his mid-thirties. A friendly conversation soon ensued between them both. The stranger mentioned that he was a salesman at a local jewelry store, but suffered from retinitis pigmentosa. He said he had been taking injections of vitamins A and C from his doctor as well as oral doses of beta-carotene (25,000 units) and rosehip C (3 tablets daily). He also took olive oil (1 tsp.), granulated lecithin (1 tsp. in juice), wheat germ oil (1 tsp.), and Wakunaga's Kyo-Green (1 glass) each day. He claimed that this program had at least staved off further deterioration of his retina for the last several years, so that at least he had managed to retain some of his sight.

Shingles (Herpes Zoster). If blisters appear on the forehead near the eyes or on the tip of the nose, seek immediate medical treatment from a qualified opthalmologist of your choice. Take an all-purpose vitamin-mineral complex (6 tablets daily), injections of vitamin B-12 from your doctor, and vitamin E (600 units daily). Apply some zinc oxide cream to the blisters. After they've cleared up, apply aloe vera gel and vitamin E to the same area. Also ask your doctor to give you 25 grams of vitamin C intravenously.

Styes. Wash the eye with a combined solution of boric acid and eyebright herb tea made with distilled water.

Ulcerated Eyelids. Poultice the eye with a wash cloth soaked in yellow dock tea. Change frequently. Drink the tea as well.

Xeropthalmia. Vitamin A (50,000. IU), D (400 IU), E (600 IU), C (3,500 mg.) and zinc (50 mg.) daily recommended.

FAINTING

Symptoms

Fainting is a short-lived condition in which there is a temporary loss of consciousness. Subject may suddenly collapse or if the fainting spell is more gradual, be inclined to lay down. Palpitation of the heart, sweating, nausea, blackout, and dizziness often accompany fainting. It is usually due to a lack of adequate blood supply to the brain.

A number of factors can cause fainting: emotional upset or hysteria; prolonged standing in hot weather (as when viewing a 4th of July parade, for instance); pregnancy, especially when the mother feels the baby first begin to move inside her belly; diseases like anemia or diabetes; sickness due to acute infection; overheated, poorly ventilated room with stale air; extreme pain; total exhaustion; and arteriosclerosis.

Relief Measures

Subject should be placed in a flat, horizontal position on his or her back. Placing some smelling salts, asafoetida, burning sulphur, or household ammonia cleaner beneath the nostrils and splashing some ice cold water on the face, should definitely help to revive the person. If due to anxiety or trauma, gently massaging the brow, forehead and face will be of great assistance. If due to a disease like diabetes, a small glass of orange or apple juice should help bring the individual out of it. If due to epilepsy, the person will automatically recover of his or her own accord.

Foods and Nutrients

An amino acid complex (2 tablets), iron (35 mg.), and magnesium (600 mg.) taken each day may help to prevent this.

FATIGUE

(See under **CHRONIC FATIGUE SYNDROME**)

FEVER

Symptoms

Fever is the elevation in body temperature beyond what is considered within normal range (97° to 99°F.). If the body temperature reaches 102°F then there is genuine cause for concern; otherwise, it should be considered as a natural manifestation of the body trying to heal itself from some infectious ordeal through which it has just passed.

Serious fever accompanies a wide variety of diseases, and in its more aggressive forms should be taken as a warning that something is terribly wrong within the system. Common symptoms include flushed face, headache, nausea, body aches, little or no appetite, and sometimes, diarrhea or vomiting. The skin may be either hot and dry or warm to the touch with some degree of perspiring. Perspiration is the natural result of the body's attempt to lower its own temperature.

Relief Measures

Intake of adequate fluids is one of the first measures to be employed in any fever, since it tends to dehydrate the body. Liquids low in sugar content are preferable to those with a lot in them. Liquids should be cool and not excessively cold and *very slowly sipped* through a straw if possible. Cool water is the best thing to drink.

The brow and forehead should be covered with damp, cool washcloths and changed every few minutes when they become warm. An airy room through which a light breeze can pass is also recommended; or an electric floor fan placed on a chair at the foot of the bed and allowed to blow across the subject is advised.

Sometimes a fever may be due to constipation. If so, a warm catnip-garlic tea enema should suffice for this purpose. Bring a pint of water to a boil; add one table-spoonful of coarsely chopped garlic. Cover, and simmer on low heat for five minutes. Remove from heat, uncover and add one tablespoonful of catnip herb. Stir, cover and steep for half-an-hour. Uncover and strain into a hot water bottle. Plug one end and connect a small rubber hose to the other end. Hang up on the inside of your bathroom door. Lay down, lubricate plastic syringe end with some Vaseline or olive oil, carefully insert into the rectum, and slowly let some of the solution trickle into your bowels. Shut off momentarily until more fluid can be taken in. Continue this procedure until the body is unable to retain any more. Shut off syringe end, hang up the hose, get up and sit down on the toilet. Repeat this procedure as often as necessary until impacted feces is removed and fever subsides.

Foods and Nutrients

Liquid protein and carbohydrates in the form of simple soups and broths are essential to restoring energy. Some chicken soup made with Pontiac (red) potatoes, turnips, and celery is very good. Kelp tablets or capsules (4 daily) should be taken to replace lost sodium. Potassium (1,200 mg.) also needs to be taken at the same time.

But *avoid* taking iron or zinc during a fever, as they will put an additional strain on the body, which it certainly doesn't need. The body will attempt to throw off extra iron to lower the fever, while zinc won't be absorbed at all and just wasted.

FLU

Symptoms

Popularly called the flu, but more properly known as influenza, this is a highly contagious viral infection which can be easily transmitted through the air by sneezing or coughing or from person to person by shaking hands or handling food or eating utensils that someone else will be using. It affects mostly the respiratory system and if left unattended can prove to be very fatal, as was the case in 1918 when an estimated 30 million people died worldwide of this epidemic, reported the January, 1989 issue of *Smithsonian* magazine.

In most flu epidemics, usually the very old and the very young are hit first and worst. But just the opposite was true in 1918; the first to fall ill and the most cruelly afflicted, were those aged 20 to 40. Flu and flu-induced pneumonia rank among the ten leading causes of death in the United States. Even in a non-epidemic year, the flu claims 10,000 lives nationally, and 30,000 to 40,000 in a bad epidemic year.

Although flu vaccines are readily available, they seldom ever do much good, since the virus keeps mutating into something very different from the most recent vaccine. As epidemiologist Nancy Arden of the Centers of Disease Control in Atlanta, Georgia, told one of the authors sometime ago, "The flu remains terribly elusive and notoriously unpredictable. Anyone who tries to predict anything about the next flu season is going to be wrong a good proportion of the time."

The early signs of flu are similar to those of the common cold, namely having a pounding headache, physical weakness, runny nose, sore throat, and aching in the arms, legs, and back. A dry, hacking cough and a sullen disposition to not eat or do anything else also prevails. In more severe cases, nausea and vomiting are likely to occur.

Relief Measures

Two things immediately come to mind which can be done for anyone who has the flu. Yet they are both so simple as to be generally ignored by the majority of the populace at large. Plenty of sleep and curtailment of one's entire routine daily agenda head the list. Both of us have repeatedly seen many, many people struggle to keep up with their busy schedules on just a few hours of rest, while popping pills of all kinds including vitamin supplements and antibiotics in the hopes of getting rid of their flus. But this never works out. Only by stopping *everything* and going to bed for long hours at a time, can the body expect to fully recuperate as it should.

The second thing is that all heavy types of food, which are difficult to digest — greasy or sugary foods—should be totally eliminated from the diet. Also all dairy products and white flour substances should be stopped as well. Instead, clear broths or soups which are consumed hot and generously flavored with pungent spices like garlic, onion, ginger root, horseradish, black pepper, and cayenne, should be the order of the day until complete recovery has resulted. They will definitely help to clear up plugged sinuses, a stuffy nose, and congested lungs.

Along with this there should be some brief visits to a sauna, steamroom or Indian sweat lodge to help dislodge internal toxins from body tissue. During this period, warm herbal teas like catnip or peppermint should be copiously drunk. They not only reduce fever but also help to kill flu viruses on account of their strong antiviral activities.

Rubbing the body immediately after such a sweat with a dry, natural bristle brush or loofah sponge will help to increase circulation and bring a warm glow of health to the skin and make the body feel a thousand times better.

Keeping the bowels open and the bladder and kidneys functioning is also important. Drinking prune juice with some pulp in it in the morning and cranberry juice periodically throughout the rest of the day will accomplish both of these tasks effectively enough.

Gargling with the right solution can make all the difference in the world to relieving a sore throat. A 6 fluid ounce glass of equal parts of hot lemonade to which has been added a teaspoonful of honey, 1/4 teaspoonful of salt, and a few shakes of Tabasco sauce, makes a terrific throat remedy. Also chewing on a couple of cloves helps, as does squeezing a few drops of Propolis Tincture in the back of the throat for quick and sure relief.

Foods and Nutrients

Nutritional supplements are crucial to fast recovery from the flu. But they work even quicker if taken with certain herbs or spices. For instance, vitamin A (50,000 IU) performs better with Kyolic liquid garlic (3 capsules) than by itself. And vitamin C (10,000 mg.) activity is enhanced when taken with cayenne pepper (2 capsules) and ginger root (2 capsules). A zinc gluconate lozenge can be sucked on during a cold or flu, but has its effectiveness speeded up if a horehound cough drop is slowly dissolved immediately following it. Vitamin E (800 IU) is useful, but becomes more improved when taken with mullein capsules (2).

Some homeopathic preparations from any local health food store are of value in treating stubborn cases of the flu. A tincture of echinacea and goldenseal (10 drops 3 times daily) possesses antibiotic properties. Gelsemium is useful for aches and chills, while oscillococcinum is helpful for nasal discharge or obstruction, sneezing, shivers, earache, and frontal sinus pain. Nux vomica will stop vomiting, diarrhea and chills, while sulphur is helpful for night sweats and fever.

Chinese astragalus (3 capsules), pantothenic acid (100 mg. three times) and Kyolic garlic extract with selenium and vitamins A and E make a delightful trio of remedies to boost energy levels when the system has been ravaged and weakened by influenza.

Because the immune system is closely intertwined with the nervous system, we recommend herbal tranquilizers like *warm* catnip tea (2 cupsules) or valerian root (3 capsules) and a high-potency B-complex (3 tablets) every day.

FOOD POISONING

Symptoms

Food poisoning is a very unpleasant and miserable condition usually induced by pathogenic and toxic organisms such as Salmonella bacteria. Common symptoms include nausea, vomiting, and cramps that can last from several hours to several days. In more serious types of food poisoning, like botulism, death can result in the elderly or the very young. Abdominal S pain, diarrhea, dehydration, and typhoid-like fever are frequent as well.

Most Salmonella poisoning is contracted from contaminated foods, especially chicken, eggs, beef and pork products. Rare or poorly cooked meats are a far greater risk for Salmonella poisoning than is medium or well-done meat. Contaminated milk, eggs, ice cream, hollandaise sauce, eggnog, Caesar salad dressing and potato salad have all caused Salmonella food poisoning in the past in various parts of the country.

Next to Salmonella, Staphylococcus Aureus is the second most frequent cause of food-borne illnesses. Since this tiny microorganism is most frequently found in the nose and throat, any sneezing and coughing on or near food can contaminate it immediately. Salad bars are a common source for this type of nasty bacterial poisoning. Staphylococcus aureus accounts for about 25% of all food-borne illnesses. Symptoms of food contamination by it include diarrhea, nausea, and vomiting within 2-6 hours after eating. These responses occur because the body is trying to rid itself of the toxins produced in the presence of this bacterium. For this reason it may be good to induce vomiting as soon as possible.

Relief Measures

Preventing food poisoning from ever happening is more important than ways to treat it. Food should be kept either hot or cold, but never left at room temperature for very long. Perishables should be refrigerated at all times, as well as any leftovers. Meat of any kind should be thoroughly cooked. Hands need to be washed after going to the toilet, blowing your nose or scratching certain anatomical parts of the body *before* handling food.

When shopping, don't dilly-dally too long from home in hot weather. Certain purchases need immediate freezing or refrigeration and unnecessary delays in getting them where they properly belong, might cause spoilage. Never use the contents of any cans that are bulging, rusted, bent or sticky! Beware of cracks in fruit jars and leaks in paper packaging, too. Set your refrigerator at 40°F. and your freezer at 0°F. See that reheated leftovers are *well* cooked before serving.

Thaw out all frozen foods, especially meats and poultry *in the refrigerator* rather than in the sink or on the table or stove. *Do not use* any of the following foods if mold has formed on them: bacon, white bread, cured luncheon meats, soft dairy products, flour, canned ham, hot dogs, roasted nuts, peanut butter, roast poultry, soft vegetables, and whole grains. Picnic items like mayonnaise, salad dressing, mustard, and milk products spell trouble with a big T if they are left in the sun or at room temperature for very long.

It is not a good idea to eat iceberg lettuce in salads or sandwiches, because the risk of serious contamination is very high. An investigative article in the May/June 1991 issue of *Eating Well* spelled out in great detail what led to the alarming and sudden outbreak of hepatitis A in the Louisville, Kentucky area which affected hundreds of people. One restaurant alone accounted for a whopping 64 cases of this deadly disease. The culprit eventually turned out to be lettuce shipped in from Mexico or some of the border towns in Texas, Arizona and California. The article also reported that many migrant field workers harvesting American lettuce, have often been seen going to the bathroom out in the open fields and using leaves from you-know-what to wipe with afterwards.

One of the authors has a friend who is a Dallas police officer. He gave permission for his name to be used here. Officer Wesley Johnson and his partner had been out on a routine patrol during June, 1991, and decided to stop at a local fast-food Mexican restaurant for a quick bite to eat. About a week later, both of them became dangerously ill with infectious hepatitis, which was eventually traced to some very old guacamole sauce they had with their meals. In recounting his own ordeal with this disease, Officer Johnson related, "I thought for awhile there that I was going to die. I have never been so damn sick in all my life. I figured that since no bullets from the guns of bad guys that I've arrested ever got me, that this Mexican food for sure would do me in. I'm just lucky to be here!" It took him and his partner at least five months to regain back all of their former strength and energy.

One of the authors is also acquainted with nutrition expert Jeffrey

Bland of Gig Harbor, Washington. A few years ago, Dr. Bland had to suddenly cancel some important speaking engagements when he became mysteriously ill and had to be temporarily hospitalized. As it turned out, some raw sushi he had consumed in a local Japanese restaurant, gave him a bad case of food poisoning, which took him some time to recover from.

There is very little which can be done to remedy such serious cases as these. Prompt medical attention in a hospital emergency room is absolutely essential! For some cases of poisoning, induced vomiting may be desirable. Syrup of Ipecac sold at most local drugstores is available for this purpose. On the other hand, taking charcoal tablets along with a coffee retention enema may help to get rid of the poisonous toxins that shouldn't be vomited up.

Foods and Nutrients

Kyolic liquid garlic extract (4 capsules 3 times daily), Kyo-Dophilus (2 capsules 3 times daily), superoxide dismutase (SOD) (5,000 mg. daily), vitamin C plus bioflavonoids (10,000 mg. daily), oat bran capsules (4 daily), and kelp tablets (10 a day) are all useful to some degree. (See Appendix under Wakunaga for the first two products.)

FRACTURES

Symptoms

A fracture is a break in a bone. A fracture is closed or simple when the skin remains intact, or else open or compound when the bone penetrates through the skin.

Fractures may occur as the result of an accident, a disease process or a mineral deficiency. Symptoms include limb deformities, limited limb functioning, shortening of the limb in fractures of long bones, terrible pain, a grating sensation if the broken bone ends rub together, and considerable swelling and discoloration of the skin overlaying the region of said fracture.

Relief Measures

No attempt should be made to set a fracture by yourself. This should always be left to doctors to do, unless one is in such a remote area that it is physically impossible to get immediate medical assistance. Then it should only be done with considerable care, much patience, and a great deal of forethought. For leg and arm fractures, newspapers tightly rolled around the limb and two flat sticks laid on either side and everything secured in place with duck or electrician's tape has sometimes been used with good success. Still, we feel to advise individuals, however, to consult a doctor as soon as possible, as this suggestion should only be temporary.

A program of bone-building herbs is required here: alfalfa (8 capsules daily), horsetail (3 capsules daily), comfrey (4 capsules daily), slippery elm bark (5 capsules daily), and kelp (6 capsules daily).

Mineral supplements to include would be: calcium (2,000 mg.), phosphorus (1,200 mg.), potassium (2,000 mg.), magnesium (1,000 mg.), and zinc (150 mg.) every day for at least a month. Vitamins to take would be A (50,000 I.U.), pantothenic acid (150 mg.), C (10,000 mg.), D (400 I.U. and plenty of sunshine, too), E (800 I.U.), and the bioflavonoids rutin and hesperidin (1,500 mg. each).

The diet should include some body-building soy protein shakes and fish, as well as plenty of pasta foods.

FREE RADICAL DETERIORATION

Symptoms

Free radical deterioration begins at a cellular level, when oxgyen-free radicals that are in other ways crucial to body chemistry, spin out of control. Immediate and obvious results are wrinkled skin, gray hair, premature senility, and stiff joints. More subtle ailments down the road include Alzheimer's, schizophrenia, Parkinson's, Down's syndrome, cancer, heart disease, stroke, paralysis, cataracts, and emphysema.

Free radicals result when molecules are torn apart and thrown out of electrical balance. In chemical terms, a free radical is a molecule with an unpaired electron; put more simply, it is a confused particle that has lost its mate.

While helpful for some immune functions, too many of them all at once can wreak biochemical havoc within the system in much the same way that those angry mobs did when they burned down several square miles of southcentral Los Angeles in late April and early May of 1992. In their frenetic search for new mates, free radicals explode the fragile equilibrium of cells. They shatter the intricate process in which the messages

of genes are transcribed into proteins. They demolish enzymes and other molecules.

Even as you're reading these very words right now, free radicals are being mass-produced within your body. More are added if you eat a lot of fried or deep-fried foods or refrigerated leftover meats. But most will be squelched by one of nature's most ferocious protective systems. Antioxidants are the things that hunt and control these molecular "sharks" that zip madly through your cellular sea.

Relief Measures

Certain spices are powerful antioxidants. They include garlic, onion, thyme, rosemary, sage, tarragon and oregano. Of these, garlic and onions are the most potent. An aged garlic extract that includes certain fish oil made by Wakunaga of America and sold as Kyolic EPA is one of the very best nutritional supplements on the market today for curbing free radical activity at all levels. This product doesn't necessarily destroy them, for without free radicals certain bodily functions would become seriously impaired, as it provides *strong management* of their activities.

Think of these herbal antioxidants and others like chaparral and pau d'arco as efficient units of national guardsmen or police enforcing law and order within your system. Without their presence, as was the case for the first few hours in the Los Angeles riots of recent memory, chaos and violence reigns which can cause terrible destruction at a cellular level. Now some of them can be taken in capsule form (about 3 a day), while others can be used in food preparation.

Quitting the habit of smoking or avoiding second-hand smoke altogether is another way to avoid any further increase of free radicals. Keeping fit through exercise also helps the body to hold them in check. The natural supplement, superoxide dismutase (SOD) helps to revitalize tired cells and reduces the rate of their destruction.

Foods and Nutrients

Believe it or not, one of the most harmful foods to the body because of the terrific amount of free radicals in it, is a plain fried hamburger! So claimed the authors of the million-copy plus best-seller, *Life Extension*. Both the fat content, the grinding of the meat and its rapid cooking on a grill or charbroiler makes it "a particularly rich source of free radicals," they wrote on page 382. So this kind of food should be greatly minimized in the diet. And when it becomes necessary to eat a burger on the spur of the moment, ask for plenty of sliced onions and hold the lettuce, mayo, catsup, mustard and other garbage they like to slap on it. At least this way you will be controlling most of those bad molecules being taken into your system.

Char-broiled meat, fried bacon, fried or deep-fried chicken, and anything barbecued, while obviously tasting lip-smacking delicious, in truth isn't doing your body very much good. We suggest that the way such meats, including fish ought to be properly prepared, is by baking, boiling or steaming them where the least contact with air is possible. A recent device currently being advertized on television boasts a new type of jet-air oven that can cook food in just minutes instead of hours. It's similar to a big blow-dryer laid on its side with a lid put over it. Such a thing may make cooking speedier,

but it's guaranteed to add tons of free radicals to your body.

Vitamin C with bioflavonoids (3,500 mg.), SOD, vitamin E (800 I.U.), beta-carotene (25,000 IU), L-Cystine, evening primrose oil (with GLA), and selenium can be taken on a regular basis to help control your body's mischievous free radicals.

FRIGIDITY

Symptoms

Frigidity is of psychological origin, usually stemming from fear, guilt and an inferiority complex, that prevents women from experiencing sensual pleasure during intercourse with their male companions.

Relief Measures

Psychological counseling may be necessary. A positive mental attitude is certainly warranted. Use bee pollen, damiana, saw palmetto, and ginseng frequently for this. The diet should include plenty of alfalfa sprouts, avocados, fertile eggs, olive oil, pumpkin and sunflower seeds, raw nuts, and whole grains.

Foods and Nutrients

Not too much red meat, chicken or turkey and sweet things should be consumed. Keep soft drink and cola intakes to a minimum. Stay away from second-hand smoke and smog.

Take kelp (6 tablets daily), high-potency B-complex (4 tablets), vitamin E oil

(800 IU), liquid lecithin (1 tsp. daily), vitamin C with bioflavonoids (3,500 mg.), and zinc (50 mg. twice daily).

FROSTBITE

Symptoms

Frostbite is a condition brought on by long-term exposure to excessive cold without adequate protection of the fingers, toes and feet, ears and nose. Dusky red, oval swellings that have an intense itch about them usually result.

Relief Measures

The best protection is to wear warm gloves or woolen mittens, a long scarf, a ski mask that pulls down over the face, several pairs of woolen stockings and boots or galoshes over regular shoes.

In the event frostbite does occur, it is best to soak limb extremities in a warm Epsom salts solution for about 20 minutes. An interal remedy which can be taken and works wonders for fast recovery, consists of two-thirds of a cup of warm brandy to which has been added the emptied contents of 3 cayenne and 3 ginger root capsules and * tsp. of grated horseradish juice or pulp.

Foods and Nutrients

Vitamins A (50,000 I.U. fish oil), C with bioflavonoids (5,000 mg.), E (800 IU), panthothenic acid (100 mg.), PABA (100 mg.), and zinc (75 mg.) work well here. The application of a cream rich in PABA and herbs like calendula, comfrey and/or chamomile to fingertips, toes, ears and nose brings some relief, too.

FUNGAL INFECTIONS

(See also under CANDIDIASIS)

Symptoms

A yeast or mold may infect the skin, mouth or vagina, and grow under the nails, between the toes, or on internal surfaces. A fungus under the nails or between the toes may cause discoloration and swelling, and the nails may raise above the surface of the nail bed resulting in infection.

Moist red patches anywhere on the body usually is a sign of a fungus (yeast) infection. When in the vagina, a cheesy discharge is present.

Relief Measures

Various suggestions for specific Candida albicans infections may be found elsewhere in this book under CANDIDIASIS. Those offered here are more for general fungus problems of an external nature.

Infected hands and feet can be soaked in a strong solution of goldenseal root and pau d'arco bark tea (equal parts or 2 tbsps. each in 2 quarts of boiling water). After this, dry hands and feet thoroughly, first with a towel and then with an electric blow dryer if necessary to remove all moisture.

Some peeled and crushed garlic or onion mixed with a little honey and applied in between the skin webs of the fingers or toes or around the nails, is handy for getting rid of fungus.

Another remedy employing garlic was mentioned in a short medical article in the *Indian Journal of Dermatology* for January, 1983. A young Indian solider, aged 30 years, was posted for some time in the Assam region in the northeastern part of that country. He reported to his army hospital unit "with a warty lesion on the ring finger of his left hand and six ulcers on the left forearm and arm of eight months duration.... Before being referred to the Air Force Hospital, he had been treated with various systemic antibiotics and local antiseptics without improvement." Doctors ran some tests and diagnosed his condition as sporotrichosis, a type of fungi that enters the body by way of minute abrasions or puncture wounds from thorny bushes, sphagum moss, and soil.

Doctors decided to try some garlic on him instead. The "natural garlic juice was prepared by crushing garlic pods in an electric blender and blended to a paste with chilled water.... A sterile gauze was soaked in this juice" and applied "on the largest ulcer and kept in position with a light bandage.

"An irritant reaction was noticed within 24 hours which made the ulcer look more angry and therefore, a second application was not done. The ulcer was kept covered with dry sterile gauze. Within 3 days however the ulcer showed remarkable improvement. A second application done after 4 days produced mild irritation again. The ulcer healed completely within ten days. On account of the satisfactory results

obtained, the garlic juice was applied on the remaining lesions similarly and kept in position for 24 hours. The patient tolerated the mild irritation well. No second application was required on most of the lesions which healed over a period of 6 to 13 days after a single application.

"The patient was kept in the hospital for two weeks to see if there was any recurrence. He was again reviewed after 6 weeks, 3 months and 6 months, during which there was no further evidence of any recurrence." Coming from a medical journal as it were, we believe that this remedy had considerable merit and has been proven to be very effective with all types of fungus, including athlete's foot, jock itch, and the fungus often accompanying AIDS.

Lutretia Starr of Hayward, California sent this remedy to one of the authors in October, 1978:

At the beginning of July, I suffered for two days with a yeast infection. I took a clove of fresh garlic, put it in the blender with four ounces of water, and liquefied it. I then strained the mixture through some close-woven cheese cloth. Adding enough water to make 24 ounces, I douched with 8 ounces every night before bedtime, for three nights.

On the fourth night I douched with a cooled tea (room temperature) made from oat straw.

Little by little the terrible itching subsided. By the fourth night it was almost gone and by the fifth night it was completely cleared up.

Foods and Nutrients

We recommend Wakunaga's Kyolic liquid aged garlic extract (4 capsules daily) and Kyo-Dophilus (3 capsules daily) and Kyo-Green (1 glass each day) until the fungus disappears.

Vitamin A (25,000 units of fish oil and 25,000 units of beta-carotene) and C (5,000 mg.) are both very good. And some vitamin E (about 800 I.U. daily) and zinc (25 mg. daily) should be included with the other items.

GALLSTONES

Symptoms

Gallstones develop when deposits of cholesterol or calcium combine with bile. Bile is a secretion produced by the liver to emulsify fats so that they can be digested. Most of the bile manufactured by the liver is stored in the gallbladder until the small intestine calls for it when fat has been ingested. However, some bile travels directly from the liver to the small intestine. Gallstones form in the passages between liver and gallbladder, between liver and intestine, or in the gallbladder itself. Gallstones are usually found in diabetics, obese and elderly people; and females, especially those who've had children.

Gallstone formation begins to appear when cholesterol crystallizes out of solution and forms stones. Nearly half of all gallstone patients are without symptoms. It is when a stone obstructs any of the bile passages that symptoms occur. These symptoms generally include nausea, vomiting, and severe right upper abdominal pain that may radiate to the right shoulder or back. The symptoms commonly occur a few hours after eating a heavy meal of fatty or fried foods. If the stone totally obstructs one of the bile passages, jaundice (a yellowish cast to the skin and eyeballs), dark urine, clay-colored stools, and itching of the skin may also occur.

Relief Measures

For removal of gallstones, one of the most favorite and successful treatments has been the so-called "oil cure." Raw, natural, unrefined vegetable oils of olive, sunflower, or walnut are used, olive being the most common. Oil cure should be preceded by a two-day cleansing diet of vegetables and fruits (preferably pears) plus soaked prunes, figs and psyllium seeds. Before beginning the cure, take a good enema to cleanse the bowels with. Take 1/2 to 3/4 of a pint of oil at a time. After taking the oil, lay down on your right side and remain in this position for two hours. Putting a pillow under your right armpit helps to keep the gallbladder in a downward position so that the stones can be evacuated more easily.

Another remedy for gallstones is this: First thing in the morning, on an empty stomach, take one ounce of olive oil, and follow next with four ounces of grapefruit juice. Take this treatment each morning for several weeks, if necessary.

Foods and Nutrients

In acute cases of gallstone attacks, *a three-day fast* should be immediately imposed if a person's health condition allows it. Those who are diabetics or hypoglycemics may need to modify this a little according to their own individual needs.

The person should go on juices first of all, preferably pear and beet greens or carrot and pineapple juices. Kefir, yogurt, homemade cottage cheese, raw *organic and fertile* eggs, olive oil, and ripe avocados are some of the foods which can be consumed safely enough without further aggravating the situation.

Useful herbs include horsetail (3 capsules daily), dandelion (4 capsules daily), comfréy tea (2 cups daily), fennel tea (I cup daily), parsley (up to 50 sprigs daily), evening primrose oil (6 capsules daily), and peppermint oil (10 drops in a glass of *warm* distilled water).

Lecithin is very useful for *preventing* the formation of gallstones. Up to 3 tablespoonfuls of the granules may be taken each day, either sprinkled on morning breakfast cereal, on a luncheon salad, or in a snack health shake or juice of some kind. Or the liquid lecithin can be taken every morning and evening (1 tbsp.) with some water.

In conjunction with this, a high-potency B-complex vitamin (4 tablets daily), vitamin E oil capsules (2 daily), vitamin D (1,500 lU daily), and vitamin A (25,000 I.U. daily) should be taken. Wakunaga's Kyo-Dophilus capsules (1 per meal each day) is also very good (see Appendix).

GANGRENE

Symptoms

Gangrene is the pathological death of body tissue due to obstruction, loss or reduction of the blood supply. It may be localized to a small area or involve an entire extremity or organ, and may be wet or dry in nature.

Relief Measures

While not too common, gangrene can still occur, especially in older people, the homeless who may be deprived of medical care, and diabetics. In such instances, hospitalization becomes mandatory. But a few remedies may prove useful in some cases where adequate medical care isn't readily available.

In India, berberine sulphate has been used to treat gangrene and related tissue necrosis problems. The alkaloid itself, berberine, is found in different plant root or bark systems. Two herbs indigenous to North America which are rich in berberine content are goldenseal root and wild Oregon grape bark and rootbark.

The fine powdered roots can be sprinkled directly on a gangrenous mass of flesh or else made into a strong solution and the same infection thoroughly cleansed out.

Foods and Nutrients

Vitamin A (100,000 I.U. daily), vitamin C (20,000 mg. intramuscular injection), and zinc (100 mg.) are valuable here.

Foods consumed should be antibiotic (garlic, onions, horseradish, and thyme) and cleansing (citrus and leafy green vegetable juices) as well as healing (papaya and mango juice, bananas) in nature.

GASTRITIS & GASTROENTERITIS

Symptoms

Gastritis is a sudden disturbance of digestion usually due to inflammation of the stomach mucosal lining. Symptoms include stomach discomfort rather than pain, nausea and sometimes vomiting, tenderness of the upper abdomen, headache, lack of appetite, and occasional fever.

Gastroenteritis is essentially the same inflammation disorder, but which affects both the stomach as well as the intestine. Can be a forerunner of peptic ulcer sometimes. Symptoms similar to gastritis, but also include higher chances of vomiting mucus and fluid *in the morning*, but showing improvement later in the day. A feeling of fullness, drowsiness, furred tongue, headache, and undue fatigue after meals is common. Forms of gastroenteritis, unlike gastritis, can be invoked by invasion into the body of the highly communicable Norwalk virus, which has a duration of 1 to 2 days and can cause fever, abdominal cramps, and diarrhea, besides the other aforementioned symptoms.

Relief Measures.

Taking the time to chew your food in smaller bites and mixing *every single*

mouthful with adequate saliva is very important. Next is to drink herbal teas like slippery elm, comfrey root, fenugreek seed, or marshmallow root and fruit juices like papaya or mango with banana which all help to coat the mucosal lining and reduce inflammation.

The addition of other herbal teas such as chamomile, peppermint or lemonbalm are helpful not only to soothe the stomach, but also to diminish the activity of the virus itself because of their antibiotic strength.

Foods and Nutrients

Many types of foods must be avoided when these conditions prevail. Rich foods (sugary and greasy kinds), red meat, chicken and turkey (because of the skin), spicy foods (like Mexican and Oriental), and acidic foods (citrus juices, coffee and black or green teas, soft drinks and colas, ice cream, sauerkraut, vinegar, catsup, mustard, pickles and mayonnaise) will only aggravate matters more. So will deep-fried foods like salted peanuts, doughnuts, and French fries.

Frequent smaller meals in which just one item is consumed in moderate portions is recommended instead. Cream-o-Wheat cereal or cooked millet with a little goat or soybean milk is right for breakfast. Some clear vegetable soup with unsalted crackers is nice for lunch. Munching on some grapes or an apple or a ripe peach or pear or melon is helpful for snacks. Dinner might consist of a plain baked potato with the skin intact and flavored with just a little yogurt and granulated kelp.

Supplements should include brewer's yeast (1 tsp. daily), extra vitamin B-

6 from blackstrap molasses (1/2 tsp. daily), inoistol (500 mg.), pantothenic acid (100 mg.), PABA (100 mg.), non-acidic vitamin C (calcium ascorbate or ascorbyl palmitate should be on the label somewhere; 3,500 mg.), liquid lecithin (1 tsp. daily), manganese (25 mg.), arid zinc (100 mg. daily).

GIARDIA

Symptoms

This is a genus of parasite with only 2 or 3 species involved in the intestinal discomforts produced in most domestic animals and man. These include considerable gas, passage of fat in large amounts in the feces, diarrhea, dyspepsia, and occasionally malabsorption of ingested foods.

Relief Measures

Dr. Singh Lampur, who worked for the International Centre for Diarrhoel Disease Research in Bangladesh has trained mothers in many villages on how best to cope with diarrhea caused by bacterial infection in the gastrointestinal system. His method calls for them to prepare rice-salt oral rehydration solutions for this problem. It consists of two handfuls of white rice, one level teaspoon of salt and one liter of water. The watery rice solution is slowly sipped when warm. It reduces diarrhea, rehydrates, decreases stool volume, and appears to villagers to "cure" diarrhea.

The use of antibiotic herbs like gold-enseal (4 capsules daily) or Kyolic liquid garlic (4 capsules daily) can also be very useful. Especially if taken on an empty stomach.

Foods and Nutrients

Vitamin A (50,000 I.U. divided equally between fish oil and beta-carotene) and vitamin C (3,500 mg.), calcium (800 mg.), magnesium (1,200 mg.) and potassium (2,500 mg.) each day until diarrhea stops is suggested.

GINGIVITIS

See under GUM DISEASE for more information on this.

GLAUCOMA

Symptoms

Glaucoma is characterized by an increase in pressure of the fluid within the eyeball and a hardening of the surface of the eyeball. The cause of glaucoma isn't known, but usually it occurs after forty and can be attributed to tumor, trauma, infection, and in one type, hereditary. This disease is usually associated with anxiety and stress, allergy or hormone problems. Symptoms include eye discomfort or pain, especially in the morning, blurred vision, halos around lights, inability to adjust to a darkened room, and loss of vision at the sides.

Relief Measures

Since glaucoma is considered a "stress disease," a person should try to avoid emotional and mental traumas of any kind. Instead inner tranquility and a more restful lifestyle should be sought for.

Climate with great temperature changes (north) is detrimental. A southern climate which is more even and temperate is much better for those with glaucoma.

Prolonged eye strain should be avoided. This means that watching a lot of television or long movies or doing excessive reading should be curtailed.

Air pollution bothers glaucoma. Smoking and second-hand smoke from those who do smoke, should be avoided. City smog and chlorinated water from public swimming pools both aggravate this condition.

Sunglasses should not be used unless the eyes are particularly sensitive to bright sunlight.

The Johns Hopkins Medical Letter for April, 1991 reported on an effective medical treatment for glaucoma. In the Glaucoma Laser Trial involving 11 medical centers across the country, 271 patients with early glaucoma were treated for a couple of years by two different methods. In one eye, each of the patients received medicated eye drops, the standard treatment for this disease. In the other, they were treated with argon laser surgery first, to "clear" the blockage. After two years, the eyes treated with lasers had lower intraocular pressures than the eyes treated with drops alone.

Foods and Nutrients

Certain fruit and vegetable juices are very helpful for this disorder: citrus, carrot, beet root and beet top, tomato and cranberry. They help to promote blood circulation within the eyeball and relieve some of the pressure that damages the optic nerve and can result in loss of vision.

Herbs like eyebright (4 capsules daily), red clover tea (2 cups daily), and alfalfa (8 capsules daily) are helpful, too. Vitamins A (25,000 IU), choline (2 grams), vitamin C. (7,0000 mg. 3 times daily), vitamin D (600 IU), the bioflavonoid rutin (1,000 mg.), chromium (150 mcg.) and potassium gluconate (2,000 mg.) are suggested on a regular basis.

GOITERS

Symptoms

A goiter is an enlargement of the thyroid gland, which is located at the base of the neck. This gland regulates metabolism, or the burning of food, growth, and body temperature, and influences mental and emotional balance and the performance of the reproductive system.

Thyroid disorders like goiter are due to an inadequate amount of iodine in the body. Symptoms of goiter are a swelling at the base of the neck, hoarseness, change in the rate of metabolism, and in some cases, difficulty in swallowing and breathing.

Relief Measures/Foods and Nutrients

Excessive consumption of cabbage and soybean products can deplete iodine from the system. Generous consumption of fish and kelp tablets (4 daily) is encouraged. Vitamin E (800 IU) increases the utilization of iodine within the body. Food should be flavored with sea salt for additional iodine, and potassium (2,000 mg.) taken to offset the large amount of sodium in the sea salt.

GONORRHEA

Symptoms

Known vulgarly also as "the clap," this venereal disease is usually transmitted by sexual intercourse and affects the reproductive organs of men and women who contract it. Because of widespread promiscuity these days, gonorrhea and other sexually transmissible diseases like syphilis and chiamydiosis are in near epidemic proportions in many parts of the country, particularly in inner city ghettos and slum neighborhoods.

In the first stage, a single, painless sore appears 3-4 weeks after intercourse with an infected person, usually on a man's penis or on the entrance to a woman's vagina or just inside of it, but can also be on the lip, nipple, anus, or finger as well. This chancre gradually becomes an oozing ulcer with a hard red surrounding, and the glands in the groin may become painlessly enlarged.

A month or two later, a mild general illness, with sore throat, sometimes "snail-track" ulcers in the mouth, a headache, mild fever and a pink non-itchy rash are evident. Sometimes the voice can become husky due to laryngitis.

With gonorrhea there is also the occurrence of scalding urine in 3 to 10 days after general infection. Then a discharge of pus from the urinary outlet and vagina occurs.

Relief Measures

The late Rabbi Wolfe Kelman, a major leader of Conservative Judaism, firmly believed that abstinence from sexual activity among young people was the best prevention of all against acquiring gonorrhea or any of its related infections. But more often than not, this is easier said than done.

Focusing one's sexual energies in other directions can be very useful. One male college student especially noted for his aggressive hormonal behavior with the opposite sex, discovered that karate was an outlet for all of his pent-up anxieties and drives. Another young man took up boxing as a way to channel his sexual needs into more healthy activity.

Internally, the best natural remedies to administer when gonorrhea is present are these: goldenseal root (3 capsules daily), Kyolic liquid garlic (6 capsules daily), chaparral (5 capsules daily), yellow dock and burdock (3 capsules each daily), red clover (4 capsules daily) and sarsaparilla (6 capsules daily). While this might seem to be a lot of capsules to be taking each day, yet a stubborn infection such as gonorrhea which is often resistant to conventional antibiotics, requires an arsenal of herbs to tackle it successfully.

Foods and Nutrients

The intake of any kind of junk food which is greasy or sugary ought to be greatly minimized, if not altogether avoided, since they tend to greatly weaken the immune system. And reduced immunity simply can't cope with such a mean adversary as this.

Vitamin A (100,000 I.U., divided equally between fish oil and beta-carotene), vitamin C (15,000. mg.), selenium (200 mcg.) and zinc (100 mg.) are the chief nutrients to be taken each day for as long as necessary until a regression of this nasty infection becomes evident.

GOUT

Symptoms

Gout is a metabolic disturbance characterized by an excess of uric acid in the blood and deposits of uric acid salts in the tissue around the joints, especially in the fingers and the toes. It can also occur in the heel, knee, hand, ear, or any joint in the body. Gout results when certain crystals are formed as an end product of improper protein metabolism. These crystals are deposited in a joint, forming a bump or growth that irritates the joint, causing it to become inflamed; thus an attack of gout occurs.

Relief Measures/Foods and Nutrients

The basic diet for gout is the same as it would be for arthritis, namely one that is a low-uric acid, low-purine diet. Foods high in potassium are protective against gout: pota-

toes, bananas, leafy green vegetables, beans, and raw vegetable juices. Purine and uric acid producing foods like red meat and poultry, dairy products and eggs should be avoided. Raw or canned goat's milk or goat's cheese is an exception to this.

Red sour cherries, red raspberries and strawberries are of specific value in the treatment of gout. Black cherry juice is available in many health food stores and should be taken (1 cup twice daily). Frozen cherries are good to use when the fresh ones aren't in season or available. Cherries have an exceptional ability to alkalize the sytem and neutralize uric acid.

Alfalfa capsules (6 daily) or tea (2 cups daily), parsley and celery juice (1/2 cup 3 times daily), cooked parsnip water (2 cups daily), juniper berries (4 capsules daily), potassium (2,000 mg.) and B-complex (4 tablets daily) should be used regularly.

GRAVES' DISEASE

See under HYPERTHYROIDISM for more information on this.

GRAY HAIR

Symptoms

Gray hair is a condition when the normal color of the hair changes and starts becoming somewhat dull or turning a dishwater white. Hereditary graying can't be prevented by nutritional means, but certainly a well-balanced diet will help to maintain normal hair color a lot longer.

Relief Measures/Foods and Nutrients

Foods high in free radicals should not be consumed too much as they tend to hasten the aging processes, of which graying hair is one of these. Fried, deep-fried and sugary foods need to curtailed as much as possible.

A return to natural hair color has been achieved by some people with supplements of copper (4 mg.), folic acid (400 mcg.), pantothenic acid (100 mg.), PABA (100 mg.), and vitamin E (800 I.U.) on a daily basis.

GUM DISEASE (GINGIVITIS)

Symptoms

Gum disease (also known as gingivitis or peridontal disease) occurs when stagnant food remains in between the teeth and causes infection around them. Gum margins become smooth, glossy, slightly swollen, tender, red and bleed at the touch of the toothbrush. If these things are left unattended for very long, pockets of pus soon form around the teeth, the gums begin receding, and the teeth become loose.

Relief Measures

Regularly brushing and flossing will help to keep teeth adequately clean. Emptying a capsule of powdered goldenseal on a moistened soft bristle toothbrush and

brushing the teeth and gum with it, will reduce gingivitis. Flushing the mouth with Listerine antiseptic also helps. Brushing the gums with powdered white oak bark or rinsing the mouth good with black or green tea will help to prevent loose teeth.

Foods and Nutrients

Vitamin A (25,000 I.U.), vitamin C with bioflavonoids (3,500 mg.), calcium (800 mg.), magnesium (1,200 mg.) and phosphorus (1,000 mg.) are useful for protecting both teeth and gums against infection.

Soft foods that don't require much chewing and sugary foods that stick to the teeth, contribute much towards gum disease as well as soft drinks and colas. Foods such as apples, celery or carrot sticks, nuts, seeds, corn chips and whole grain breads and cereals are good items to snack on.

HALITOSIS

See under BAD BREATH for more information on this.

HANGOVER

Symptoms

A hangover usually comes the next morning following a late night of excessive consumption of alcohol. Alcohol causes dilatation of the blood vessels within the skull and face, resulting in a pounding headache and flushed features hours later.

Relief Measures/Foods and Nutrients

Eating some bread, doughnuts or pasta before retiring will help to absorb some of the alcohol from the bloodstream. Drinking hot coffee, black or green tea, or herbal teas such as chamomile or catnip will help the headache to diminish. So will taking a hot shower followed by a quick cold one.

Brewer's yeast (1 tsp.) and vitamin C (3,500 mg.) and the bioflavonoid rutin (500 mg.) will help, too.

HAY FEVER

Symptoms

Hay fever (also called allergic rhinitis) affects the mucous membranes of the nose, eyes, and air passages. Dust, pollen, feathers, and animal hair are often the cause; however allergies could also be the underlying cause. Symptoms include itchy eyes, watery discharge from the nose and eyes, sneezing, and nervous irritability.

Relief Measures

A periodic cleansing fast is helpful for the body. Usually done on a weekend when physical activity and stress can be held to a minimum, it consists of eating mild foods (avoiding starches, animal protein, alcohol, sweets, and caffeine) such as clear soups or broths and gruel (cooked watery cereal) as well as drinking plenty of fruit and vegetable juices. All of these fluid foods have a wonderful flushing action on the system and can help to remove accumulated poisons from the body.

Wearing a protective mask over the mouth and nose in the Spring and early Fall when pollen and dust are the most prevalent, will help to reduce symptoms somewhat. Also drinking plenty of *hot* black or green tea during these periods seems to be of benefit as well, since their high tannic acid contents will reduce watery discharges from the eyes and nose.

Foods and Nutrients

The authors have discovered that simply by omitting sugar and sweet foods entirely from the diet or as much as possible, will curtail by at least 50% or better the symptoms common to hay fever sufferers. Dairy products and especially ice cream, pastries, soft drinks and colas should be avoided, too.

Regular supplementation should include Kyolic liquid garlic extract (4 capsules), vitamin A (50,000 I.U. fish oil and 50,000 I.U. beta-carotene), brewer's yeast (1 tsp.), pantothenic acid (300 mg.), vitamin C with bioflavonoids (5,000 mg.), extra rutin bioflavonoid (750 mg.), and Kyo-Green (1 glass) on a daily basis. (See Appendix under Wakunaga for Kyolic products.)

HEADACHE

Symptoms

A headache is a pain or ache in any portion of the head.

It's a symptom rather than a disease in itself. Most commonly, headaches fall into 1 of 3 categories: tension headaches, due to a contraction of the neck, scalp, or forehead muscles; vascular headaches, produced by uneven dilation rates of the blood vessels in the brain; and sinus headaches, caused by inflamed mucous membranes of the nose. Sinus headaches are often attributed to changes in the weather, the onset of menstruation, or a bad head cold.

There are many possible causes for a headache. Food allergies can be one of them. Another can be diseases of the eyes, nose, or throat. A trauma to the head, an injury to the neck (such as whiplash), misalignment of the spinal vertebrae, misalignment of the jaw, a bad tooth, perfume, hypoglycemia, vitamin or mineral deficiencies, "crash" diets, anger or frustration, loud sounds, and bright lights are other possibilities.

A rule of thumb to remember is this: If your headache persists for any *great* length of time and fails to respond to remedial treatments, by all means see a doctor as soon as you can! It could be something serious or even life-threatening!

Relief Measures

Lucy W. of Ventura, California is an executive secretary for the CEO of a large insurance firm located there. The many demands made upon her time and the numerous responsiblities in her charge, are enough to give anyone a headache. Or at least that's what she told one of the authors a year ago at a health convention in Los Angeles. She herself had suffered from recurring headaches because of the stressful office environment in which she has to work for a decent living.

But Lucy got smart and did something about her problem. Here's the program she devised for herself which she freely shared with one of the authors. "First thing, I do," she said, "when I get off of work is to go some place where the area is pretty good and do some deep breathing exercises, bending, and a little vigorous walking. I've found that this really eases the pounding sensations inside my head quite a bit.

"Next thing I'll do when I get home is to soak in a tub of *hot* water filled with Epsom salts. I add about 3 tablespoonfuls to half a tub of water. Sometimes I'll put in ten drops of peppermint oil. You talk about a nice way to relax and unwind. Listen! this *is* the cat's meow when it comes to getting rid of tension headaches!

"After I towel myself off good, then I'll spend about ten minutes going over my body with a luffa sponge. It really gets the circulation going like mad, and gives your whole body a healthy tingling feeling, too. Once in awhile I'll have my boyfriend massage my legs and back for me. But I'll usually spend a few minutes on the floor in a squatting position and rub the soles of my feet. I'll then do the same thing to each of my palms. I've found that massaging those key pressure points really gets the nerves relaxed."

Foods and Nutrients

Lucy drinks a cup of warm chamomile or catnip tea right after her tub soaking. "It helps me to unwind quite nicely," she adds. "I also take Schiff B-complex vitamins (4 tablets daily). I use some of the Kyo-Dophilus (4 capsules daily with meals) that I get from Mrs. Gooch's (a local chain of health food stores in southern California). I also take iron (35 mg.) and magnesium (1,200) supplements as well."

HEART ATTACK

Symptoms

When the coronary arteries that supply the heart with oxygen thicken, harden and narrow, the heart is deprived of needed oxygen. This deprivation of oxygen often results in chest pain, called angina pectoris. When damage to the heart muscle is incurred, the person suffers a heart attack. And since the coronary arteries cannot provide the heart with sufficient oxygen, doctors usually refer to a heart attack as a "coronary."

Typical symptoms of an impending coronary include chest pains radiating out to the left arms, the neck or jaw, or the area between the shoulder blades; heavy, substernal pressure that feels as if the chest is being squeezed; shortness of breath; sweating; nausea; and vomiting.

Relief Measures

Plenty of exercise is imperative. Walking, jogging,,climbing, swimming, rope jumping, horseback riding, bicycling, dancing, playing tennis, or bouncing on a mini-trampoline are the best forms of aerobic exercise to pursue.

Mental and emotional stresses should be avoided or else held to an absolute minimum. Medical research has amply demonstrated that negative thoughts and bad feelings can really injure the heart if not quickly corrected.

Those who smoke should stop this filthy habit once and for all! And those who don't but are around smokers should avoid second-hand smoke by asking the others to please put out their cigarettes. This type of smoke can hurt the heart a lot!

Hawthorn berries make a wonderful heart rejuvenant. At least 4 capsules a day should be taken with meals. Add to this 2 capsules of cayenne pepper to improve blood circulation.

Foods and Nutrients

Intake of red meat should be greatly minimized. If poultry has to be consumed, it should be done so on an infrequent basis and then only if the skin has been removed. Pork products should be avoided at all costs, since they are high in fat as well as being an inferior meat. Wild game, lamb, veal, chevon (young goat), and rabbit are preferable for those who must have some red meat.

Fish is the most ideal meat to consume. Either salt-water or fresh-water will suffice, just so long as it has fins and scales. Any other kind of seafood should be avoided, because the meat is inferior, possibly contaminated, and not fit for the body to properly utilize for energy needs. (Readers are encouraged to consult Leviticus 11:9-12 on this matter.) Such fish ought to be boiled, steamed or baked rather than fried, deep-fried or broiled.

Foods high in lecithin should be consumed more often. These include raw seeds and nuts, whole grains, and unrefined vegetable oils (olive, sunflower, sesame). Lecithin can also be taken in liquid or granules (1 tbsp. daily).

Leafy green, red, orange and yellow vegetables are high in calcium, iron and beta-carotene. Romaine lettuce, parsley, zucchini, tomatoes, carrots, pumpkin and squash are good to eat and high in these important nutrients for the heart.

Additional supplementation should include: Kyolic garlic (4 capsules daily), vitamin C (3,500 mg.), magnesium (1,200 mg.), niacin (150 mg.), vitamin B-6 (100 mg.), vitamin E (800 I.U.), Kelp (3 tablets), and black strap molasses (1 tsp.). These need to be taken on a fairly consistent basis for a healthy heart.

HEARTBURN

Symptoms

Heartburn is a burning sensation in the stomach. It often occurs when hydrochloric acid, which is used by the stomach for digestive purposes, backs up into the esophagus. It can be caused by excessive consumption of spicy or fatty and fried foods, alcohol, oranges, grapefruits, lemons, limes, chocolate, catsup, mustard, pickles, mayonnaise, salsa, and potato chips. Problems like hiatal hernia, peptic ulcers, gallbladder disorders, stress, allergies and enzyme deficiency can also contribute to it. Not chewing your food properly and eating in a hurry definitely will cause heartburn!

Relief Measures

Chuck Stewart from Minneapolis is a computer salesman. He has a quota to meet every month, and unfortunately spends more of his time to meet it than to give proper attention to his health. He eats "on the run" as he describes it, and jokingly claims to "eat everything and anything that isn't moving or wiggling on my plate." The result is classic heartburn every time!

But Chuck discovered that by taking two capsules of Wakunaga's Kyo-Dophilus and one capsule each of powdered alfalfa and comfrey, "makes the heartburn go away just like that" (at the same time snapping his fingers in mid-air for emphasis).

Foods and Nutrients

Slowly sipping some 7-Up, Perrier water or apple cider vinegar will also make heartburn disappear very quickly. So too will warm catnip, peppermint or chamomile teas. Antacids should be avoided since they contain aluminum and sodium which can aggravate high blood pressure and cause Alzheimer's disease.

HEMORRHAGING

See under BLEEDING for more information on this.

HEMORRHOIDS

Symptoms

Hemorrhoids or piles are ruptured or distended veins located around the anus. The most common cause of hemorrhoids is strain on the abdominal muscles due to factors such as heavy or improper lifting, pregnancy, overweight, constipation, or a sedentary lifestyle. The flow of blood through the vessels of the anus is especially sensitive to the pressure and strain of pregnancy and constipation. The blood collects in these vessels and the pressure against the weakest sections causes tiny bulges or piles. They may itch, tear, and bleed, causing pain.

Relief Measures

One of the authors has a younger brother who has been bothered with hemorrhoids for years. He finds relief every night before retiring by applying a little Vaseline petroleum jelly to his hemorrhoids with his fingers, after which his hands are thoroughly washed with soap and water. Another person one of the authors knows, uses witch hazel tincture instead, which he claims shrinks them. He saturates several cotton balls with the liquid and dabs it on that way. A woman we know has found relief by applying vitamin E oil to her piles.

Foods and Nutrients

Fiber is the key here to clearing them up. Whole grain cereals and breads, and raw vegetable salads and some fruits are necessary. Daily walking is a must. Keeping the rectum clean after every bowel movement is advisable. Vitamin A (25,000 I.U.), B-6 (100 mg.), C (3,500 mg.) and calcium (600 mg.) also help.

HEPATITIS

Symptoms

Hepatitis is an inflammation of the liver caused by infection or poisons. It starts with flulike symptoms of fever, weakness, drowsiness, abdominal discomfort, and headache, possibly accompanied by jaundice. Soon extreme fatigue and loss of appetite set in. The liver is unable to eliminate the toxins, allowing them to build up in the system; and it cannot store and process certain nutrients that are vital for the body.

There are two types of viral hepatitis: infectious hepatitis (the A and non A kinds, and non B type) is caused by the ingestion of contaminated shellfish, polluted water, the inhalation of airborne germs from infected persons, or by injections, or body secretions. Serum hepatitis, the second type (hepatitis B) is far more serious and can be deadly. It's contracted from contaminated blood transfusions, injections using unsterilized needles, or from contaminated chemicals taken into the system by injection.

Relief Measures

Fresh green juice enemas should be administered at least 5 times a week. Best vegetables for this are celery, endive, and parsley. Some Kyolic liquid aged-garlic extract can be added (2 tablespoonfuls per enema).

Hot peppermint oil packs should be placed over the liver and gallbladder, and changed when they become cool. With a pair of ice tongs, immerse a clean wash cloth in boiling water. On a flat cookie sheet, remove excess water with the aid of a rolling pin. Fold wash cloth in half and apply several drops of concentrated peppermint oil over a wide area of the side that will go face *down* on the skin. Place into position over the liver and cover with a heavy hand towel to retain the heat longer.

Foods and Nutrients

Tom Allen (not his real name) is a high-powered Houston divorce lawyer. Once he was in the border town of Brownsville to the south representing a client in a particularly nasty custody battle for, of all things, *not* the kids but the couple's pair of prize show poodles! Anyway, while eating in a Mexican restaurant, he contracted you-know-what and in a week's time became "as sick as a yellow hound dog," as he aptly described it for one of us.

A local nutritionist whom his wife knew quite well, put Tom on the following supplement program. Within just six weeks, he was well and recovered enough to tackle another big divorce case with his usual speed and flamboyant style! Every day he took these things: Thisilyn (4 capsules), Wakunaga's Kyolic 102 Formula (4 capsules), Wakunaga's liquid Kyolic with B-1 and B-l2 (6 capsules), goldenseal root (4 capsules), Kyo-Green (2 glasses every day with meals), an evening primrose oil (4 capsules), vitamin A (75,000 I.U.), beet root (1 tsp. in some water or juice), iron (25 mg.), vitamin C (10,000 mg.), and brewer's yeast (1 tbsp. every morning in milk).

HERNIA

Symptoms

A hernia or rupture is a bulge of the abdominal contents, usually a loop of intestines, through a weak spot in the muscular wall. It occurs more frequently in males than it does in females. Fairly common from birth to old age, less in the middle years. Caused primarily by a weak part in the muscle wall itself, especially where the testis descends in the man. Secondary causes can be attributed to conditions that raise the abdominal pressure and put a strain on that weak place: chronic coughing, straining during a bowel movement, heavy manual labor, pregnancy, abdominal tumors. Or a hernia can be due to conditions that weaken the abdominal wall: old age, prolonged stays in bed due to illness or laziness, and lack of regular exercise.

Such a hernia can be readily identified by a lump under the pubic hair by the groin on one or both sides. Coughing and straining make it larger, but it may disappear on lying down. Also there is usually pain in the groin on exertion, and sometimes in the testicle. There tends to be a dragging sensation or heavy feeling if the hernia is very big.

Relief Measures

Surgery, of course, is the first sensible elective that most men choose. But for some there are other satisfactory options which can at least help to manage the situation for many years with reasonable success, though not cure it. One of the authors' 78-year-old father has worn not one but two appliances (rupture belts) for close to 50 years now and gotten along very nicely without having any operations on them. Of course, we certainly don't recommend this procedure for everybody. But at least in the case of those who don't want surgery, this is another alternative available.

Foods and Nutrients

Comfrey root or slippery elm bark teas (2 cups of either each day) should help to some extent in the knitting process of torn muscle tissue if taken early enough right after the hernia has occurred. Calcium (600 mg.), magnesium (1,200 mg.), manganese (50 mg.), zinc (25 mg. three times daily), vitamin B-6 (100 mg.) and vitamin E (800 I.U.) help expedite the healing process after surgery or may assist in the knitting together of injured tissue within the body.

HERPES

Symptoms

Herpes is one of the oldest viruses known to man. It's been around since the time of the pharoahs and probably even longer, possibly even dating back to the dinosaur era millions of aeons ago. *Advanced Ophthalmology Journal* (38:17) pointed out some years ago (1979) that there were more than 60 types of this virus known to infect over 30 different vertebrates. But just four kinds infect the human race: herpes simplex (Type I), genital herpes (Type II), herpes zoster (shingles), and the Epstein Barr Virus (EBV).

Herpes is simply recognized by the presence of cold sores around the corners of the mouth and lips and inside the mouth, as well as skin eruptions elsewhere on the body. It can cause blindness if it gets into the cornea of the eye and cause serious neurological damage in the form of encephalitis if it gets into the brain.

Genital herpes is sexually transmitted and is the most widespread of the four. It can range in acuteness from a silent infection to a very serious inflammation of the liver including fever, severe brain damage, and stillbirths. Once it enters the body, it never leaves. It can only be kept under control so that it won't recur later on. Fluid-filled blisters and open sores around, on and inside the reproductive organs of both men and women is the most evident sign of its presence. Also low-grade fevers and muscular aches and pains are typically experienced by both sexes.

Herpes zoster occurs in young children as chicken pox and in elderly people as shingles. It usually breaks out on the surface of the belly just beneath the ribs leading over to the navel, but can appear anywhere else on the body if it so chooses. An attack of shingles is usually preceded by 3-4 days of intense pain in the affected area. Then numerous and very painful and itchy blisters appear, lasting upwards for one to two weeks or more. They eventually become crusty scabs and in time, drop off. If left unattended, shingles can be fatal.

The Epstein-Barr Virus is usually linked with malignant lymphoma, a solid cancer tumor that occurs most often in the lymph nodes, neck, face, spleen, ovaries, and abdomen.

One thing which can be said about all four herpes viruses is this: they can certainly initiate the cancer process in many people if immediate measures aren't taken to control them. Over 20 years ago, Dr. Fred Rapp wrote a landmark article in *Advances in Cancer Research* (19:265-66, 1974) entitled, "Herpes viruses and Cancer" in which he explored the real possibilities of this very thing at some length.

Relief Measures

Herbal treatments should include a full complement of the following high-powered antibiotic herbs: Kyolic garlic (6 capsules daily), echinacea (4 capsules daily), myrrh gum (4 capsules daily), goldenseal root (4 capsules daily), and red clover tea (2 cups daily). Also pau d'arco is helpful as well.

To relieve swelling and pain, apply ice packs. To relieve itching and pain apply fluid extracts of hyssop or witch hazel tincture. Use a small hand-held hairdryer to dry the skin off with.

Get plenty of rest. At least 8 hours is recommended. Try very hard to avoid stress. Don't let yourself become upset by things. Drink catnip or chamomile teas to keep your system relaxed, since Types I & II and the herpes zoster virus like to hide out in the ganglion nerves of our bodies. Too much mental and emotional stress will soon have them breaking out of their hibernation periods.

Foods and Nutrients

A full supplement program should include all of the following: Vitamin A (75,000 I.U. daily), vitamin C (10,000 mg.), the bioflavonoid rutin (150 mg.), L-Lysine (750 mg.), zinc (100 mg.), vitamin E (800

I.U.), magnesium (1,200 mg.), phosphorus (800 mg.), and vitamin D (400 I.U.).

Junk food should be avoided by all means. This includes abstaining from alcoholic beverages, colas, soft drinks, coffee, fried and deep-fried foods, and anything with white sugar or natural sugars in it. This can range from the obvious no-no's like Twinkies to less obvious things like. figs and dates .

Dairy products and citrus fruits and juices should be held to an absolute minimum while the herpes viruses are active, since they, like all of the other foods above, create an acid condition within the blood which is favorable to these viruses. Foods high in mineral salts, which includes most organic vegetables, should be liberally consumed, since they create an alkaline environment which the herpes family doesn't like.

HIATAL HERNIA

Symptoms

Hiatal hernia is a condition which arises when an opening or hole occurs in the diaphragm muscles through which the stomach pushes, or herniates. Ulcers generally accompany this malady. The heartburn is due to the leakage of stomach acid back into the lower esophagus. Symptoms include heartburn and belching. Often the acid comes up into the throat, causing a burning sensation, and there is great discomfort behind the breastbone. About 50% of the population over 40 suffers from this.

Relief Measures

George W. is an engineer for the railroad. For some time had been suffering from an unexplained burning in the back of his throat, which he described to one of the authors as being "like I'd drunk battery acid or something similar."

He was advised to drink one full cup of *warm* marshmallow root tea or fenugreek seed tea with every meal. He soon discovered that his problem cleared up and remained that way as long as he kept drinking his tea three times a day.

Foods and Nutrients

Alice N. is 49 and is a telephone switchboard operator. She, too, suffered from constant heartburn and belching, which her doctor diagnosed as being a hiatal hernia. She started drinking papaya juice with every meal, which she reconstituted from the pulpy concentrate she bought in a health food store, according to the directions on the bottle label. After this, she was no longer troubled with her problem. She said that mango juice works very well, too. Some have even tried aloe vera juice (1/2 cup with each meal) with good success.

HICCUPS

Symptoms

Hiccups is a disturbance in the normal synchronization between the movements of the lid that shuts off the airways during swallowing, and the diaphragm (the muscular sheet between chest and abdomen that is used in breathing). It is this diaphragm which gets out of step.

Relief Measures

Most hiccups go away within an hour or so after they occur. Tradition maneuvers to stop the spasm and make the diaphragm function properly include sipping warm water, sucking on a cube of sugar, holding the breath, or doing deep breathing exercises. Some people try breathing into a paper bag to produce air with a high concentration of carbon dioxide, which stimulates the breathing easier. One of the authors has tried this himself and knows that it works. Hiccups due to indigestion can be quickly remedied by stirring one teaspoonful of Arm & Hammer Baking Soda into a glass of warm water and sipping it slowly. Hiccups isn't serious in itself, but consult a physician if it persists for more than 3 hours.

HIVES

Symptoms

Hives or urticaria are weals with unendurable itching that appear suddenly for no reason at all and may last for hours or even days on end. Hives is usually a manifestation of special sensitivity to something or someone. Some allergies may trigger hives. Insect and plant stings, certain foods (like chocolate), some drugs and serum injections (aspirin and penicillin are common offenders), and mental and emotional traumas can raise weals in a hurry.

Relief Measures

Detoxifying the body and relaxing the mind are the two best approaches to this problem. Burdock, yellow dock, sarsaparilla, or red clover teas are good for this. Meditation is good for emptying the mind, and cups of *warm* catnip or chamomile tea do a nice job of relaxing the nerves.

Foods and Nutrients

High-potency B-complex (6 tablets daily), magnesium (2,000 mg.), liquid lecithin (1 tsp. daily), and vitamin E oil (1,200 I.U.) are useful internally, while externally, tincture of witch hazel, or any creams or salves with panthothenic acid, PABA, zinc or calendula in them will relieve the itching considerably if left on overnight.

HOARSENESS

Symptoms

A condition arising in the extreme back of the throat wherein the pharynx, soft palate and tonsils (if intact) become inflamed to the extent that normal loss of tone voice is evident and the victim can barely manage to speak in audible whispers, and then only with considerable difficulty.

This may be due to excessive use of one's voice because of present occupation (school teacher, professional singer, auctioneer, stockbroker, clergyman) or due to a viral infection in the back of the throat.

Relief Measures

Years ago, the famous Italian opera singer of the 1920's, Enrico Caruso (often called "the Great Caruso" because of his majestic voice), was asked by a reporter what he did to keep his throat in good shape. He replied that before every performance he gave and immediately after it was over, he would gargle with and slowly sip a warm glass of port wine or burgundy into which he had squeezed the juice of half a lemon and added 1/2 teaspoon of white sugar. One of the authors of this book, who uses his voice a lot in lecturing and teaching, has tried this for himself and can swear to its success just like Caruso did.

Foods and Nutrients

Here are two other things which may be helpful. Slowly suck on a zinc lozenge or piece of horehound candy for awhile. Another method is to drop some 40% bee proposal tincture in the bottom of the throat with the head tilted backwards.

HOOKWORM

Symptoms

Hookworm infestation caused by Necator Americanus or Ancylostoma Duodenale was once a widely distributed disorder in the southeastern United States. But for many decades it was effectively controlled by simple sanitary measures and the recognition of the common method of infection by walking barefoot in contaminated soil. Now, however, because of the growing economic plight affecting millions of America's poor and unemployed in many of her inner cities, hookworm is making a rapid comeback, particularly among young children.

Larval forms pierce the skin and migrate to the lung or liver and intestinal tract if swallowed. The chief manifestations are a profound anemia produced by blood sucking and some symptoms similar to jaundice (see under JAUNDICE for a more complete description).

Relief Measures/Foods and Nutrients

Rosa B. is Hispanic and lives in Jamaica, New York in a crowded tenement with her four children and five other people. Her seven-year-old son Alvarez exhibited a change in his skin color and breathing rhythm, heart palpitations, becoming easily tired, and given to frequent periods of slumber. A doctor at a neighborhood clinic diagnosed the problem as being hookworm.

Rosa consulted her aged grandmother who was well acquainted with herbs. She suggested giving the child some boiled garlic and onion soup in small amounts, some wormwood tea (only 1/4 cup twice daily), and a little hot sauce on some corn chips. In three days, the kid was up and about being his usual energetic self again.

HOT FLASHES

Symptoms

Hot flashes are a part of the constitutional upset which sometimes accompanies the menopause period of a woman's life when her periods cease and major glandular changes occur. They are comparable to the easy blushing of a sixteen-year-old girl: reddening of the face and neck, accompanied by sweating, and followed by a cold shiver, brought on by nervousness, and a hot atmosphere, but sometimes occurs in bed at night.

Accompanying symptoms include headaches, dizzy spells, moodiness, including depression and crying without much reason, an inability to concentrate, grumpiness, loneliness, an increase in appetite, intestinal gas, constipation, irregular periods, etc.

Relief Measures/Food and Nutrients

A retired nurse one of the authors casually knows, who lives in Seattle, Washington, encountered her own hot flashes when she reached menopause. But being quite nutritionally-minded, she did some things about it and soon alleviated her condition entirely.

For one thing she omitted all sugary foods from her diet. This included anything with a high amount of sugar in it, be it processed or natural foods. Besides pie and ice cream, she also omitted carrot, apple, and citrus juices from her diet as well. Secondly, she reduced her intake of red meat and chicken, substituting soy protein foods, nuts, and legumes instead. Thirdly, she omitted coffee, tea, alcohol, colas and soft drinks. Fourthly, she omitted catsup, mustard, pickles, mayonnaise, fried and deep-fried foods.

She took brewer's yeast (1 tsp.), lecithin (1 tsp.), vitamin E oil (800 mg.), calcium, iron and zinc every day with her meals.

HYPERACIDITY

Symptoms

Hyperacidity is a condition in which the stomach secretes an abnormally high degree of gastric juice. Belching, heartburn, intestinal discomfort and gas are the most common symptoms.

Relief Measures/Foods and Nutrients

A guy named "Bubba" that one of the authors knows, lives in Galveston, Texas. He is a real, honest-to-goodness Southern "redneck," and likes his chili dogs heavy with jalepeños and the beer to wash them down with light and ice-cold. Considering this as being typical of his diet, it's no wonder he suffers from repeated hyperacidity.

But a local chiropractor whom Bubba visits from time to time to get an adjustment, suggested that he start drinking some peppermint tea whenever it seems as if his gut were about to "boil over" with an excess production of hydrochloric acid.

He made himself some tea by bringing a quart of water to a boil, then turning the heat off and adding two table-spoonfuls of dried peppermint leaves. He covered the pot with a lid and let the brew steep for half-an-hour before straining and drinking one cup with each meal.

Bubba now claims that he can still "eat anything I like" but not have to suffer with the miseries previously associated with his problem. While this may be fine, it isn't always practical. Peppermint tea may have

cleared up one of his aggravations, but if he continues his indiscrimate dietary pattern, other problems are sure to crop up in the course of time. It seems some people never learn.

HYPERACTIVITY

Symptoms

Hyperactivity is considered by most doctors to be a disorder of certain mechanisms in the central nervous system, particularly in children, although it can occur in adults as well. One of the authors who resides in Portland, Oregon, has been a pediatrician for a number of years, during which time he has probably seen over 10,000 children, many of whom were hyperactive. From all of these cases, he has compiled a list of 20 different symptoms which easily characterize a hyperactive kid (and a hyperactive adult for that matter, too).

1. Easily stimulated in crowds or with stress.

2. Motor-driven, constantly moving, walked by ten months.

3. Responds to stimuli in a physical way; seems to touch everything.

4. Fidgeting, wiggling, foot-tapping.

5. Climbs, daredevil, accident-prone.

6. Attention deficit disorder (which also happens to be the new-fangled medical term for hyperactivity).

7. Exuberant, impatient, cannot wait his or her turn.

8. Demands nearly always met.

9. Can only attend to one command at a time.

10. No self-control, waits until last minute to urinate.

11. Ticklish, overreacts to pain, touch, heat, cold.

12. Laughs and cries easily.

13. Talks, interrupts, class clown.

14. Cheerful pest.

15. Distractible, unfinished work, jumps from one thing to another.

16. Unaware of time of day or household rhythm.

17. Throws, breaks things, toys taken apart or destroyed.

18. Bites or picks nails, twists hair, bangs head.

19. Tics, twitches, bed-rocking, sucks thumb or pacifier often.

20. Chews on clothes, blankets, buttons, and furniture.

Relief Measures

The full complement of B vitamins is certainly the first line of defense against this.

A high-potency B-complex (2 tablets daily) is suggested. The child may require extra B-6 and niacin as well, but should be administered under a doctor's supervision. Magnesium is usually lacking in adequate amounts in hyperactive kids, so the authors recommend at leat 800-1,200 mg. per day. Some vitamin E (600 I.U.) is useful too.

If you have one of those little Jekyll-and-Hyde hyperactive types as a child or grandchild, who manifests occasional flashes of normal cuteness in between frequent bouts of nasty behavior, take heart because there's hope! Just put the kid on a no-sugar, no-white-flour, no-milk, no-artificial flavors or colors routine for a couple of weeks. You'll be totally amazed at the B-I-G difference this makes! At the same time give the kid an amino acid complex along with a children's chewable vitamin C; they seem to work great together.

HYPERTENSION

Symptoms

Hypertension is an abnormal elevation of blood pressure. While the cause is still unknown, this malady frequently accompanies arteriosclerosis or kidney disease. Blood pressure is the force exerted by the blood against the walls of the blood vessels. The pressure can temporarily rise after physical activity or emotional tension but after a period of relaxation will return to normal. An abnormal condition arises when the pressure does not return to normal and remains high.

Symptoms of hypertension may be nonexistent, or they may include headache, nervousness, insomnia, nosebleeds, blurred vision, edema, shortness of breath, dizziness, ringing in the ears, and eventually hemorrhaging in the eyes.

Relief Measures

Exercise is essential in preventing high blood pressure since it keeps the circulatory system healthy. Walking is the very best thing to do for this—at least two miles a day is recommended. Striving for internal peace and a more tranquil environment are also absolutely essential. Anger and noise, just like sodium, can really aggravate hypertension.

Ed Weber of Pasadena, California had a blood pressure reading of 230 over 120. He started taking Wakunaga's Kyolic EPA garlic (1 capsule three times daily). In just ten days, after another blood pressure check, his reading was 190/115.

Foods and Nutrients

One glass of Wakunaga's Kyo-Green each day, along with magnesium (2,000 mg.) and calcium (600 mg.) helps to control hypertension.

HYPERTHYROIDISM

Symptoms

Hyperthyroidism is a condition in which the thyroid gland produces too much hormone, resulting in an overactive metabolism. It's also called Graves' disease, which former U.S. President George Bush and his wife, Barbara have and control with prescription medication.

Typical symptoms include dry skin, stiff muscles and cramps, hair loss, elevated cholesterol, abnormal menstrual periods, infertility, headache and dizziness, slowed heart rate, and a hoarse voice, reported the January, 1991 issue of *Pharmacy Times* (57:43).

Relief Measures

Those who suffer from this should be wary of rushing into surgery or submitting to radioactive iodine (1-131), since there the adverse side effects from both can be much worse than the symptoms themselves are.

Sulphur is the key here to suppressing overproduction of thyroid hormone. Herbs high in sulphur content should be consumed regularly, such as garlic and onions.

Foods and Nutrients

Other foods rich in sulphur include: cabbage, kale, kohlrabi, brussel sprouts, cauliflower, mustard greens, horseradish, and spinach. Peaches, pears, soybeans, turnips, and rutabagas are also helpful.

Dairy products should be avoided for up to 3 months, as well as coffee, tea, soft drinks, and anything containing nicotine.

Brewer's yeast (1 tbsp. daily), a multivitamin-mineral supplement (4 tablets daily), vitamin C (3, 500 mg.) and essential fatty acids work well together here.

HYPOGLYCEMIA

(See also **BLOOD SUGAR PROBLEMS**)

Symptoms

Hypoglycemia is a health condition which has puzzled doctors for over a hundred years. Hypoglycemia can mimic many different diseases; in decades past, many hypoglycemics were committed to insane asylums because doctors thought they were lunatics. The standard treatments for a long time in such dark and dreary places were electric shock therapy, prescription medications, and sometimes prefrontal lobotomies (an extant surgical procedure in which one or more nerve tracts in the front portion of the brain were severed to reduce hysteria and pain).

An overproduction of insulin by the pancreas results in low blood sugar or hypoglycemia. Poor diet and badly managed stress are the key factors here responsible for such a problem. The late chain-smoking but very knowledgeable nutritionist and radio talk show host, Dr. Canton Fredericks was an expert on this disease. With the cooperation of several New York City physicians who treated thousands of cases of hypoglycemia each year, he made a list of those particular symptoms of which such patients complained the most. They are ranked below according to their frequency of occurence:

Nervousness	94%
Irritability	89%
Exhaustion	87%

Faintness, dizziness, tremor, cold sweats, weak spells	86%
Depression	77%
Vertigo, dizziness	73%
Drowsiness	72%
Headaches	71%
Digestive disturbances	69%
Forgetfulness	67%
Insomnia (awakening and inability to return to sleep)	62%
Constant worrying, unprovoked anxieties	62%
Mental confusion	57%
Internal trembling	57%
Palpitation of heart, rapid pulse	54%
Muscle pains	53%
Numbness	51%
Indecisiveness	50%
Unsocial, asocial, antisocial behavior	47%
Crying spells	46%
Lack of sex drive (females)	44%
Allergies	43%

Lack of coordination	43%
Leg cramps	43%
Lack of concentration	42%
Blurred vision	40%
Twitching and jerking of muscles	40%
Itching and crawling sensations on the skin	39%
Gasping for breath	37%
Smothering spells	34%
Staggering	34%
Sighing and yawning	30%
Impotence (males)	29%
Unconsciousness	27%
Night terrors, nightmares	27%
Rheumatoid arthritis	24%
Phobias, fears	23%
Neurodermatitis	21%
Suicidal intent	20%
Nervous breakdown	17%
Convulsions	2%

Relief Measures

A lot can be written about ways to treat this blood sugar disorder. But a summary of the most important things will be mentioned here.

The first is to become more familiar with the disease itself. This is achieved by talking to those who have the problem already and find out what they're doing about it, talking with doctors who treat this condition and learning what they may recommend for it, and also reading various books about hypoglycemia.

The second thing is to become very aware that any food with sugar in it is liable to spell disaster for a hypoglycemic's sense of balance and well-being. We recommend William Duffy's book, *Sugar Blues* as an introduction to this. Another book is *Psychodietetics: Food as the Key to Emotional Health* by by Arline Brecher and Drs. Emmanueal Cheraskin and W. M. Ringsdorf. And Carlton Fredericks' own book, *Eating Right For You* should also be added to the list as well. Most of these titles were published a few decades ago, but can probably be found at your local library.

The third thing is to stay away from specific foods that plunge blood sugar levels like crazy. They are garlic and onions, cayenne pepper, pau d'arco, and goldenseal. There is some clinical evidence in the medical literature to support this claim for the first four herbs, and plenty of anecdotal proof for the latter. Now all five herbs are excellent for diabetics, but should be avoided by those suffering from low-blood sugar. (An exception to the rule would be using aged garlic extract. Benjamin Lau, M.D., Ph.D. of

Loma Linda Medical School in Loma Linda, Calif. informed one of the authors awhile back that his own research with Kyolic aged-garlic extract showed that there was no adverse reactions to this supplement in hypoglycemics. There can be, however, with regular raw garlic or other garlic preparations.)

Various types of stress is a fourth indicator to familiarize yourself with. Cold weather is harder on hypoglycemics than warm weather is. Loud or long talking can also wear down the systems of hypoglycemics. Anger and frustration only plunge their blood sugar levels lower and worsen their conditions.

Fifthly, those with hypoglycemia should avoid the traditional three big meals of the day, and instead opt for seven or eight smaller ones divided up in 2-3 hour segments throughout the waking hours of each day. Eating a small snack before bedtime also seems to help many of them rest better. In addition, the diet should be frequently rotated so that food allergies don't develop. Carefully chewing the food and enjoying each meal in tranquil surroundings are also very important.

Foods and Nutrients

A high-fiber diet will help to stabilize the blood sugar swings. During a low blood sugar reaction, combine fiber with a protein food (i.e., bran or rice crackers with raw cheese or almond butter). Instead of eating applesauce, choose a whole apple. The fiber in the apple will act as a braking mechanism in slowing down the absorption of the fructose in it, thereby preventing fluctuations in blood sugar levels. Add a glass of fruit juice for a rapid rise in the blood sugar if necessary. Fiber alone (found in unsalted, unbuttered popcorn, oat bran, rice bran, crackers, and guar gum) will slow down a hypoglycemic reaction. Fiber should be consumed 30 minutes before meals to avoid a reaction. A glass of Wakunaga's Kyo-Green in between meals will further stabilize the blood sugar. (See Appendix under Wakunaga.)

Supplements are an important part of any prudent treatment program for hypoglycemia. Without them, only marginal success can be achieved, even with an improved diet. But by including them in an overall plan, hypoglycemia can be safely and easily managed. While we could mention a lot of them here, only seven of them will be mentioned here, ranked in order of their nutritional importance and suggested intakes:

chromium	300 mcg daily
manganese	50 mg. daily
zinc	50 mg. daily
vitamin B-1	100 mg. daily
vitamin B-S	
(pantothenic acid)	500 mg. daily
vitamin C	3,500 mg. daily
rutin	1,000 mg. daily

To show just how important a single vitamin can be in the health and well-being of an individual, we cite the obscure but fascinating experiment conducted many years ago by Dr. Wilder of the Mayo Clinic. He asked a group of his patients to eat a diet low in thiamin or vitamin B-l to permit researchers to study the personality disorders common to hypoglycemia that can originate with a degree of deficiency not severe enough to cause beriberi. The diet used in that famous experiment consisted of lean meat, cheese, skim milk, fruits and vegetables. It was supplemented with brewer's yeast, from which vitamin B-1 had been completely removed, plus vitamins A, C, and D. The food plan was deceptive in that it nearly approximated the reducing diet voluntarily consumed by millions of obese women who take no supplements with it and yet blame their irritability and nervousness on the frustrations of weight-loss menus. We present a condensed history of one of the volunteers in the experiment, whose reactions were typical of the group as a whole.

Prior to the experiment, "Ethel" (as we'll call her) had no obvious symptoms of hypoglycemia. She was appraised by the consulting psychiatrists as well adjusted, congenial, industrious, efficient, and vigorous. After two months on the deficient diet, Ethel worked slowly and negligently, followed instructions inaccurately and became forgetful, irritable, and quarrelsome. Her appetite flickered. Three months more and the doctor noted in his report: "Ethel wept and laughed alternately. She was critical of herself. She displayed apathy, confusion, and fatigue. She complained of indigestion and of numbness of the hands and feet." Two months later, she was unable to work because of dizziness and weakness. She described herself as feeling "helpless." She was confused and bewildered, and said decisions were difficult to make. Here the experimental diet was ended, and the missing vitamin intake supplied. "The improvement," the doctor's diary noted, "was gradual. Ethel still tired easily and was alternately cheerful and apathetic, sleeping poorly." At the end of four months of correct diet with two months of supplementation with thiamine, Ethel "became congenial, cooperative, and industrious. She no longer complained."

This case study demonstrates just how much difference the presence or absence of a single nutrient can make in the lives of ordinary individuals, not to mention hypoglycemics.

A final word of caution about the frequent use of fresh-made juices. There is a big advertizing campaign right now on late night television and in magazine ads for people to invest in various types of commercial juicers. These are fine in their place. But drinking too much fruit or vegetable juice *without* the benefit of the fiber sends way too much sugar too quickly into the system, which can by very detrimental to the health of those with hypoglycemia.

HYPOTHERMIA

Symptoms

Hypothermia is any unexpected and significant decrease in body temperature below the normal 98.6° F. (37° C.). Internal organs and extremities are affected the most. The most evident sign is a feeling of coldness even when the body may be well insulated with clothing at the time. Also lethargy, swollen hands and feet, and cold, clammy skin are other symptoms of it.

Relief Measures

A very gradual rewarming is called for lest gangrene set in somewhere. Preferably this ought to be done in a hospital environment so proper procedures can be followed.

Intake of cayenne pepper (6 capsules daily), grated horseradish root (1/2 tsp. twice daily in 1 glass of Kyo-Green) (see Appendix under Wakunaga), ginger root (4 capsules), beet root powder (1 tsp. twice daily in 6 fl. oz. of water), and red clover tea (1 cup warm tea twice daily with meals) all help to promote greater circulation. (See under **FROSTBITE** for additional suggestions.).

Foods and Nutrients

Supplements to be used are vitamin C (10, 000 mg.), rutin and hesperidin (300 mg. each), calcium (1,400 mg.), chromium (300 mcg.), copper (4 mg.), and zinc (25 mg.).

HYSTERECTOMY

Symptoms

This year about 650,00 American women will undergo a hysterectomy, or complete removal of the uterus. About 45% of them will be castrated, the medical term for removing the ovaries—a practice that still continues despite a growing body of evidence that shows it may do more harm than good.

Today, one American woman in three has had a hysterectomy by age 60. By 1995, the National Center for Health Statistics projects that about 783,000 such operations will be performed, mostly on women in their late thirties and forties. Hysterectomy right now is the second most frequent operation for women in the United States, outranked only by caesarean section.

The most dramatic consequences of hysterectomy occur when the ovaries are removed, depriving a woman of her natural supply of estrogen. One obvious result is instant menopause, including hot flashes and vaginal dryness. Other possible side-effects include:

- A vastly increased risk of bone-mass loss, often leading to osteoporosis.

- Depression related to estrogen deprivation (although evidence here is conflicting), in addition to psychological depression.

- An increased risk of heart disease—again, the evidence is inconclusive.

- Fatigue, insomnia, urinary tract problems, joint pain, headaches, and dizziness. Some of these ailments may be due to menopause induced by surgery.

- A lack of sexual interest and desire after surgery.

Relief Measures

No longer do women need to suffer the "unkindest cut of all." Recent advances in medicine now offer women better alternatives. One is a new minor surgical procedure called endometrial ablation. For several years Joan Petersil's menstrual periods were ruining her life. "I would have them sometimes for 18 days in a row," the 43-year-old legal secretary from Los Angeles said. Hormonal therapy and a D&C—a scraping of the uterus—failed to correct her problem. Petersil was facing a hysterectomy when her gynecologist, Phillip Brooks, told her about this alternative. She checked into L.A.'s Cedars-Sinai Medical Center and received general anesthesia. Then Dr. Brooks inserted an instrument about the size of a pen through her cervix and cauterized the inner lining of her uterus in less than 20 minutes. Petersil returned home that afternoon, and resumed work a few days later. She hasn't bled a drop since. "I'm an entirely new person," she joyfully exclaimed.

Dr. Vicki Georges Hufnagel, surgeon/medical director of the Center for Female Reconstructive Surgery in Los Angeles, offers women still another alternative. Author of the highly popular book, *No More Hysterectomies*, she has pioneered a unique way of saving the female reproductive organs instead of taking them out. All of her surgeries are videotaped and patients' familes are encouraged to watch the surgeries as they happen or else review them later on with her.

Foods and Nutrients

Before and after surgery, avoid dairy products, coffee, colas, soft drinks, sweet things, red meat, and processed foods. Take boron (3 mg. daily), chelated calcium (2,000 mg. daily), magnesium (1,600 mg. daily), eveing primrose oil (4 capsules daily), Kyolic EPA (6 capsules daily), brewer's yeast (1 tbsp.

daily), vitamin C (3,500 mg. daily) and vitamin E oil (800 I.U.) daily.

HYSTERIA

See under **BLOOD SUGAR PROBLEMS, HYPOGLYCEMIA,** and **NERVOUSNESS** for more information on this.

HYPERVENTILATION

Symptoms

Hyperventilation is a condition in which the breathing rate becomes speeded up, either through excitement, anxiety, lung disease, a blood infection, pneumonia, and even poisoning. It can feel like a heart attack is coming on, when it really isn't.

Symptoms include a pounding heart, tingling fingers, sweaty palms, and a *combined* psychological and physiological feeling as if you're going to die. More than likely though, you'll be around to pay next year's federal income and property taxes.

Relief Measures

Breathe into a paper bag. The theory to this being that it will allow you to replace the carbon dioxide "blown off" while hyperventilating.

Sit down, be calm and relax. Practice breathing naturally. Think beyond yourself and get your mind away from your current breathing patterns. In other words, become *detached* from the problem mentally. Do some simple walking or jogging. Avoid uncomfortable situations that may fill you with anxiety or fear. Cut down or out your intake of coffee, tea, colas, and chocolate, all of which have caffeine in them. Don't smoke and avoid second-hand smoke as well.

Foods and Nutrients

Drink a cup of *warm* peppermint or chamomile herbal tea. Take a high-potency B-complex (2 tablets daily). Drink papaya or mango juice. Snack on melons. Drink *cool* catnip tea.

IMPOTENCY

Symptoms

Impotency is the inability of the average adult male to get or keep an erection or to experience premature ejaculation. This inability to ejaculate makes impregnation of a woman's ovum with male sperm virtually impossible. Some reasons for this may be diseases such as diabetes, use of prescription, over-the-counter or illicit drugs, drinking alcohol, smoking, low sperm count, low self-esteem, and depression.

Relief Measures

About ten years ago (December 6, 1983 to be exact) one of the authors was in Houston, Texas to speak at a large holistic health convention. He appeared on The Ben Baldwin Show on KPRC radio for two hours. In between commercials, this author and Mr. Baldwin had a lot of off-the-air discussion about specific things relating to herbs.

Mr. Baldwin mentioned that he had suffered from impotency and had tried just about everything there was without much result. He heard about yohimbine bark increasing the sexual prowess of male rats and decided to give it a try for himself. He made a fluid extract from some fresh yohimbine bark and Johnny Walker Whiskey. (He never specified the amounts used.) He would shake the contents kept in a glass fruit jar and sealed with a Mason ring lid several times daily for two weeks. After which time, he strained the mixture out and drank 1 cup an hour before engaging in lovemaking with his female companion. He swore that it gave him an erection *every single time* without fail.

Foods and Nutrients

Supplements which are useful here include the amino acids L-Arginine (500 mg.) and L-Tyrosine (500 mg.), vitamin E (800 I.U.), vitamin A (25,000 I.U. fish oil), vitamin C (3,500 mg.), and zinc (100 mg.) daily.

INCONTINENCE

Symptoms

Incontinence is the inability to prevent the discharge of any of the usual bodily excretions, especially of urine or feces. When police sometimes have to administer a temporary choke-hold on an uncooperative suspect they're about to handcuff and arrest, this action will often result in immediate incontinence of that individual. One of the authors who has rode on patrol in the past with members of the Dallas Police Department, remembers this happening more than once with suspects who had to be restrained in this rough manner. Also in frontier times when criminals were hung from the gallows, a nervous reaction triggered immediately after the neck was broken was the quick discharge of urine and feces into the corpse's trousers.

Relief Measures

Keeping a daily diary of what one eats or drinks that may cause leakage, will help to track down the dietary cause better. Going easy on fluids several hours before bedtime will alleviate bedwetting at night. Stay away from alcohol, coffee, and citrus juices—they are fantastic diuretics but not intended for those with incontinence by any means.

Drink cranberry juice (1 cup) and take some white oak bark capsules (3) twice daily. Both will help to slow the undesired dribbling of urine. Daily helpings of unbuttered and unsalted popcorn also helps, or anything with a lot of fiber in it.

Losing weight, even by a few pounds, can cut down the incontinence problem quite abit. Walking when the bladder has been emptied just before bedtime should curtail much of this during sleep.

Go when you have to go. Don't make excuses or try to hold it. And when you do urinate, stay on the toilet until you feel your bladder is empty. Then, stand up and sit down again, lean forward slightly at the knees and try again. This should squeeze out any extra urine that might remain behind.

Realize that there are now available special supplies for those who continue to have such a problem. There are several brands of absorbent products in the form of underpants or pads and shields. These new products absorb 50 to 500 times their weight in water, neutralize odor, and congeal fluid to prevent leakage. The type you may require depends, of course, on your own individual anatomy and the kind and degree of incontinence you have. Don't feel embarrassed about buying them or asking your pharmacist to assist in your purchase of some.

Incontinence often comes with old age when men and women have lost their ability to tighten the pelvic muscles around the neck of the bladder. Without the ability to do this, some urine will be lost every time the abdominal pressure rises. One remedy is to strengthen the pelvic muscles with Kegel Exercises. But first, an elderly person (particularly older women) must be examined to rule out the need for the surgical correction of a ruptured pelvic floor, or some other type of treatment.

Kegel exercises involve tensing the pelvic floor (as in holding back a stool) for 10 seconds, followed by 10 seconds of relaxation. This must be done at least 90 times a day (i.e., for at least 10 minutes, 3 times daily) for about 3 months before evident benefit occurs. Many older people give up too soon when they don't see results right away. The medical journal *Geriatrics* (46 (12):70, 1991; and 47 (1):78, 1992) mentioned this in several of its recent issues.

Foods and Nutrients

Certain acidic foods such as sauerkraut, apple cider vinegar, and tomato juice as well as some fermented foods (yogurt, buttermilk, tofu, aged garlic extract) seem to hold urine longer in the system. These should be incorporated into the diet more often. But fried or deep-fried, barbecued, broiled, and sugary foods, including a lot of red meat, will tend to increase urination; therefore, their intake should be limited.

INDIGESTION

Symptoms

Indigestion is often more a symptom of a particular problem in the stomach or intestines than it is a disorder in itself. But sometimes it can be an actual problem, too.

Symptoms include belching, abdominal pain, heartburn, intestinal gas, a bloated feeling, nausea, vomiting, and a burning sensation after finishing a meal.

Relief Measures

Herbal teas seem to help a lot here. A cup of warm spearmint, peppermint, lemon balm, lavender, or chamomile helps to relieve such after-dinner miseries.

Also eating more slowly and methodically and thoroughly chewing every mouthful so it mixes well with saliva, definitely will reduce your chances of getting indigestion.

Right food combinations is another way to help prevent indigestion from happening to you. Learn what foods can be properly combined with others and what cannot be. Some trial-and-error testing on

your own helps, too. For instance, milk does not go with tomatos or tomato-based products such as canned soup, catsup, and salsa. Nor does cake or pie and ice cream go well with a meat-and-potatoes dinner.

Keep meals simple. Allow no more than two dishes at the most at any given meal. Eating several smaller meals periodically throughout the day instead of the standard two or three big ones, keeps the stomach from becoming upset.

Consume meals *without* the benefit of beverages. Let the saliva glands provide the necessary enzymes for every mouthful of food chewed and swallowed, so that digestion can be improved. Drinking liquids with any meal only dilutes these enzymes and renders them fairly useless.

Foods and Nutrients

One-quarter cup of aloe vera juice every morning and evening on an empty stomach relieves heartburn and other gastrointestinal symptoms. Take Wakunaga's Kyo-Dophilus (2-3 capsules) with each meal or some papaya juice or some *warm* catnip tea or some pancreatin (a digestive enzyme)—all will help promote better digestion.

INFECTION

Symptoms

Infections are the starting point of many illnesses and often are not serious enough for medical attention. However, they can result in a wide variety of serious illnesses including swollen glands or tonsils, sore throat, colds, hay fever, encephalitis, and viral pneumonia. White blood cells, lymph cells, and antibodies mobilize to prevent any bacteria, virus, or toxin from entering the body. An adequate diet is essential for the maintenance and reinforcement of these defenses.

Relief Measures

The herbs echinacea, goldenseal and aged garlic help to prevent, as well as treat, existing infections. They can be taken in capsules or fluid extracts. For preventive purposes less is required: echinacea (1 capsule or 10 drops), goldenseal (1 capsule or 8 drops), Kyolic aged-garlic extract (2 capsules). On the other hand, present infections demand more of them: echinacea (3 capsules or 30 drops), goldenseal (2 capsules or 16 drops), Kyolic aged-garlic extract (6 capsules).

Foods and Nutrients

Vitamin A (100,000 I.U.), vitamin C with bioflavonoids (15,000 mg.), pantothenic acid (500 mg.), high-potency B-complex (4 tablets), zinc (100 mg.) and Wakunaga's Kyo-Dophilus (3 capsules) and Kyo-Green (1 glass twice daily) should be taken every day while the infection persists.

INFERTILITY

Symptoms

Infertility is the inability to become pregnant after a year or more of regular sexual activity during the time of ovulation.

It's also the inability to carry a pregnancy full-term. Infertility is generally due to a hormonal imbalance, pelvic inflammatory disease, or more often the sexually transmissible disease called chlamydia.

Relief Measures/Foods and Nutrients

A combination of several things taken or done at the same time seems to be effective in helping to bring about conception. During the first few days of every month when a woman is fertile, she should take royal jelly, bee pollen, vitamin E (800 I.U.), vitamin C (3, 500 mg.), and dong quai. He should take royal jelly, bee pollen, Korean ginseng, vitamin E (1,200 I.U.), vitamin C (5,000 mg.), and Mexican damiana. The same amount of dong quai or damiana is taken by each one, namely four capsules daily.

Then before sexual intercourse the couple should use egg white as a vaginal lubricant to induce conception. Andrew Toledo, M.D., an assistant professor of the Dept. of Gynecology and Obstetrics at Emory University in Atlanta, Georgia, believes that egg white has the least effect on sperm motility and survival simply because it's pure protein just like sperm is. "Sperm doesn't do well in a carrier different from its own structure," reasons Dr. Toledo, except maybe for egg white.

Other recommendations: ease up on your work schedule; stop smoking; don't over exercise; don't douche; go easy on colas and coffee; avoid steroids, drugs and alcohol.

INFLAMMATION

Symptoms

Inflammation occurs when a part of the body reacts to trauma or infection. It can be caused by arthritis, bacterial infection, or strain. The symptoms are swelling, heat, and pain. Sometimes the afflicted area turns red. Any organ or tissue of the body, whether internal or external, can become inflamed.

Relief Measures

Any mucilaginous herb made into a tea for external use or else taken internally in tea or capsule forms helps bring relief to inflammation. Such herbs would be marshmallow root, comfrey root or leaf, fenugreek seed, and slippery elm. Poultices can be of the cool tea and applied to the skin throughout the day. Or several cups can be drunk for internal relief.

Yarrow is also an excellent antiinflammatory herb. The August, 1969 *Journal of Pharmaceutical Sciences* (58:938-41) contained a lengthy report on how this herb reduced tissue and joint inflammation by 35% in rats. This action was attributed to the protein-carbohydrate complex in the flowers.

Another outstanding herb is calendula. A Bulgarian medical journal, *Acta Physiologica et Pharmacologica Bulgarica* (8:163-67, 1982) reported that an ointment of calendula extract was applied to surgically induced wounds in Wister albino rats and promoted rapid healing of the tissue, including reduction of inflammation. And an American trade publication, *Cosmetics & Toiletries* (100:45) reported in its October,

1985 issue that calendula accelerated healing and reduced tissue inflammation nicely.

Foods and Nutrients

Coffee, colas, soft drinks, white flour products, sugary foods, fried and deep-fried foods all aggravate cases of inflammation. Consume organic fruits and vegetables, whole grains, fish, juices, and mineral or spring water.

Supplements should include vitamin C (10, 000 mg.), rut n (300 mg.), SOD (superoxide dismutase), zinc (100 mg.), horsetail (2 capsules), vitamin A (25,000 I.U. fish oil) and vitamin E (800 I.U.).

INFLUENZA

See under the FLU for more information on this.

INSECT BITES

See under BITES for more information on this.

INSOMNIA

(See also SLEEPWALKING)

Symptoms

Insomnia is a condition of habitual sleeplessness, occurring with repetition. It can result from stress, drugs, low blood sugar, muscle aches and pains, anxiety, stomach upset, asthma, and allergies.

Relief Measures

Equal parts of catnip and hops made into a tea (1 tsp. of each steeped in 1.5 pints of boiling water for 30 minutes) will help an insomniac get a good night's rest. So will skullcap and valerian (2 capsules each).

Foods and Nutrients

Foods rich in the amino acid tryptophan induce sleep: cashew butter, warm milk, goat cheese, and black mission figs. Avoid caffeine-containing foods, alcohol, sugary foods, candy, pork products, potatoes, spinach and tomatoes close to bedtime as they tend to stimulate brain activity. Supplements should include calcium (800 mg.), magnesium (1,600 mg.), and a high-potency B-complex vitamin (2 tablets) several hours before retiring.

IRRITABLE BOWEL SYNDROME

Symptoms

Irritable bowel syndrome is a common abdominal complaint, probably the most common reason for visits to gastroenterologists. It's also called spastic colon, mucus colitis, or nervous bowels. It usually develops in late adolescence or early adulthood, and affects twice as many women as men. It does not lead to cancer, does not require surgery, is not caused by any known physical abnormality, and is not the same thing as inflammatory bowel disease—a much more serious disorder that may produce ulceration of the intestinal wall.

The symptoms typically include cramping (often on the left side of the abdomen, but it may mimic heartburn or backache), bloating, and an urgent need to move your bowels. The stool may be loose and watery, and you may notice white mucus in it. Eating may make you feel worse, and defecation or passing gas brings relief. You have no fever or bleeding, and you can't think of anything you've consumed or done to have brought this condition on. Mysteriously, the diarrhea may give way to constipation, but you may still have abdominal pain and a lot of gas as well. The condition may correct itself in the course of time, but then return again when you least expect or want it to.

Relief Measures

Emotional stress and anxiety are certainly associated with irritable bowel syndrome. Dr. William Whitehead of the Johns Hopkins University School of Medicine believes that emotional upset can make such intestinal symptoms worse. He advises people with this problem to keep their minds at ease and hearts free of frustration and anger.

Charcoal tablets from any local healthfood store or drugstore will relieve gas and bloating. Use only on an as-needed basis (5 tablets daily), since they are highly absorbent and will also absorb nutrients the body depends on. Or take ginger root (4 capsules) or chamomile or peppermint teas (1 cup) to relieve this problem.

Foods and Nutrients

When an intestinal upset occurs, eat a bland diet. Fruit and vegetable juices are preferred in such instances instead of in their whole states. Gerber or Heinz baby food is another alternative to use.

Stay away from animal fats, butter, margarine, milk, cheese, fried and deep-fried foods, spicy foods, wheat bran and wheat products, nuts, seeds, junk foods, sugary foods, colas, soft drinks, beer, wine, coffee, citrus juices, and pastries.

Alfalfa tea (2 cups daily) or capsules (6-8 daily) and Wakunaga Kyo-Dophilus (3 capsules daily) are advised. Aloe vera juice (1 cup daily) and an enzyme complex that is low in hydrochloric acid (HCl) and high in pancreatin is another remedy combination worth using.

ITCHING

Symptoms

Itching is a nervous or allergenic response to irritating emotions or substances. This response usually provokes an urge to scratch the skin like crazy for temporary relief.

Itching can be due to synthetic or natural fibers (rayon or wool), nervous and skin disorders (hives and eczema), noxious or toxic plants (stinging nettle or poison ivy), peeling sunburned skin, food allergies, insect bites and stings, medication, soap and household cleaners, and infectious diseases (fungus and chickenpox).

Relief Measures

Lightly rubbing some tincture of witch hazel on the skin and then drying it in front of a small rotating fan brings surprising relief in minutes. So does running an ice cube over the skin. Or an itch can be lightly rubbed with a chicken feather.

Older people commonly suffer from itching due to excessively dry skin, and may benefit by adding humidity to the air, and from the use of a bath oil. An alternative to using bath oil is to soak in a warm tub of baking soda solution (half a cupful of soda in a tub of warm water).

Sometimes herbs can cause an allergic, itching reaction. Raw garlic and concentrated peppermint oil are two of these and care should be taken in how they are handled or applied. And if itching persists for more than a week's time and fails to respond to an antihistamine or to simple treatment, by all means, we encourage you to see your doctor soon!

Foods and Nutrients

Pantothenic acid (100 mg.), PABA (100 mg.), vitamin E oil (400 I.U.), and zinc (100 mg.) taken orally and also included in a salve application, will give considerable relief to a very frustrating and often annoying health dilemma.

JAUNDICE

Symptoms

Jaundice is a condition in which the skin, whites of the eyes, and urine become abnormally yellow due to the presence of pigments from worn-out red blood cells. Ordinarily such cells are excreted in bile as waste products; however, in jaundice they accumulate in the blood and are deposited in the tissues.

The disease can be caused by a condition that prevents the bile from entering the intestines; surgical trauma, swelling or spasms of the bile duct, or obstruction of the duct by a stone, cyst, or cancer.

Anemia can often result in jaundice; severe liver damage or cirrhosis can also occur as a result of jaundice. Jaundice could indicate blood, kidney, or liver disturbances. By all means, consult a physician in such cases. Self treatment may be fine, but medical care is also required!

Relief Measures/Foods and Nutrients

There are several herbs and foods which are excellent for this condition. Milk thistle extract in the form of Thisilyn and Efamol Evening Primrose Oil (both from Nature's Way and available at health food stores) can be taken every day (3 capsules of each). Also Kyolic EPA and goldenseal root should be taken as well (two capsules of each with meals).

Fresh juice made every day from your kitchen juicer is a must: beet tops, beet root, parsley, dandelion greens, peeled lime, and tomatoes. This concoction is *terrific* for an ailing liver. Follow up with brewer's yeast (2 tsp. daily) and vitamin C (15,000 mg. every day).

KIDNEY STONES

Symptoms

Kidney stones are abnormal accumulations of mineral salts, which form in the kidney but may lodge anywhere in the urinary tract. They can be the size of sand or gravel or as large as bird eggs. Often removed surgically, they can reappear if the diet isn't substantially improved. The stones are composed mainly of calcium phosphate or oxalate. They form most rapidly in urine that is alkaline as opposed to urine that is more acidic in content.

Relief Measures

Phyllis C. is a housewife from Houston, who attended a lecture which one of the authors gave there some years ago. She had been plagued with a large kidney stone travelling around inside of her body, which gave her a great deal of pain. She consulted a local curandera (Spanish folk healer) who instructed her to drink a lot of manzanita tea, which she procured from a local herb shop catering to the Hispanic community. Within five days, the stone had dissolved and passed through her system without further problems. The author told her that catnip tea (3 cups daily) would have worked just as well if she had not been able to get the other.

Foods and Nutrients

Magnesium (1,200 mg. daily), vitamin B-6 (200 mg. daily), and vitamin C with bioflavonoids (7,000 mg. daily) are essential. Do not drink soft drinks, colas, coffee, or black or green teas during this period, until the stone(s) are gone.

LARYNGITIS

See under HOARSENESS for more information on this.

LEAD POISONING

Symptoms

Until only qite recently, lead poisoning had been a public health problem of very low priority for the news media to even bother considering. But as more fatalities turned up in many inner city housing projects of young children eating old paint peelings from the walls, this was eventually

pushed to the forefront and has received widespread publicity ever since.

Investigations by public health officials and scientists soon expanded into other areas for potential lead poisoning: auto exhaust, ceramic glazes, auto lead-acid batteries, tobacco, canned fruit (packed in lead-soldered cans), bone meal, insecticides, and water distributed through lead piping.

Lead poisoning is a very subtle and progressively slow health problem that generally doesn't show up in full magnitude until some years later. Children born from mothers with high levels of lead in their placentas, usually register severe reading problems, learning disabilities, and poor eye-hand coordination by the time they're ready to start school. Others may suffer from growth retardation and nervous system disorders. Extreme and prolonged hyperactivity in younger children may also be traced to lead poisoning.

Lead builds up in body tissue and could ultimately lead to severe gastrointestinal colic, paralysis of the extremities, blindness, mental imbalances, loss of memory, and even insanity in some instances. It also causes male impotency, reproductive disorders and infertility in both sexes, and nemia.

Relief Measures

Three things which can be done very quickly to insure that your environment becomes more lead-free are these:

(A). Avoid cans sealed with lead solder, which leaches into foods. A lead-soldered can will often have remnants of solder and indentations along the seam. Generally, canned products from Third World countries are of this type and should be avoided entirely.

(B). Have your water tested to insure a safe level of lead and other minerals. Your state health department usually provides a service that will test your water for such contaminants at a reasonable fee.

(C). Do not buy any imported ceramic ware from Mexico, Spain, or other countries, as these have been found by the Food and Drug Administration to release minute but potentially harmful amounts of lead into the food cooked in them or served upon them.

Getting a hair analysis or blood workup can help determine if your body has a higher-than-normal lead content.

Drinking alfalfa tea (3 cups daily) and alternating it with liquid aloe vera (two half-cupfuls daily) every day can help to flush some of this lead out of the system. So can tomato juice, and burdock or yellow dock teas (2 cups of any of them daily).

Foods and Nutrients

Loading your diet with legumes such as navy beans and chickpeas, whole grain cereals and breads, potatoes, eggs, soybean products, apples, garlic, and onion helps considerably. Calcium (900 mg.) and magnesium (2,000 mg.), Kyolic EPA (3 capsules), an amino acid complex (3 tablets), rutin (300 mg.),and vilamin C (3,500 mg.).

LEG CRAMPS

Symptoms

A leg cramp (also called a "Charley horse") is an involuntary contraction, or spasm, of a muscle in the leg or foot. Cramps most commonly occur at night, when the limbs are cool, especially after a day of hard physical exertion, and more often in the elderly, the young, and people with hardening of the arteries. Such cramps appear to be brought on by unnatural positions which impair the blood supply to the lower extremities, causing the muscles to abnormally contract, thus bringing about cramps. A cramp usually lasts only a few seconds or minutes.

A cramp that is a "Charley horse" is a pulled and bruised muscle that results in soreness and stiffness. It's usually induced by a blow or a forceful stretch of the leg during athletic activity.

Relief Measures

One of the very best things for getting rid of this type of cramping, is to stretch the leg or foot out as far as possible and hold it in that position for a few seconds before relaxing the limb. Then repeat the procedure 15 seconds later, and relax. Keep this up for several minutes at a time. Sometimes the application of hot and cold packs or a gentle massaging of the muscle itself often clears the problem up.

Foods and Nutrients

A high intake of protein (preferably fish and soybean) is recommended for those experiencing "Charley horses." High intakes of calcium (1,000 mg.), magnesium (2,000 mg.), potassium (2,500 mg.), and phosphorus (800 mg.) are advised for routine cramping situations.

LEG ULCERS

Symptom!

Leg ulcers are open sores which develop on deteriorated patches of skin, usually in the elderly and more often in diabetic cases. When poor circulation in the legs restricts blood flow, the skin tissue begins to erode. When this happens it becomes more susceptible to the development of a running sore. The broken skin seldom ever heals itself. Leg ulcers can also be found in those with varicose veins.

Relief Measures

A retired army colonel who resides in an out-of-the-way place called Brilliant, Alabama, told one of the authors about a most unusual herbal formulation he takes for his circulatory problems, and testified that it helped to clear up more than one leg ulcer and several varicose veins from which he had been apparently suffering for some time. He took 4 capsules daily.

The contents of this fairly simple formula are as follows: red beet root, wheat grass, barley grass, red clover blossoms, and spinach leaf.

Other treatments for leg ulcers include soaking a poultice in some Wakunaga Kyo-Green solution and applying it to the sore. Also making an ointment out of some crushed zinc tablets, a little powdered goldenseal root from Wakunaga, a little Kyolic liquid aged-garlic extract, some vitamin E oil, and a little honey, and then applying it to the sore helps heal it a lot faster.

Foods and Nutrients

Vitamin A (25,000 I.U.), vitamin E (800 I.U.), vitamin C (3,500 mg.), rutin (300 mg.), alfalfa tablets (6-8), zinc (100 mg.), and Wakunaga's Kyo-Green (one 8 fl. oz. glass) on a daily basis is recommended.

LEPROSY

Symptoms

Leprosy is a chronic skin disease endemic to tropical and subtropical parts of the world. While virtually nonexistent in the Western Hemisphere or Europe, it still is quite pervasive elsewhere. We felt to include it here for the benefit of those travelling abroad who may be unlucky enough to acquire it or for health care providers overseas who may get a copy of this book for their own clinical use.

Leprosy is caused by Mycobacterium leprae and has the potential to produce mutilation of the extremities and disfigurement of the face, but is rarely ever fatal. Also called Hansen's disease, it is of Biblical origins and was made famous in the film epic Ben-Hur, when the mother and sister of *Ben-Hur* contracted the disease during their long imprisonment by the Romans. Seen in two forms or as an intermediate between the two, the tuberculoid type may be limited to a few nerves and skin areas, whereas the lepromatous type is disseminated throughout the entire body.

Relief Measures/Foods and Nutrients

The recently popularized tea tree oil from Australia has found favor with some doctors in Indonesia and the Philippines. They apply very small amounts of this very potent antiseptic oil to the most serious skin eruptions with very good results. They've told one of the authors on some of his previous visits to such countries that tea tree oil seems to kill the bacteria causing leprosy better than anything else they've tried mt the past, including such standard drugs of choice as dapsone (DDS or 4,4'—diaminodiphenyl sulfone), clofazimine, or rifampin.

In India one of the authors has seen some Ayurvedic doctors wash the skin of their leper patients with lime juice, as well as giving strong doses of lime juice internally. They also provide their patients with a lot of garlic and onions and turmeric in the form of the traditional curry powder in foods which they believe are good for lepers to eat.

The authors would like to add vitamin A (100,000 I.U.), vitamin C (15-20 grams by intravenous injection), goldenseal root (5 capsules), and dandelion root (5 capsules) to this regimen, although such aren't usually available in many Third World countries on a ready basis.

The tropical weed, gotu kola, has found much favor from India to Indonesia for the treatment of leprosy. And is used topically as well as internally for the recovery from this disease with moderate-to-good success.

LEUKEMIA

See under CANCER for more information on this.

LEUKORRHEA

Symptoms

Leukorrhea is a nonbloody white vaginal discharge. Leukorrhea is often caused by a one-celled microorganism known by the popular name of chlamydia, and is sometimes caused by a fungal infection like Candida albicans. Other causes may be excessive douching, vitamin B-complex deficiency, heavy use of prescription antibiotics or oral contraceptives, or intestinal parasites. Leukorrhea is more frequent in diabetic and pregnant women. Symptoms include burning, itching, and vaginal discharge.

Relief Measures

Several herbal teas with strong antimicrobial actions to them are suggested here. The person should drink one cup each of chaparral, red clover and pau d'arco tea, morning, noon and night on an empty stomach. It doesn't matter at what time which tea is drunk, just so long as they are taken about four hours apart.

A woman should douche with equal parts of chaparral and goldenseal tea twice daily, and make sure her vagina is always kept clean and dry.

Foods and Nutrients

Kyo-Dophilus (6 capsules daily), high-potency B-complex (4 tablets daily), and vitamin C (3,500 mg. daily) are advised.

Also see under **CANDIDIASIS** for more information.

LICE

Symptoms

Lice are members of the ectoparasitic insect orders Anoplura (the sucking lice) and Mallophaga (the biting lice). The sucking kind possess nipper-like, heavily scierotized jaws and a characteristic broad head, while the sucking type are characterized by a narrow head with piercing and sucking mouthparts that lie in a sac concealed in the head.

Lice generally inhabit the scalp and pubic areas, and sometimes even beneath the armpits of their human hosts or wherever there is a lot of hair. They will lay their eggs in such places, which usually appear as tiny grayish-white lumps. These are the blood-sucking kind as a rule and can cause considerable skin irritation that leads to scratching, which in turn leads to an epidermal infection resulting in pustular spots.

Relief Measures

The very best remedies for getting rid of lice are strong soaps. A good pine-tar soap from any veterinary or animal supply house works well in such conditions. Also the scalp may even be rinsed with a weak solution of Lysol cleaning detergent with equally good results, making sure *none of it gets into the eyes*! Prevention is very simple: practice good hygiene on a daily basis by bathing regularly and wearing clean clothes.

Foods and Nutrients

For some reason, lice *cannot* tolerate sweaty odor of garlic or brewer's yeast. High amounts of Kyolic (6 capsules) and the latter (2 tbsp.) each day will send them somewhere else.

LUMBAGO

See under BACKACHE for more information on this.

LUPUS ERHTHEMATOSUS

Symptoms

Lupus is a chronic inflammatory disease that affects many different organs throughout the body. It is an auto-immune disorder meaning that the body's own immune defenses turn on itself. The vast majority of sufferers are older women.

There are two types of lupus: systemic lupus erthyematosus and discoid lupus erythematosus. The systemic kind affects the organs and joints of the body, and the discoid type is a much less serious skin disorder. Both can flare up and then go into remission.

It's believed that both types of lupus are viral induced and prompt the immune system to produce special antibodies that in turn attack the body's own organs and tissues. This produces inflammation of the blood vessels and/or joints, thereby affecting many parts of the body. The kidneys are often involved; 50% of those with lupus develop nephritis as well.

Lupus comes from the word meaning wolf, since the rash that this disease produces appears on the faces of those infected, thereby giving them a wolflike appearance. At least half of the following eight symptoms must be present simultaneously or following one another before a correct diagnosis for lupus can be made: abnormal cells in the urine; arthritis; butterfly rash on the cheeks; sun sensitivity; mouth sores; seizures or psychosis; low white blood cell count, low platelet count, or hemolytic anemia; or a specific antibody found in 50% of lupus sufferers or lupus cells in the blood.

Relief Measures

Strong sunlight should be avoided. Wear protective clothing and dark sunglasses if you have lupus. Rest and exercise are important. Get plenty of sleep and walk regularly. Don't get into arguments or situations which create anxiety and frustration within you. Remain calm, have a happy and positive outlook on life in general and strive for peace and quiet at all times.

Echinacea (4 capsules daily), goldenseal root (2 capsules daily), wild Oregon graperoot (4 capsules daily), red clover tea (2 cups daily), sarsaparilla tea (2 cups daily), and pau d'arco fluid extract (25 drops daily) are all useful herbs to take for this condition.

Foods and Nutrients

The diet should consist of very little fried or deep-fried foods, red meat, and salty snack foods (canned or packaged nuts, potato chips). In fact, the use of salt in the diet should be held to an absolute minimum; the same goes for white sugar and honey, too.

It seems that those foods which are heavily sprayed (leafy green vegetables and some fruits like grapes) or packaged and contain a lot of chemical additives (luncheon meats and bakery goods) are harmful to lupus victims, and should, therefore, be avoided. Organically grown food which is pesticide-free and foods with very little chemical preservatives in them should be consumed instead.

An amino acid complex (3 tablets daily), a high-potency B-complex (3 tablets daily), a calcium/magnesium supplement (3 tablets daily), Korean and Siberian ginsengs (3 capsules of each daily), an unsaturated fatty acid coirplex (3 capsules daily), vitamin E oil (800 I.U. daily), and zinc (100 mg. daily) constitute a very good nutritional program to help send this disease into remission.

MALABSORPTION SYNDROME

Symptoms

This is a fairly recent health problem of growing magnitude within the American population. It is essentially the body's inability to properly absorb protein and key minerals and vitamins that are a requisite part of optimal health. Poor malabsorption may be due to diseases of certain digestive and metabolic organs (stomach, pancreas, liver, and gallbladder). It may be due to an imbalance of intestinal bacterial flora which helps to break food down. It could be due to an intolerance for certain things in specific foods (the gluten in grains). Or it could be attributed to an excessive use of alcohol, drugs, antacids, or laxatives.

Whatever the causes are, the symptoms become visibly apparent: weight loss, diarrhea, dry skin, hair loss, muscle weakness, fatigue, and anemia. Those suffering from malabsorption of some kind require more nutrients than the average person to treat and correct their problems. Many victims are unable to break down health food supplements in tablet form. Encapsulated supplements should be taken instead. And a change of diet and thorough cleansing program can heal and clean the colon.

Relief Measures

Mucilaginous herbs such as comfrey, marshmallow, fenugreek and slippery elm bark are very helpful in promoting good absorption of ingested nutrients. These first three herbs can be taken in capsule form (about two per meal); the latter, slippery elm can be taken in capsules (3 per meal) or else as a tea (1 cup per meal).

Wakunaga's Kyo-Dophilus has proven itself to be an effective product in helping to promote better assimilation within the body. About two capsules per meal are advised. (See Appendix under Wakunaga for more information.)

People with malabsorption syndrome should avoid consuming greasy, sugary, salty, or very acidic processed foods. These are hard to digest and interfere with the normal distribution of assimilated nutrients.

Foods to eat more often include well-cooked brown rice, oatmeal, steamed vegetables, cooked millet, steamed or baked fish, barley malt, nut and soy milks, papaya juice, mineral or spring water, and chamomile or peppermint teas with each meal.

The authors recommend injections of B-complex vitamins, including B-12 by a physician (1 cc of B-12 three times weekly is standard therapy for such a problem).

Occasional weekend fasting on mild foods only (preferably liquids) and a modest intestinal cleansing program will help renew the digestive powers of the entire gastrointestinal tract. It's comparable to a monthly house-cleaning project, and makes the body feel suprisingly invigorated again.

MALARIA

See under FEVER for more information on this.

MALNUTRITION

Symptoms

Malnutrition occurs when sound nutrition is in serious default. This may be due to malabsorption, poor diet, over eating, and oft times starvation. While the pathetic sights of children with distended abdomens and spindly legs and arms from such faraway places as Ethiopia, may greet our eyes in a televised news documentary or ad campaign from some world hunger relief organization asking for donations, such pictures don't tell us the whole story. In fact, many of America's well-fed middle and high-school kids suffer from varying levels of malnutrition, but usually in the form of vitamin and mineral deficiencies which don't always show up so dramatically as outright starvation does.

Symptoms don't always have to be a gaunt skeleton with sunken eyes and tight skin over a bony frame to indicate malnutrition. They can also be traced to fleshy features that have a gray pallor in them or seemingly chubby bodies that lack the energy and stamina to which youth is so accustomed.

Relief Measures

Some of the same herbs proposed for malabsorption syndrome apply here as well. But the one we like the best is powdered slippery elm bark: at least four capsules should be taken twice daily with meals on a regular basis.

Also a very nourishing grain drink made out of boiled barley broth and some slivered cashew milk whipped up in a food processor, is ideal for correcting malnourishment. Some powdered whey or soy milk can also be added to this mixture, and flavored with a little pure vanilla and pure maple syrup to taste.

Foods and Nutrients

The same dietary do's and don'ts given for malabsorption apply here as well. But brewer's yeast (one tsp. every morning) can be taken in some juice or milk to help boost critical B-vitamin needs. An enzyme complex and Wakunaga's Kyo-Dophilus (1 capsule each per meal) work well together here.

MANIC-DEPRESSIVE DISORDER

Symptoms

This is a psychosis that is characterized by extreme mood swings. The typical manic-depressive individual will go from a period of unrealistic enthusiasm and elation to misery and the depths of depression. When he is in the depressive stage, he will demonstrate low self-esteem and have feelings of hopelessness. He will lack motivation to do anything, even to get out of bed. Some people in this stage sleep for weeks. They withdraw from social activities, avoid relationships with others, and are unable to work.

When in the mania stage, the manic-depressive person will have what appears to be unlimited energy. He or she may go for 24 or even 36 hours without a wink of sleep.

These periods of mania come and go at random, quite suddenly and without prior notice. Some have them often and others may go for years between such abnormal occurrences. Symptoms include changes in sleep pattern, withdrawal from society, extreme pessimism, failure to finish projects that were started with enthusiasm, chronic irritability, sudden attacks of rage, and lack of inhibition, especially in sexual behavior.

Relief Measures/Foods and Nutrients

Amino acid supplements are very important here. L-Taurine (250 mg. six times daily) should be taken with vitamin B-6 (25 mg. three times daily) and vitamin C (500 mg. twice daily). L-Tyrosine (250 mg. six times daily) should be taken with the same vitamins also. Magnesium (1,200 mg.), calcium (400 mg.), potassium (1,600 mg.), and brewer's yeast (2 tbsps. daily) are all necessary. Sugary foods are to be excluded from the diet.

MEASLES

Symptoms

Measles is a viral infection that attacks the lungs and produces a nasty skin rash. Although most common to elementary school children, adults can also contract it as well. It is highly infectious and is distributed through the air by coughing and sneezing.

There are two kinds: German (rubella) and red (rubeola). The first is caused by a virus which induces a mild fever, some sneezing, runny nose, slight cough, red eyes, and a rash of small, flat, pink spots appearing all over the body, which usually last for a couple of days. Glands at the back of the neck usually become tender and swollen, but subside within about four days.

The second kind is also viral induced and often occurs in epidemic proportions across the country in the winter and spring. Initial reactions before the main illness sets in are elevated temperature (up to 103° F.), runny nose, occasional vomiting, and an ill feeling. Main symptoms include sore, red eyes and a dislike for light; an apparent bad cold; miserable outlook; a hacking cough; and a blotchy rash that is dark red in color, which begins behind the ears, then spreads out over the chest, body and limbs.

Relief Measures

Two of the very best herbs to give children who have this are mullein and catnip teas. Bring a quart of water to a boil and add two tablespoons of each herb. Stir, cover, set aside, and let steep for 45 minutes..When moderately warm, strain, sweeten with some pure maple syrup, and have the sick child drink as much of this as he or she wants to.

If the child's temperature becomes excessive, then give him or her some warm peppermint tea to drink in small, measured (1/4 cup) doses every couple of hours. When an intolerable itching sets in making the child want to scratch, bathe the skin with some hyssop tea (made the same way as the other teas) or some tincture of witch hazel purchased from a nearby drugstore.

The child should also be given some Kyolic liquid garlic in the capsule form (2 every four hours). But if the child is unable to swallow the capsules, then put the liquid (1/2 tsp.) into a little applesauce or fruit juice and have the youngster swallow it that way.

Foods and Nutrients

The sick child should be given slippery elm tea (1 cup twice daily) and powdered or liquid vitamin C (equivalent to 3,500 mg.) instead of tablets. Some cod liver oil (1 tsp.) mixed in with a little applesauce will make it more palatable to a child's fussy and discriminating taste buds.

A sick child should also be given a garlic enema as well. Boil up a pint of water into which has been added a coarsely chopped garlic clove. Simmer for 20 minutes. Cool and strain. Put into a hot water bottle with a hose and syringe attachment and administer through the rectum while said child is laying down on the bathroom floor.

MEMORY IMPAIRMENT

See under MENTAL RETARDATION for more information on this.

MENIERE'S SYNDROME

See under BLOOD CIRCULATION and ARTERIOSCLEROSIS/ATHEROSCLE-ROSIS and EAR DISORDERS for more information on this.

MENINGITIS

Symptoms

Meningitis is an infection by either bacteria, viruses, or fungi of the three layers of membranes which lay between the skull and the brain. These infecting organisms are routinely spread via the bloodstream from acute infections of the nose and throat.

Children seem to be more likely candidates for this disease than adults do. Typical symptoms are headache, stiff neck, high fever, chills, nausea, vomiting, changes in mood, and drowsiness (which sometimes turns into a coma).

Relief Measures/Foods and Nutrients

One of the authors has previously toured mainland China with the American Medical Students' Association (1980) and more recently Japan with other scientists (1990). In both countries he found that garlic was the main treatment of choice by doctors for this disease. Recovery success was high, being anywhere from 80-95% as a rule.

Kyolic liquid aged-garlic extract (4 capsules every 5 hours) is necessary. The trace element germanium (100 mg. three times daily) should be taken in conjunction with this garlic extract, seeing as how both work quite well together. A vegetable broth well flavored with cooked garlic and onion should also be consumed each day by the individual.

An amino acid complex and a high-potency B-vitamin complex (two tablets of each daily) should also be taken. Vitamin A (25,000 I.U. fish oil), vitamin E (1,200 I.U.)

and vitamin C (7,500 mg.) are additionally helpful.

MENOPAUSE

Symptoms

Menopause is that point in a woman's life when she stops ovulating. It's also commonly referred to as "the change of life" phase. An "All in the Family" 1972 segment had the cantankerous Archie Bunker saying to his wife: "Edith, you're gonna have a change of life, you gotta do it right now. I'm gonna give you just 30 seconds. Now come on, CHANGE!" His wife, Edith, gave him a somewhat embarrassed look from the dinner table where both were sitting, and asked in slow, measured tones of humility: "Can I at least finish my soup first?"

For generations of women of a certain age, Edith's classic rejoinder said it all. Husbands might joke or misunderstand, but menopause was something women themselves didn't want to discuss—not with their mothers, their daughters, their doctors or their closest friends. It was like shaving your legs—something you did in private. Even women who wanted to know more about what was happening to their bodies were squeamish about asking questions. After all, it had to do with plumbing, and worse, it carried the unspoken stigma: *you're getting old!*

Menopause affects each woman differently. Some start early, some start and stop, but most experience the change around the age of 50. The transition can last up to 5 years. Typical symptoms include hot flashes, dizziness, headache, difficulty breathing, shortness of breath, heart palpitations, and depression. If a woman has low blood sugar, rest assured that these symptoms will be a lot more pronounced. Between 1992 and the year 2010 almost 40 million American women will have passed through menopause.

Relief Measures

Two things which seem to make the menopausal experience a lot harder on women is constant dieting and the cultural association in this country with youth and beauty. There is evidence available now that women who diet excessively to stay thin have a harder time with menopause. Part of that is biological: since estrogen is stored in fat cells, women who are a bit chubby retain more of it than those still struggling into a size 6 as they turn 50.

But it's the psychological factor of turning old which often makes menopause such a dreaded thing to look forward to with a majority of women. As a Santa Fe, New Mexico art gallery director, Anne Schleider (age 54) put it, after going through menopause in 1984: "With every hot flash that I experienced, it seemed to be blinking to my sub-conscious 'old-old.' I used to be noticed a lot when I was younger. At a point around 50, it started to slow down and then it stopped. I think that the prettier a woman is in her youth, the more insecure she is. When the looks start to go, she's not left with very much else."

So the obvious solution to both problems is a change of attitudes in how a woman feels about herself physically. If a woman in her late twenties or early thirties begins adding a little more weight to her hips, buttocks and thighs, she needs to carefully weigh in her mind the pluses and minuses of going on a weight loss program of some kind. Surely she will look more svelte after shedding those unwanted pounds, but is it worth the risk of enduring greater miseries when menopause hits a few more years down the road? Wouldn't she be better off instead *retaining* that extra weight (unless it's excessive and life-threatening) and learning to live with it psychologically, so the menopause years can glide by more smoothly? Can't a plump woman turn her acquired obesity into a positive image without going through self-imposed physical torture to get rid of it now and then really suffer when menopause comes? Only a woman faced with such present and future dilemmas can really answer these questions herself. But common sense suggests unless the obesity is of serious medical consequence, it might be better for her not to try so hard to lose it in order that her change of life passes pleasantly enough without becoming the dreaded ordeal which it now seems to be.

Studies of other cultures have noticed that the more women are revered in aging, the *less* trouble they seem to have with menopause—physically or psychologically. A University of California (San Francisco) anthropologist, Yewoubdar Beyene, a native of Ethiopia, studied women in Mayan villages and discovered they *actually looked forward* to menopause, because it brought them considerable freedom from years of intensive childbearing. She drew mostly blank stares when she asked many Maya women about their hot flashes. "People thought I was out of my mind going around asking such questions," she said. In fact, in the majority of such instances, as she and one of the authors of this book (who is himself an anthropologist) have discovered, there are virtually no

cases of hot flashes to speak of among most women of Third World cultures who live in humble material circumstances.

And even when she did find some cultures on the Greek island of Evia where a small number of the women had suffered hot flashes, the negative feelings about menopause were *totally absent!* Again, she attributed it to the *lack* of social stress on remaining as youthful looking as possible. Overall, she concluded in her studies, "Menopause is part of being a woman, but the menopausal experience is definitely shaped by culture."

Under such circumstances then, women living in an American society such as ours, must not allow themselves to become intimidated by all of the television and magazine ads emphasizing youth so much these days. They must begin to psychologically prepare themselves with the unpleasant but realistic fact that *everyone* grows older sooner or later. They must start in their *early* thirties to view the onset of old age more like a graduation from high school into college, than a transition of superficial beauty into wrinkles and gray hair. Through mental conditioning in the present, they can begin to appreciate the value of expensive antiques, not because such collectibles are young but rather due to their *old age!* Then in the very near future when menopause finally rolls around for them, they will actually welcome it in a sense, knowing full well that because of their attained maturity they have increased in *self* worth and *public* value!

Once women have managed to cross that important threshhold of their lives, they seem to experience something the late anthropologist Margaret Mead termed "postmenopausal zest!" There are legions of women who hit their professional strides or forged new careers in their 50's, from Eleanor Roosevelt to Margaret Thatcher to Golda Meir. Even women who suffered terrible symptoms during menopause all claim they emerged on the other side with a new sense of purpose and vigor.

Germaine Greer, who once abandoned her own hormonal therapy because of bad effects upon her health, described her personal transition through menopause as almost like dying and going to heaven: "It came to me as a great surprise that on the other side of all that turmoil, there is the most wonderful moment in one's entire life—really, the most golden, the most extraordinary, luminous instant that will last forever!" This is the mental and emotional reward for all women who make the ultimate transition and come out of it stronger, wiser, and usually better off because of it.

Foods and Nutrients

The authors recommend for women going through menopause the following herbs and nutritional supplements which will be of definite assistance to them. Black cohosh (3 capsules daily), licorice root (2 capsules daily), squaw vine (3 capsules daily), Siberian ginseng (4 capsules daily), and dong quai (3 capsules daily) are all helpful and should be taken together during the worst parts of the menopausal experience.

Wakunaga's Kyo-Dophilus (3 capsules), lecithin (2 capsules daily), vitamin B-6 (150 mg. daily), vitamin E oil (1,200 I.U.), vitamin D (500 I.U. daily), an amino acid complex (3 capsules daily), magnesium (1,200 mg. daily), calcium (600 mg. daily),

and a multiglandular supplement (2 tablets daily) should also be included as well.

Dairy products, sugary foods, red meat, and greasy food causes hot flashes. Therefore, their intakes should be greatly reduced or eliminated altogether.

MENTAL RETARDATION

Symptoms

Mental retardation or deficiency is a subaverage general intellectual functioning that originates during the developmental period and is associated with impairment in adaptive behavior. The American Association on Mental Deficiency lists eight medical classifications and five psychological classifications; the latter five replace the three former classifications of moron, imbecile, and idiot. Mental retardation classification requires assignment of an index for performance relative to a person's peers on two interrelated criteria: measured intelligence (IQ) and overall socio-adaptive behavior (a judgemental rating of the individual's relative level of performance in school, at work, at home, and in the community).

Psychological classifications of mental retardation

Classification	Stanford-Binet IQ	Wechsler IQ
Borderline	68-83	70-84
Mild	52-67	55-69

Moderate	36-51	40-54
Severe	20-35	25-39
Profound	below 20	below 25

Symptoms

In today's more sophisticated society, humanitarian-minded people like to use the term "mentally handicapped" instead of what they perceive to be a more regressive and negative "mental retardation." But for practical intents and purposes, the authors don't feel to share in this game of semantics and have elected to continue using the medical term which has been in vogue for many decades now.

MENTAL RETARDATION

Relief Measures

A small amount of evidence exists in the clinical literature from other countries to show that at least one herb, in particular, may be of some modest benefit in helping to improve the IQ status of those who are mentally handicapped. The herb is gotu kola and is a pervasive and common weed throughout much of Southeast Asia.

An Indian doctor, M.V.R. Appa Rao, M.D. and some of his associates, tested this herb—called Mandookaparni in Sanskrit—on "30 children of both sexes and free from epilepsy and all other neurological defects, from a local home for the mentally retarded, at Madras" during 1972. The subjects ranged in age from 7 to 18 years. Before and after taking gotu kola extract, "all the children were tested with the Binet-Kamat test and their Intelligence Quotients recorded." Dr. Rao stated in his report which appeared in the *Journal of Research in Indian Medicine* (8:4-13, 1973) that "all of them were within the mental age of 9." The equivalent of a 500 mg. tablet of gotu kola was given to one group of retarded children once a day, while a vegetable-colored starch tablet serving as the placebo was administered to the others.

Results were dramatic to say the least! A definite improvement in the IQ's of the gotu kola group was evidenced, when compared to that of the children taking the placebo. Gotu kola increased the IQ by nearly 10% as compared to a measly 3% increase with the colored starch tablet. The following table gives the IQ's for each group, before and after the experiment.

Intelligent quotients of retarded children

Gotu Kola Group

Initial	Final
31.90	35.37
45.20	49.12
17.70	28.41
21.90	25.16
43.60	54.10
40.00	49.18
47.60	52.87

Initial	Final
37.00	46.50
27.70	34.01
16.70	18.58
41.60	53.06
33.30	43.54
24.00	31.05
33.00	47.15
23.10	30.14

Placebo Group

Initial	Final
37.80	48.89
22.20	24.04
26.60	28.04
44.04	48.09
37.50	38.09
76.60	76.42
41.60	46.26
39.30	43.27
24.40	27.32
41.60	44.90

Initial	Final
33.30	35.37
38.00	38.60
51.40	55.78
19.80	21.54

Other benefits were also noticed in the herb drug group. "Those children, who were very restless and fidgety became expressive, communicative and cooperative, after drug administration. The drug was also noted to have increased powers of concentration and attention."

Several possible explanations for the success of gotu kola in mental retardation may be found in other literature. *Medicinal Plants of the Philippines* by Eduardo Quisumbing mentions that gotu kola is "very rich in vitamin B" (p. 685). Some of the B vitamins such as thiamine, inositol, and niacin are especially helpful in the brain, where they seem to strengthen the memory. An earlier study by Dr. Rao published in another Indian medical journal, *Nagarjun* (120:33-41, June 1969) showed how gotu kola "brought about a steady increase in blood sugar levels" in normal healthy adults. This rise in blood sugar helps to provide the brain with more nourishment to function better. And an article published in the Italian medical journal *Minerva Cardioangiologica* (30:201-7, April 1982) told how gotu kola remarkably improved blood circulation in elderly patients suffering from chronic venous insufficiency. When the brain receives more blood, it gets an increase of oxygen, sugar, and B vitamins, all of which are vital for learning and thinking.

For general memory impairment, about 2-3 capsules of gotu kola are suggested each day with meals. But for more severe retardation problems, double or triple this amount may be necessary. In his first cited article, Dr. Rao also spoke of vitamin B-1 (15 mg. daily), vitamin E (1,200 I.U.) and glutamic acid. In regard to this particular glutamate amino acid, Drs. Eric R. Braverman and Carl C. Pfeiffer tell of 12 grams of glutamic acid given orally per day, helping a group of mentally retarded patients improve their "intellectual performance, alertness and attentiveness" in their book, *The Healing Nutrients Within*.

So we can gather from this information that when gotu kola is used either by itself or more preferably in conjunction with other nutrients, that dramatic improvements in the mental capabilities of retarded persons is evident.

Foods and Nutrients

Because blood sugar plays such a vital role in the maintenance of a strong memory, those junk or processed foods which are high in refined sugar should be eliminated from the diet, as they're liable to induce a state of hypoglycemia which is known to depress mental functions. (Consult the entry under HYPOGLYCEMIA in this book for additional dietary advice.)

MIGRAINES

See under HEADACHE for more information on this.

MISCARRIAGE

See under PREGNANCY for more information on this.

MOLES

Symptoms

Moles are dark or light brown, slightly raised spots, like permanent freckles, which usually start in youth and can eventually become large, hairy and rather unsightly.

Most of us have several moles all our lives, and they do no harm whatever. The best advice in such cases is to *leave them alone*! However, when a bluish-black mole starts growing or a normal one begins expanding in size, then *immediate* medical attention should be sought in promptly dealing with them, as they are often an early warning sign of skin cancer.

Relief Measures

Because of the unpredictable nature of moles, we suggest either leaving them alone if no growths are evident, or else letting a doctor look at them. *Under no circumstances should self-treatment of moles be attempted!*

Foods and Nutrients

Yellow dock, burdock, or sarsaparilla (3 capsules of any of these daily), vitamin C (3,500 mg.), niacin (100 mg. daily), potassium (1,600 mg. daily), and zinc (50 mg.

daily) may be of some assistance in preventing further moles from occurring.

MONONUCLEOSIS

See under FEVER, FLU, and INFECTION for more information on this.

MORNING AND MOTION SICKNESS

See under NAUSEA for more information on this.

MULTIPLE SCLEROSIS

Symptoms

Multiple Sclerosis or MS is a progressive, degenerative disorder of the central nervous system. The disease is variable in its progression and affects various parts of the nervous system by destroying the myelin sheaths which cover the nerves, causing an inflammatory response. Its symptoms include a staggering gait, blurred vision, dizziness, numbness, breathing difficulty, weakness, tremors, slurred speech, bladder and bowel problems, emotional problems, sexual impotence in men, and paralysis. MS usually occurs in persons between the ages of 25 and 40. The disease progresses slowly and may disappear for periods of time but usually returns intermittently, often in a more severe form.

Relief Measures/Foods and Nutrients

Sulphur is one of the key elements in the successful treatment of this malady. Foods high in this mineral should be consumed with frequency: cabbage, kale, kohlrabi, brussel sprouts, cauliflower, mustard greens, spinach, garlic, and onion. Wakunaga's Kyolic liquid aged-garlic extract (8 capsules daily) should be taken.

Evening primrose capsules (4 daily) are quite helpful, too.

The B vitamins are helpful, particularly in the form of brewer's yeast (1 tsp. twice daily). So is vitamin A (25,000 I.U.), D (600 I.U.), and E (1,200 I.U.). A non-acidic vitamin C (3,500 mg.) is useful, too. Long-term sufferers of MS won't do as well on supplements as young patients will.

Massage and exercise (swimming and stretching) are important for MS sufferers to have and practice.

MUMPS

Symptoms

Mumps is a viral infection that typically infects children between the ages of 3 and 16. However, it can occur after puberty. When it does, it often causes complications (such as sterility) in the ovaries and testes. The average incubation period of the virus is 18 days. The mumps patient is contagious any time from 48 hours before the symptoms commence to nearly a week after they've started. Symptoms include swelling of one or both of the parotid glands at the jaw angles below the ears, fever, sore throat, headache, and pain when swallowing or chewing..If the testicles are affected, they become swollen and painful; if the ovaries or pancreas are affected, abdominal pain results.

Relief Measures

One of the very best herbal treatments for mumps, measles, and chickenpox is mullein tea. Half cupfuls of the warm tea should be administered to a sick child every couple of hours. Additionally, warm and cool packs of this same herbal tea can be laid on the forehead, across the throat and chest, and under the back of the neck, to reduce swelling, inflammation, and fever.

The sick child should also be given copious amounts of cold catnip tea flavored with some honey and pure vanilla. A warm garlic enema is also advisable.

Foods and Nutrients

The sick child or teenager should be given liquid nourishment in the form of clear soups and juices. No solid foods such as red meat, bread, potatoes, or dairy products should be consumed during the peak of sickness. The stomach needs to rest and should be given only light, mild food to digest. No greasy, salty, or sugary foods should be consumed either as they will only hinder recovery.

Vitamin C is helpful here. A liquid or powdered vitamin C is preferable, although children's chewables may be given. Figure on administering about 500 mg. every 3 hours.

A young child should be given a zinc lozenge to suck on but not chew. If the child

is very young, make sure he or she doesn't swallow it whole and possibly choke on it.

Vitamins A (25,000 I.U. beta-carotene) and E (400 I.U.) are useful, too. Especially when taken with some Kyo-Dophilus (1 capsule twice daily) from Wakunaga (see Appendix).

MUSCLE CRAMPS

See under ABDOMINAL CRAMPS-PAIN AND SWELLING and LEG CRAMPS for more information on this.

MUSCULAR DYSTROPHY

Symptoms

There are five major and three less common types of muscular dystrophy, each with its own pathology; one form may affect persons at a specific age, another involves the degeneration of a specific muscle area in the body. Some forms may stop progressing, but so far none have gone into total remission. The disease is currently considered to be largely hereditary except for one type that occurs in adults around the age of 40 or 50.

Until the last decade (1980's), no one really understood why muscular dystrophy could be passed on from generation to generation. One speculation was that it could be due to an abnormally high genetic requirement for vitamin E, which is essential for the formation of the nucleus of every cell. But in late 1987, a Boston research team headed by Louis Kunkel of Harvard Medical

School identified the missing *protein* (called dystrophin) which starts a cascade of events leading to the characteristic muscle weakness of one type of this disease, Duchenne Muscular Dystrophy (DMD). DMD is an inherited disease carried by women and passed down to sons. Affected males experience progressive muscle wasting and usually die in their 20s.

Then just a year later, Israeli scientists discovered two different forms of this dystrophin protein: one in the muscle cells and another located in brain cells. Writing in the January 5, 1989 journal *Nature*, they pointed out that about 30% of DMD victims also suffer mental retardation as well. Several years later in the February 6, 1992 issue of *Nature,* three separate teams of gene hunters reported having found a gene defect responsible for adult muscular dystrophy. That condition is marked by muscle loss and weakness in early adulthood and results in death in their 50's or 60's when the heart and lungs fail. The defect causes a segment of gene coding to be repeated—much like repeating a word over and over in the middle of a sentence. The repeat causes instability of gene function; the more often the repeat, the more severe the symptoms. And the effect is magnified in succeeding generations.

Sometime before muscular dystrophy can be detected, amino acids and a substance called creatine are lost in the urine. This indicates that muscle tissue is breaking down. The major symptom is great weakness in the legs and back, so that the patient has trouble walking. The weakness gradually progresses throughout the muscles of the body, creating partial, then total paralysis.

Relief Measures/Foods and Nutrients

The diet of a person with muscular dystrophy should be adequate in all the essential nutrients including proteins and vegetable oils most of all. In the early stages, muscular wasting can be arrested and remissions prolonged. In others, the disease may not worsen and often improvement, including muscle strength, can be observed without complete recovery.

Nuts, seeds, and legumes are very rich in the proteins needed for the partial remission of MD. Among these, the authors recommend nuts like almonds, Brazils, cashews, and pecans, seeds such as sunflower, and legumes like lentils. Certain seed oils (olive, sunflower and sesame) are very helpful if taken each day (1 tbsp. of any of these).

Two nutrients which work very well together for MD are selenium and vitamin E oil. According to the journal, *Acta Medica Scandinavica* (219:407-14, No. 4, 1986), MD patients treated with daily doses of selenium (0.2-1.3 mg.) and vitamin E oil (100-600 I.U.) for almost 2-3 years showed remarkable improvements in their grip strength and ability to perform physical tasks, as well as an increased capacity for exercise.

The B vitamin choline (500 mg.), liquid lecithin (1 tsp.), and an unsaturated fatty acids complex (3 capsules) taken each day is essential for muscle improvement.

MYASTHENIA GRAVIS

Symptoms

Myasthenia Gravis affects muscles in any part of the body but most often the muscles of the face and neck. In the disease, there is an underproduction of acetylcholine, a compound that transmits nerve impulses to the muscles. It is characterized by exhaustion and progressive paralysis. Symptoms include double vision, drooping eyelids, choking, and difficulty in breathing, swallowing, and talking (imperfect articulation, stammering, and stuttering).

Relief Measures/Food and Nutrients

The following supplement program was worked out independently by one of the authors, who is a medical doctor for this disorder. But the other author, who is a medical anthropologist has made a couple of contributions of his own. When put together, it represents an excellent nutritional therapy for Myasthenia Gravis sufferers.

Manganese	15 mg.
Vitamin E	400-800 I.U.
Vitamin C	2,500 mg.
Brewer's yeast	1 tsp.
Vitamin B	2 tablets
Rex's wheat germ oil	1 tsp.
Vitamin D	400 I.U.
Liquid lecithin	1 tbsp.
Calcium	600 mg.
Unsaturated fatty acids	3 tablets

Everything can be purchased in any healthfood store or nutrition center, with the exception of the Rex's wheat germ oil. This is only available at a veterinary or animal livestock supply house.

Avocados are particularly suited for this type of ailment.

MYOCARDIAL INFARCTION

See under **HEART ATTACK** for more information on this.

NAIL PROBLEMS

Symptoms

Nails are composed almost entirely of protein. Abnormal or unhealthy nails may be the result of a local injury, a glandular deficiency such as hypothyroidism, or a deficiency of certain nutrients.

A protein deficiency can cause opaque white bands to appear on the nails or cause them to become dry, brittle, and very thin. Insufficient amounts of complete proteins and/or vitamin A slow down the rate of nail growth (which is also affected by various drugs). A shortage of vitamin A or calcium in the diet may also cause dryness and brittleness. A lack of the B vitamins causes nails to become fragile, with horizontal or vertical ridges appearing. The B complex is also a factor in fungus infestation found underneath the nails. Frequent hangnails usually indicate an inadequate intake of vitamins C and folic acid and protein. An iron deficiency can disturb the growth of the nails, causing dryness, brittleness, thinning, flattening, and eventually the appearance of moon-shaped nails. White spots can be caused by a zinc deficiency.

Oriental doctors have long looked at the nails of their patients for signs to indicate metabolic disturbances within their bodies. Such changes in nail appearance could mean the presence of a disease long before it shows up in the rest of the system. The following table gives readers a brief rundown on what various changes could indicate.

THICK NAILS—Weakened vascular system and poor blood circulation.

BLUE ON WHITE MOON AREA OF THE NAIL—Possible overexposure to silver or lung difficulties.

RED ON WHITE MOON AREA OF THE NAIL—Possible coronary problems.

BRITTLE NAILS—Iron deficiency; thyroid problems; impaired kidney function; circulatory disorders.

FLAT NAILS—Raynaud's disease.

YELLOW NAILS—Lymphatic system congestion; respiratory disorders; diabetes; liver trouble.

WHITE NAILS—Liver or kidney dysfuctions; possible anemia.

DARK NAILS THIN, FLAT, SPOON-SHAPED NAILS—Vitamin anemia; B-1 2 deficiency.

DEEP BLUE NAIL BEDS—Pulmonary obstruction like asthma or emphysema.

NAIL BEADING—Rheumatoid arthritis.

PITTED RED-BROWN SPOTS FRAYED AND SPLIT ENDS —Psoriasis.

CHIPPED, PEELED, CRACKED, OR EASILY BROKEN NAILS—Nutritional deficiency; insufficient hydrochloric acid, protein, minerals.

BRITTLE, SOFT, SHINY NAILS WITHOUT A MOON—Overactive thyroid.

WHITE LINES ACROSS THE NAIL—Liver disease.

THINNING NAILS—Itchy skin disease.

NAILS SEPARATED FROM THE NAIL BED—Thyroid disorder.

HALF-WHITE NAIL WITH DARK SPOTS ON THE TIP—Possible kidney disease.

RAISED NAILS AT BASE WITH SMALL WHITE ENDS —Respiratory disorder (emphysema or chronic bronchitis). May be hereditary nail condition.

RED SKIN AT THE BOTTOM OF THE NAIL—Connective tissue disorder.

RIDGES—Influenza.

DOWNWARD CURVED NAIL—Possible heart, liver, or respiratory problems.

WHITE LINES—Possible heart disease, elevated fever, or arsenic poisoning.

RIDGES RUNNING UP AND DOWN THE NAILS—Tendency to develop arthritis.

NAILS THAT RESEMBLE HAMMERED BRASS—Tendency toward partial or total air loss.

UNUSUALLY WIDE, SQUARE NAILS—Horrible hormonal imbalance.

WHITE NAILS WITH PINK NEAR THE TIPS—Cirrhosis of the liver.

Relief Measures

Do not expose the hands to excessive soap and water, or else the nail may become loose from the nail bed. Water causes the nails to swell, and they shrink when dry, resulting in loose and brittle nails.

Don't cut cuticles. While fashionable in some quarters, this uncovering of the nails is harsh and irritating, causing infection. Use Johnson & Johnson Baby Oil or lanolin lotion and gently push them back. If you have diabetes, consult your physician if the cuticles become inflamed, because the infection can spread.

Don't repeatedly immerse your hands in water that contains harsh detergents or unfriendly chemicals. This usually results in the splitting of the nails. Discolored nails can be caused by prolonged illness, stress, nicotine, allergies, or even diabetes.

Apply a base coat before putting on any nail polish to prevent yellowing. If nails are green, it could mean a bacterial or fungal infection has set in, which can separate the nail from the bed. Apply Wakunaga's Kyolic liquid aged-garlic extract around the finger tips.

Wear cotton-lined gloves when doing housework such as dishes and laundry or when cleaning the bathroom or using furniture polish. This protects your hands and nails against abrasive chemicals.

The herb called horsetail or shavegrass is very high in silicon. Silicon is considered to be a "beauty" mineral for maintaining the health and integrity of the nails, the hair, and the skin. About 3 capsules daily with meals is suggested where some nail problems may be prevalent.

Foods and Nutrients

One of the authors recalls a recent Jane Doe case of a woman aged 55 who came to see him about her nails. They were brittle and badly chipped. He put her on the following nutritional program, and within a couple of weeks her nails looked beautiful and healthy once more. She took: Knox unflavored gelatin (1 tsp. in juice every morning); soybean protein (1 tsp. powder in juice every afternoon); emulsified vitamin A (50,000 I.U. fish oil); brewer's yeast (1 tsp. every evening in juice); Wakunaga's Kyo-Green (1 tbsp. at noon in juice or water); oatstraw tea (1 cup in the evening with dinner); and vitamin C with bioflavonoids (3,500 mg.).

Additionally, she was instructed to consume more egg yolks, cooked oatmeal, Brazil and cashew nuts, millet, and sunflower seeds. While some advocate a calcium-magnesium supplement, in her case this author didn't feel it was necessary.

NAUSEA AND VOMITING

Symptoms

Nausea is a sick feeling produced within the stomach that leads the sufferer to want to vomit. Nausea can be due to:

- the wrong kinds of food (too much, too fatty, spicy, or hot, with too much alcohol);

- hypersensitivity to specific foods (shellfish or pork;

- prescription and over-the-counter medications (antibiotics, sulpha drugs, aspirin, emetics, expectorants);

- poisonous agents (household cleaners);

- stomach disorders (gastritis, ulcers, cancer, gastrointestinal bleeding, hiatul hernia);

- anxiety or other emotional disturbances;

- migraine headaches;

- trouble inside the skull affecting the vomiting center in the brain (injury, abscess, tumor, meningitis, bleeding);

- travel or motion sickness;

- mountain sickness due to high altitudes;

- early pregnancy;

- commencement of some feverish illness (mumps, measles);

- jaundice;

- general illnesses (pernicious anemia, Addison's disease, thyroid disorder);

- acidosis in young children.

Relief Measures

While the authors do not advocate the consumption of colas or soft drinks, because of their high sugar, phosphoric acid, and artificial additive contents, they believe there is a small therapeutic role for them when it comes to treating nausea. A pharmacist named Robert Warren, who heads the Pharmacy Services at Valley Children's Hospital in Fresno, California, uses coke syrup to help settle the upset stomachs of children (1-2 tsps.) and adults (1-2 tbsps.).

Or choose a non-cola soft drink such as 7-UP. One of the authors knows of a doctor in Phoenix, Arizona, who advises all of his patients to drink a little 7-UP, Canada Dry, or ginger ale if they feel nauseous. But he insists that they let such carbonated drinks stand until flat and lukewarm before drinking.

Certain herbal teas help bring relief to an upset stomach. Lukewarm cups of spearmint, catnip, chamomile or lemon balm will settle even the most queasy stomachs.

Powdered ginger root capsules are also good for preventing nausea and vomiting. An article in the medical journal, *Lancet* (1:655, March 20, 1982) reported how powdered ginger root proved superior over dramamine (a standard anti-nausea medicine) in reducing motion sickness in three dozen college undergraduates who had been subjected to minutes of high speed and jerking motions in a tilted rotating chair especially devised for this experiment. Two or three capsules of ginger root taken at once will calm an agitated gut nicely.

Orientals have known for many centuries that acupuncture is an effective, drugless, and painless way to treat various health problems. Acupressure is a modified version of this without the benefit of the needles. Just apply pressure to the webbing between your thumb and index finger on either hand. Use firm, deep pressure, and a rapid massaging movement for several minutes. And we don't mean to caress it either, but to exert *hard* pressure. Then using the same type of motion and pressure, rub with your thumb or thumbnail on the top of your foot between the tendons of the second and third toes.

Foods and Nutrients

Cool papaya, mango, or apple juice or apple cider will relieve nausea if *sipped* slowly through a straw.

If your stomach is suffering from the heebie-jeebies, try munching on some dry toast or graham crackers.

Take some Kyo-Dophilus capsules (3) from Wakunaga, if the nausea is due to indigestion.

But ultimately the best way to stop nausea is just to allow the body to discharge whatever is in the stomach that is making you sick. The nausea leaves at once, and after a good upchuck you'll probably be feeling a lot better for having done it, than trying to keep the irritating substance inside.

NECK PAIN

Symptoms

Neck pain is a discomfort which is often attributed to poor sitting posture. It comes about when the head is kept in an awkward position, that is, pushed forward with the ears in front of the shoulders for many hours at a time, either through driving long stretches or else typing at a desk all day.

Obviously, some people are more prone to neck pain than others because of their particular occupations. Besides secretaries and truck drivers, there are beauticians, carpenters, roofing specialists, plumbers, those who lay carpet or tile, gardeners and landscape experts, chiropractors, and surgeons. All of these professions demand quite a bit of bending over, which can make the neck hurt after a while.

Relief Measures

An ice pack or ice wrapped in a towel is a good choice when stiffness is just settling in. If your neck has been slightly injured, ice can help hold down swelling. After ice has reduced any inflammation, heat is a wonderful soother—be it from a heating pad or a hot shower.

Over-the-counter anti-inflammatories such as aspirin from your local drug store or white oak bark or white willow bark capsules (3 at a time) from any health food store should help reduce pain and swelling.

Good posture is important at all times. When walking, keep your head level but pull your chin in, as if you were making a double chin. Also avoid having your head lowered all the time when working at a desk or reading. This will prevent stressing the muscles in the back of the neck. If you work with a video display terminal all day, it's important to have it positioned at eye level. If you force yourself to look up or down hour after hour, you may cause your neck to spasm. And consider putting down the telephone. If you talk on the phone a great deal, especially while attempting to write things on a memo pad, you've got your neck in an awkward position—surely an invitation to pain and stiffness. Also, if you sit in a chair that doesn't give you good back support, you increase your chances of worsening any existing neck problems and maybe even causing new ones. Actually, you're a lot better off if you roll up a towel and then place it against the small of your back when sitting. It will better align your spine and give you much firmer support. Always be sure to sleep on a firm mattress, too, since one that sags can cause a lot of neck problems or worsen

existing conditions. If you have neck pain, you may be better off by tossing your pillow aside and sleeping with your head flat to the mattress instead. By implementing any of these suggestions, your body will have better posture, whether in an upright or reclined position.

Just as the feet need rest from constant standing, the neck needs arest from constant sitting. Your head weighs about 8 punds, and that's quite a bit of weight for the neck to support without much help from the rest of your body. So periodically stand up and walk around. Here are some simple exercises to do for combatting stiffness and preventing neck pain in the future. Do each one a minimum of five times a day. Do the first three exercises for two weeks before starting the rest.

1. Slowly tilt your head forward as far as possible. Then move your head backward as far as possible.

2. Tilt your head toward your shoulder, while keeping your shoulder stationary. Straighten up, then lean toward the other shoulder.

3. Slowly turn your head from side to side as far as possible.

4. Place your hand on one side of your head wiile you push toward it with your head. Hold for five seconds, then relax. Repeat three times. Then do the same exercise on the other side.

5. Do basically the same exercise as above, only provide slight resistance to the front of your head while you push your head forward. Then provide slight resistance to the

back of your head while you push your head backward.

6. Hold light weights—say 3 to 5 pounds—in your hands while shrugging your shoulders. Keep your arms straight as you do this.

CAUTION: The authors remind readers that any whiplash injury resulting from an auto accident, requires the immediate care of a skilled physician *first,* and then a competent and qualified chiropractor *secondly.* Such severe neck pain can be treated with an ice pack instead of heat until proper medical attention can be given to it. Ice will reduce the swelling, but heat only inflames the injury more.

Foods and Nutrients

Pantothenic acid (130 mg.) and PABA (100 mg.)—two of the B-complex vitamin group, as well as calcium (800 mg.), magnesium (1,600 mg.), manganese (75 mg.), and zinc (100 mg.) will help to relieve much of the suffering which accompanies neck pain, when they are taken on a daily basis until the problem is entirely corrected.

NEPHRITIS

See **BRIGHT'S DISEASE** for more information on this.

NERVOUSNESS

Symptoms

Nervousness is a condition brought on by stressful situations over which we have little or no control, and by anxious feelings due to worrying or to expectations not yet realized. One of the authors was personally acquainted with the late Canadian epedimiolo gist, Hans Selye, N.D. of Montreal. He said that stress can be good and, in. fact, quite useful if properly manajed. But poorly handled stress, which he termed *dis*tress, can cause profound health changes that aren't always nice.

Typical symptoms of nervousness include irritability, high blood pressure, headaches and neckaches, diarrhea, dizziness, loss of appetite, ulcers, colitis, heartburn, insomnia, and depression. A state of prolonged nervousness eventually tires the body, weakens the immune system, creates hypertension, raises serum cholesterol and triglyceride levels beyond normal, affects the performance of the heart, and can even disturb routine cell division just enough to possibly cause cancer later on.

Relief Measures

Physical activity is always good to clear the mind and keep stress under control. Running, walking, swimming, golfing, or engaging in team sports of some kind such as basketball or soccer, are good outlets for releasing nervous frustrations. Sometimes even playing those games which require a great deal of mental effort (chess, checkers, poker, Monopoly, Risk) can be effective enough to relieve pent-up tensions for a while.

Meditation with or without yoga exercises is another way to relax the nerves. Closing the eyes, laying back in a chair or on a couch or bed under quiet circumstances, and slowly focusing the mind on something wonderful and pleasant, is comparable to having your nerves "massaged."

In fact, physical massage with warm and aromatic herb oils is, indeed, a delightful treat for the body. The oils of lavender or sandalwood penetrating through the skin and the rubbing and gentle squeezing of the muscles, sends chemical signals of relief and peace to high-strung nerves, which soothe and caress them in a very special way.

Getting plenty of rest provides the body with nourishment of a different kind, just as food does for energy and stamina. Sleep causes everything within the system to slow down dramatically for a period of hours. It is during this time that the body can heal itself and recuperate from the tensions and labors of the previous day. A nervous system this well rested experiences a renewal of itself that couldn't do otherwise. It's safe to say, that restful naps in the afternoon and night-time sleep does more for the nerves than any exercise, diet, herbs, or food supplements might hope to accomplish.

More frequent and short-term weekend vacations doing things you obviously enjoy, are better for the body than the customary annual one or two weeks at the most. Also finding a hobby you like and devoting some of your spare time to it, is another way to relieve the stress that bothers your nerves.

Herbs such as catnip or chamomile make refreshing and delicious teas (2 cups daily of either) when sipped while warm; so does peppermint, spearmint, and lavender. Or valerian or hops in capsule form (3 at a time of either) can help relax the body. All of these plants have compounds within them which exert a tranquilizing influence upon the central nervous system for up to five hours at a time.

Foods and Nutrients

Around each and every nerve of your body is a fatty, protein coating called myelin sheathing. This substance insulates the nerves from infection and helps to preserve their conductive integrity. But when they are subjected to too much adrenalin, produced by an excited body, or too much sugar from an abundant consumption of sweet things, then their protective coating begins to wear away in various places. When this happens, the nerves cannot adequately transmit all of the signals which the brain sends through them to different parts of the body. They also tend to become somewhat irritated and sore much like your big or little toes would be if confined to a tight-fitting shoe for very long.

But there is a combination of several nutrients which will assist the body in rebuilding myelin sheathing that has worn away from any of the nerves. High-potency vitamin B-complex (4 tablets), liquid lecithin (2 tsps.), vitamin E oil (800 I.U.), calcium (800 mg.), magnesium (1,600 mg.), extra pantothenic acid (400 mg.), and the amino acid L-Tyrosine (1,000 mg.) taken daily with citrus or papaya or pineapple juices for better assimilation is recommended.

NEURALGIA

Symptoms

Neuralgia is a painful disease that strikes without warning, usually at middle age or older in men and women. The smallest stimuli can trigger it for no apparent reason—shaving, jarring, a cold draft, or eating very hot or cold food. Only one side of the face at a time seems to be affected by this: bouts of lancing pain in the temple, jaw, teeth or ear, accompanied by twitching of the face, occasional flushing, or infrequent watering of one eye, one nostril, or the mouth.

Relief Measures

During an attack, it's best to drink liquids through a straw. Make sure they are either lukewarm or cool, never hot or cold. Apply an analgesic such as Mentholatum Deep-Heat Rub or Ben-Gay to the affected area, but keep such materials away from the eyes. The application of warm or cool packs may also help.

Foods and Nutrients

Folic acid. (400 mg.), ziacin (400 mg.), vitamin C (1,500 mg.), rutin (200 mg.), phosphorus (1,200 mg.), copper (4 mg.), and potassium (2,000 mg.) all seem to be of definite benefit for neuralgia.

NEURITIS

Symptoms

Neuritis is the inflammation or deterioration of a nerve or set of nerves. Symptoms can usually vary with the cause. Typical symptoms include pain, tenderness, tingling and loss of the sensation of touch in the affected nerve area, redness and swelling of the affected areas, and in severe cases, convulsions.

Causes of neuritis include injury to a nerve, such as in a direct blow or a nearby bone fracture; infection involving a nerve; diseases like sugar diabetes, gout, and the blood cancer, leukemia; chemical poisoning of the system by lead, mercury, or methyl alcohol; and vitamin B deficiency, especially of thiamine.

Relief Measures/Foods and Nutrients

Organically grown foods devoid of pesticides and unprocessed foods without chemical preservatives in them should be consumed as much as possible until this condition has passed.

Those supplements with their respective Juices listed uider NERVOUS-NESS should be taken here on a regular basis.

A mild food fast on the weekend, and internal cleansing with enemas and herbal teas like sarsaparilla, red clover, burdock, or yellow dock (up to three 8 fl. oz. glasses a day) should be periodically undertaken to flush out harmful chemical residues from the body.

NIGHT BLINDNESS

Symptoms

Night blindness is the inability for some people to visually adapt to the dark within moments as the majority of us can. Such individuals, when driving along the road at night and seeing the headlights of an oncoming car in the opposite lane of traffic, will be temporarily blinded for a couple of minutes to the point of not being able to see any reassuring road stripes, reflective signs or even dimly perceived shoulders. They will have to brake and pull over until they can again make out familiar objects in the dark. Or when going into a theater after the movie has already started, they're very apt to be groping around for an empty seat, often bumping shins and spilling popcorn in the process.

Relief Measures

Back in the mid-1950s, a German medical doctor discovered that dandelion flowers were quite effective in treating night blindness in some of his patients. As reported in the *Journal of The American Medical Association*, it briefly mentioned the success he had with this herb, but said nothing about how it was administered.

The authors think that the best way to take the flowers, after picking them in the spring or Summer and washing them good, is in juice form. Either run them through a juicer or else liquefy them in a food processor with enough water. Because they're apt to be bitter, we recommend that they be mixed with a secondary juice such as carrot or pineapple. One half cup twice daily is sufficient.

Foods and Nutrients

Foods which are high in vitamin A and zinc should be consumed regularly. Vitamin A-rich foods include fresh-or saltwater fish, fish oil, green and yellow fruits and vegetables, and dairy products. Zinc-rich foods include brewer's yeast, liver, seaweed, soybeans, spinach, sunflower seeds, mushrooms, and raisins. Additional amounts of A (50,000 I.U.) and Zinc (100 mg.) should also be taken *together*.

NIGHTMARES

Symptoms

A psychologist once described your typical nightmare as "an ordinary dream gone bad about which you can do nothing except wake up and scream like hell!" Usually a physiological condition of some kind produces nightmares when you sleep—hypoglycemia, hormonal imbalances, neurosis, alcoholism, drug addiction, or junk food consumption.

Relief Measures

One of the authors remembers his Hungarian grandmother using *warm* catnip tea as an effective antidote to *prevent recurring nightmares*. He has tested this out for himself on several different subjects in the past, with satisfactory results. He recommends one cup of tea for children under twelve years of age, and two cups for an adult, about an hour before retiring.

Foods and Nutrients

Some therapists who've treated patients suffering from horrific nightmares and other psychoses have advised them to take high-potency B-complex (3 tablets) and phosphorus (500 mg.) together. This combination of nutrients is reported to have helped about 40% of the time.

NOCTURNAL EMISSIONS

Symptoms

Nocturnal emissions are infrequent discharges of semen occurring periodically with the male species, most often at night while sleeping. They are usually prompted by dreams of some kind, and generally happen after considerable time has elapsed between moments of sexual activity.

They are nature's way of helping the body to release extra accumulations of sperm. This is by far a more natural and healthier process, than anything which may be mechanically induced to achieve the same results. While most medical books today speak favorably of and even encourage the practice of masturbation, too much of it over an extended time can be very detrimental to the central nervous system.

Relief Measures/Foods and Nutrients

For practical health reasons, nocturnal emissions are certainly preferable to masturbation. As such, they should be allowed to continue whenever the body feels it's time to release more of this fluid from the reproductive organs.

Nocturnal emissions temporarily cease sometimes when there is an accumulation of too much uric acid in the bloodstream. This comes from overconsumption of red meat. Also too much phosphoric acid in the system from the excessive drinking of soft drinks and colas, can retard this natural process. Intake of such items needs to be more carefully monitored and modified.

A few homeopathic doctors think that if men took some animal glandular preparations, that this might assist them in having more frequent emissions on their own. But this is more anecdotal than clinical they say. Also the routine use of vitamin E oil (1,200 I.U.) and zinc (100 mg.) may help restore this sometimes embarrassing but very necessary part of nature to a man's physical functions.

NOSEBLEEDS

Symptoms

Nosebleeds are commonly caused by physical injury, such as a blow to the nose. Excessive dryness (causing the nasal membranes to crack, form crusts, and bleed), sudden change in atmospheric pressure, scratching with the fingernail, or blowing the nose too forcefully can also cause injury to the nasal lining.

There are two kinds of nosebleeds: anterior and posterior. A posterior type is quite common to the elderly, especially those suffering from hypertension. This nosebleed originates in the back of the nose and runs down the back of the mouth into the throat no matter what position the person is in at the time. If severe, it can flow in both directions at once. This nosebleed is critical and demands prompt medical attention.

The anterior nosebleed is the routine kind and flows from the front part of the nose. If one stands or sits, the flow of blood comes out of one or both nostrils. When lying down, it may go back into the throat. While frightening because of the obvious sight of blood, it isn't serious and can be self-treated in most cases.

Relief Measures

There are five basic steps to stopping an anterior nosebleed. First of all, blow all the clots out of both sides of the nose. Secondly, sit up in a chair and lean forward. Thirdly, put a small piece of gauze inside the nostril(s), then pinch all the soft parts of the nose together between your thumb and index finger. Hold for five minutes. Next, apply some crushed ice and cold washcloths to the nose, neck, and cheek. And finally, lay back and refrain from any activity for a few hours and any intensive exercise for at least several days.

Sometimes increasing room humidity helps to check recurring nosebleeds of this type. A vaporizer is good for this. Temporarily going off of prescription (Coumadin, or Heparin) or over-the-counter (aspirin) medications may help to stop the frequency of nosebleeds, since these items tend to thin the blood. When the nasal membranes become sore from dry air, dip a cotton Q-tip into some comfrey ointment or aloe vera gel and insert into the nostril(s). Or wet the Q-tip end and dip it into some white

oak bark powder, before putting into the nose.

Foods and Nutrients

The bioflavonoids, rutin and hesperidin, are useful for controlling nosebleeds. About 300 mg. of either every other day is suggested. Also foods rich in vitamin K are essential for blood clotting: alfalfa, kale, and all dark green leafy vegetables. Those prone to nosebleeds often should see a doctor and not use garlic or ginger, as they interfere with normal clotting action.

OBESITY

Symptoms

Since so many people are currently overweight, most doctors now consider obesity—a state of excess body fat—to be another *major disease*! Anyone who is 20% over the norm for their age, build, and height can be medically regarded as having this disease to some extent. Symptoms of this disease are more likely to be other diseases: kidney dysfunction, heart disease, diabetes, hypertension, abnormal pregnancies, depression, liver damage, colitis, diverticulitis, and constipation.

Relief Measures

The very best way to lose weight and *keep it off permanently,* is by exercising regularly. A brisk walk before breakfast turns up your "fat thermostat" inside just enough to "burn up" some excess fat. And if you work in an office building, using the stairs instead of the elevator before going to lunch, will set off another chemical combustion to "melt away" additional fat. But if you want to make an even more impressive dent in your weight loss for that day, try some bicycling, swimming or a fast game of racquetball or tennis before eating dinner.

Just 10-15 minutes a day of walking, climbing *down* stairs, and some other intensive physical activity at night, is equivalent to turning on your body furnace so more stored fat can be oxidized. Scientists who specialize in weight control find that doing these simple exercises *before* a meal resets your fat thermostat more quickly to a higher degree of combustive action.

It's not only *what* you eat that will keep you thin, but also *how* you eat as well. Fiberous foods that require a lot of chewing and take longer to digest, is what should occupy at least one-third of your daily diet. Celery, carrots, radishes, whole grain breads, nuts, seeds, and apples are some of these items. Put less food on your plate. Take smaller bites and learn to chew *very slowly*. By doing so, each mouthful will become thoroughly shredded and mixed with adequate saliva to facilitate better digestion. Saliva has tremendous enzyme action to it, which not only helps the stomach to break down food more completely but also satisfies the appetite longer so that the body doesn't become as hungry so often.

Obese people need to fast at least once a month. The best time to do this is on a weekend when you can rest and relax and not have much heavy physical activity. Mild foods such as fruit and vegetable juices, soups and broths, and cooked cereals are recommended over other foods. A lot of liquid should be consumed during this time.

Such a short fast will enable the body to discharge more of its accumulated toxins, and actually help to set the stage for even greater weight loss in the weeks to come when the proposed exercises and eating program are implemented. Diabetics need to have their doctors' advice when fasting, and hypoglycemics should never fast without using a good soybean, spirulina, or chlorella protein supplement.

One of the authors is a medical anthropologist. He ha.s a friend, Dr. Vaughn 11. Bryant, who is chairman of the Dept. of Anthropology at Texas A & M University. Some years ago Dr. Bryant received considerable media attention nationwide for his revolutionary "Cave Man Diet Program," which he himself lost over 30 lbs. on. Several unique aspects to this prehistoric "diet plan" are:

-Never eat three big meals, but divide them up into 5 or 6 smaller ones.

-Learn to live on healthy snacks instead of regular meals. Cave people were always munching on nuts or seeds and nibbling on fruit or berries.

-Develop a "cud" made from 1 or 2 small pieces of celery stick, around which have been tightly wrapped a number of parsley sprigs. Put these into the back of your mouth and *very slowly* grind them up with your molars. But instead of totally shredding and swallowing them, keep them in your mouth as long as possible, giving them an occasional chew every now and then and moving them about with your tongue. Prehistoric people observed wild animals like deer doing this, and adapted the practice for themselves; it kept them pretty trim as a result.

Foods and Nutrients

Stay away from animal fat and sweets. Studies conducted with obese-prone rats and overweight college students, have determined that not only do fats and sugars put on the pounds, but they also create *addictions* in the brain towards foods that are greasy and sweet. Such addictions prompt people to consume more of those bad things that will add to their weight, and less of what is good that will help them be slender.

Animal fat is found principally in butter, cream, ice cream, whole milk, rich dressings, mayonnaise, and fried foods. Sweets include candies, soft drinks, colas, pies, cakes, cookies, doughnuts, pastries, jams, and jellies.

And try to stay away from white flour products, salt, white rice, or processed foods as much as possible. Remember, too, that fast food restaurants contribute more towards obesity than supermarkets sometimes do.

Learn to eat more complex carbohydrates that also offer quality protein. Such foods might include fresh or salt-water fish (with fins and scales; no shellfish), whole. grain cereals and breads, brown or wild rice, beans, sunflower seeds, Idaho or Maine baked potatoes (without the sour cream, butter, cheese, or bacon bits on top), lentils, and tofu.

Get into the habit of eating *before* you go shopping. Food psychologists have learned that when people shop in a large supermarket on an empty stomach, they will be more inclined to buy those forbidden foods that send. their weight into the stratosphere.

Instead of sugar, use barley malt sweetener, pure maple syrup (from Vermont or Quebec, Canada), honey, or blackstrap molasses. These generally contain far less calories, have more vitamins and minerals in them, and are certainly a lot healthier for you, too. By the way, it may be worth mentioning in passing that rats and mice will *not* touch white sugar *at alll*! Smart rodents they are!

Herb teas (chamomile, peppermint, spearmint, linden) mixed with unsweetened fruit juices (pear, apple, papaya) are very satisfying low-calorie drinks and are also very filling. Use them between meals and whenever a desire for sweets comes over you.

Unsalted and unbuttered popcorn, raw peanuts, and raw sunflower seeds make some very fine and tasty snacks, which satisfy the appetite.

Certain foods and powdered herbs will fill you up for at least 5 or 6 hours. They are cooked oatmeal, buckwheat pancakes, seven-grain toast (lightly buttered), glucomannan (3 tablets or capsules every couple of hours), and psyllium seed hulls (4 capsules every few hours or 1 tbsp. in an 8 fl. oz. glass of water every 3 hours).

Kyo-Green from Wakunaga (1 full glass in the morning), liquid or granulated lecithin (about 1 tbsp.), amino acid complex

(2 capsules), evening primrose oil (3 capsules in the afternoon), vitamin C (3,500 mg.), B-complex (2 tablets), vitamin E oil (800 I.U.), magnesium (1,600 mg.) and calcium (800 mg.) should be used regularly.

OILY HAIR AND OILY SKIN

Symptoms

Oily hair is a scalp condition in which the sebaceous glands located at the base of every hair shaft produce an excess amount of sebum, the fatty "oil" in oily hair. Generally speaking, the more hair (or the finer the hair is), the more oil glands there are; and the more oil glands, the more oil there is apt to be.

The texture of the hair really does make a big difference. Oil sticks onto fine, straight hair quite easily. Blondes with silky, baby-fine hair tend to have the worst problems with oiliness; they may have up to 140,000 oil glands on their scalps, while redheads may average about 85,000 oil glands per head.

Oily skin is often a hereditary condition of surface greasiness, but can also be attributed to environmental considerations (protection against exposure to excessive sunlight) or vitamin deficiencies (low levels of riboflavin or B-2). Hormones can also be a factor as well. Pregnant women sometimes notice an increase in skin oil as hormonal activity changes. So do women taking certain types of birth control pills. Stress can even kick the oil glands into overdrive. The wrong cosmetics can easily aggravate an otherwise mild case of oily skin. And teenagers are very prone to oily skin, thanks in large part to their constant diet of junk food.

Relief Measures

Since intense heat and humidity can accelerate oil production, it may become necessary to shampoo hair twice a day, once in the morning and again in the evening sometime. Choose clear shampoos because they have less goo in them, and can clean oil away better without leaving a filmy residue behind. Massage the scalp during shampooing. For really oily hair, figure on doing a double-shampoo, leaving both on the scalp for at least five minutes a piece.

After rinsing with water, do a second rinse with beer or vodka, since alcohol of any kind is famous for cutting grease. Then rinse again with plain water. Afterwards, apply a mixture (equal parts) of tincture of witch hazel and Listerine antiseptic mouthwash. Work into the scalp thoroughly with the fingertips. If your scalp is especially oily, then apply this mixture each time you shampoo. It should help keep those oil glands from over-producing.

Two other terrific rinses for cutting the oiliness of your scalp is with citrus juice and apple cider vinegar. Squeeze the juice of two lemons into a quart of distilled or spring water. Or try adding a teaspoonful of vinegar in a pint of Perrier mineral water. Either one works great as a wonderful finishing rinse, removing soapy residue that can weigh down oily hair, and acting as a terrific tonic for the scalp.

Don't overbrush oily hair. Too much vigorous brushing will only carry more oil from the base roots to the ends of your hair. Learn to relax more, because mental and emotional stress of any kind tends to cause an overproduction of hormones within the body; and they, in turn, boost oil production in the scalp.

Clay masks or muds masks are useful for absorbing excess oil from the skin. Use a darker brown clay for this, because it seems to do a better job of cleansing the skin surface of any greasiness it may have at the time. Hot water to which has been added a little beer or alcohol makes a very good solvent for cutting oil when used in conjunction with plenty of soap. Two of the best skin degreasers for this are Ivory and Lava hand soaps.

After washing the face, apply an astringent of some kind to help tighten up the oil glands and remove any excess oil remaining. Acetone is a marvelous fat and grease solvent, and most astringents usually have some of it in them. If you use it regularly, you can probably remove most excess oil from your skin. One brand that contains acetone is called Seba-Nil. Ordinary rubbing alcohol or tincture of witch hazel also work well as astringents. Carry some astringent pads with you and use them throughout the day to cleanse your face, instead of always washing it with soap and water, which tends to dry and irritate the skin after a while.

Foods and Nutrients

One mineral essential for shiny hair and healthy looking skin is silicon. The herb horsetail or shave grass is rich in silicon. Take about two capsules daily with a meal for improving your hair and skin textures.

Some of the B vitamins are especially helpful for the hair and skin: B-1 (10 mg.), B-2 (10 mg.), B-6 (.50 mg.), biotin (500 mg.), choline (found in lecithin, 500 mg. or 1 tsp. liquid lecithin), inositol (500 mg.), niacin (200 mg.), pantothenic acid (100 mg.), and PABA (100 mg.).

People with oily hair or skin should cut down on their dietary intakes of fried and deep-fried foods, and chocolate (candy, milk, chips, cookies, and cake).

OSTEOPOROSIS

Symptoms

Osteoporosis is a reduction in the total mass of bone, with the remaining bone being fragile or "brittle." Osteoperoris generally affects women more than men, because the latter have 30% more bone mass than the former do. An estimated 24 million Americans currently are bothered with osteoporosis.

Estrogen deficiency is the leading cause of this deficiency in the menopausal female. Second to this is an inability to absorb sufficient amounts of calcium through the intestine or an imbalance between the ratios of calcium and phosphorus in the body.

Relief Measures

In his book *Preventing Osteoporosis*, Dallas physician and exercise authority, Kenneth Cooper, M.D., refers to osteoporosis as the "silent destroyer." He states that the weakening of bones can be going on for years or even decades without a person knowing it. Bone mass peak is achieved in the spine for most of us between the ages of 25 and 33 and in our long bones such as the hips from ages 35 to 40.

If you don't exercise regularly, you will definitely lose bone mass. In fact, some studies have shown that weight-bearing exercise can actually *increase* bone mass. Running is one of these, and walking is another; you should walk at least 20 minutes a day, 3-4 days a week to keep your bones in shape. Playing tennis or racquetball with *both* forearms instead of just the right one, will help to increase the density and size of the bones in each of them.

Dr. Cooper insists that no one is ever too old to exercise!

Foods and Nutrients

Get enough calciumin the diet! Calcium phosphate in milk is an excellent source. Low-fat cheeses and yogurts and skim milk are also high in calcium. Other calcium-rich foods include red salmon, sardines, nuts, and tofu. If you use a little apple cider vinegar—when preparing stock from bones, the vinegar will dissolve the calcium out of the bones. One pint of your soup then should equal about a quart of homogenized and pasturized milk in calcium content.

If you can't get enough calcium from these types of foods, then you may need to take a calcium supplement. Get one that has magnesium with it. Or better still, get separate supplements of each mineral and take a 2-to-1 ratio of magnesium (1,600 mg.) over calcium (800 mg.). Also be sure to include

adequate phosphorus (800-1,000 mg.) and vitamin D (400 I.U.) with them, since they are essential for the proper assimilation of calcium. Or eat foods rich in phosphorus (eggs, fish, grains, liver, yellow cheddar cheese) and vitamin D (salmon, sardines, tuna fish, egg yolks, milk and sunflower seeds).

Restrict alcohol, caffeine, red meat, fiber, and salt consumption as they tend to interfere with normal calcium utilization within the body.

PAGET'S DISEASE

Symptoms

Paget's Disease is a painful degeneration of the bones. Any bone in the body can be affected, but the most common sites are the long bones of the legs, the lower spine, the pelvis and the skull. In the early stages of the disease, calcium is removed from the bones, softening them. In later stages, the bones begin to grow again, but the new growth somehow becomes distorted. The bones remain soft and become abnormally thick.

Symptoms include a deep, dull, aching bone pain, headache, deafness, blindness, and bowed legs.

Relief Measures/Foods and Nutrients

An Australian physician, Dr. R. A. Evans of the Repatriation General Hospital in Concord, New South Wales, successfully used calcium supplements and a combination of medications designed to keep blood levels of calcium high in nine sufferers of Paget's Disease.

Searching for an alternative to expensive, hazardous drug treatment, Dr. Evans decided to try to raise the blood level of calcium in people with Paget's Disease. To do this, he gave them from 500-1,000 mg. of calcium 3 times daily between meals, an antacid tablet with meals to keep phosphorus from interfering with calcium absorption, and a drug to keep calcium from being excreted in the urine. The treatment lasted for over six months.

Dr. Evans discovered that the bone pain in his patients had either "subsided or was considerably reduced in eight of the nine after a period of 20 to 70 days..." The regimen mentioned here costs about 2% of the conventional drug treatment—injection of a thyroid hormone called calcitonin- and is certainly a lot safer because of its reduced side-effects.

PAIN

Symptoms

Pain is an unpleasant sensation associated with actual or potential tissue damage. It is mediated by specific nerve fibers to the brain where its conscious appreciation may be modified by a variety of factors.

Some of the more familiar types of pains are these:

-afterpains and birth pains—painful cramplike contractions of the uterus occur-

ring after childbirth, and uterine contractions occurring in childbirth.

-false pains—ineffective uterine contractions mimicking true labor.

-growing pains—aching pains experienced at night in the limbs of growing youngsters.

-hunger pains—cramps in the epigastrium associated with hunger.

-intermenstrual pain—pelvic discomfort occurring at the midpoint of the menstrual cycle.

-labor pains—rhythmical uterine contractions which under normal conditions increase in intensity, frequency, and duration, culminating in a vaginal delivery of an infant.

-nerve pain—neuralgia.

-organic pain—pain caused by an organic wound or injury to pathologically changed tissues; can include everything from bedsores and cysts to malignant tumors.

-phantom limb pain—an abnormal sensation often felt by amputees in which the surgically removed limb still seems to be present, and is commonly marked by burning, pricking, tickling, or tingling.

-psychogenic pain—pain which is usually correlated with a psychological, emotional, or behavioral stimulus.

-rest pain—pain occurring generally in the extremities during rest in the sitting or lying positon.

-soul pain—psychological pain of the mind or heart due to distress of some kind, noted especially in melancholia.

Relief Measures

There are different remedies for various types of pain. Any pains relating to pre or post-pregnancy conditions can be easily relieved with hot red raspberry leaf tea. About 1-2 cups every couple of hours during the last week of pregnancy and also for a week after delivery, is recommended.

Growing children may need extra magnesium, phosphorus and calcium in that order to relieve some of these pains. Foods rich in magnesium (bran, honey, green vegetables, nuts, seafood, spinach, and kelp), phosphorus (eggs, fish, grains, liver, poultry, and yellow cheese), and calcium (milk, cheese, molasses, yogurt, almonds, and liver) are suggested. Supplementation of these essential minerals for children under the age of twelve should be as follows: magnesium (300 mg.), phosphorus (600 mg.), and calcium (800 mg.).

Nerve and phantom limb pains can be best treated with those herbs in ointment or liniment form which exude a deep penetrating warmth and are highly aromatic. Eucalyptus, peppermint, and sandalwood oils come to mind, as well as tincture of witch hazel. Rubbing substances with any of these herbs in them or their respective oils on the skin or on the ends of amputated stumps, will usually bring quick relief as a rule.

Pains of the mind and heart, which are mentally and emotionally based, are best treated with a combination of herbal therapy and psychological counselling. Herbs such as chamomile or catnip, when slowly and leisurely sipped as warm teas flavored with honey, help to create more of a relaxed state in the system. And with the proper counselling from a trained therapist or even a good friend or close relative, a greater state of security can be achieved within that person who is thus disturbed.

Organic pain due to cancer may be temporarily relieved in some instances with herbs such as hops, catnip, valerian, skullcap, and white willow bark. They can be taken in liquid extract (up to 35 drops daily) or capsule (up to 8 a day) form. But their effects are somewhat limited and rather short-lived for the most part.

Foods and Nutrients

A medical research team at Temple University School of Dentistry in Philadelphia, reported over a decade ago in the medical journal, *Pain* (Vol. 11, no. 2, 1981) a definite connection between the amino acid tryptophan and pain tolerance. People who received tryptophan supplements were able to tolerate greater amounts of pain than were people who received nontherapeutic placebos. According to Samuel Seltzer, D.D.S., professor of dentistry and leader of the research team, subsequent studies have shown "very significant" increases in pain tolerance thresholds in patients with chronic pain who were placed on three-gram-daily tryptophan supplements for just one month.

"Most of these patients had suffered from dental, facial, and headache pain for years," Dr. Seltzer said. "They had made the rounds, but nobody was able to help them until we put them on tryptophan therapy. It was a 75% success. He encourages people to eat more soybeans, wheat germ, and sunflower and sesame seeds, which are high in tryptophan, but avoid corn because it is high in the amino acid leucine, which cancels out the pain-relieving effects of tryptophan.

One piece of medical research showed some years ago that when surgical patients and those with acute medical conditions, were placed on at least 1,000 mg. of magnesium each day, their levels of pain dropped drastically. And in 32 acutely ill medical patients reporting no pain, magnesium levels were normal; but in 28 patients with "pain as a major symptom," magnesium levels were well below normal. Similarly, in surgical patients undergoing elective surgery, magnesium levels were normal; however, in those undergoing acute surgery where pain was involved, magnesium levels were "significantly lower than normal" both before and after surgery, stated the August, 1980 issue of *Biochemical Medicine*.

Other things which can help to relieve pain are mental imagery, humor, Chinese acupuncture and Japanese acupressure massage or shiatsu, yoga exercises, spinal manipulation or chiropractics, swimming, bouncing on a mini-trampoline, and soaking in a hot tub for awhile.

PANCREATITIS

Symptoms

Pancreatitis is an inflammation of the pancreas. It is caused by an obstruction of the pancreatic duct from stones, scarring, or cancer. Alcoholism, viral infection, abdominal injury, obesity, poor nutrition, and drugs increase your risk of developing pancreatitis.

The disease can be either acute or chronic. Acute pancreatitis is indicated by nausea, vomiting, and pain around the umbilicus radiating to the back (an extremely critical condition). Chronic pancreatitis is often related to gallbladder infections and gallstones.

Other symptoms include abdominal swelling, excessive gas, upper abdominal pain, described as burning or stabbing, vomiting, fever, hypertension, muscle aches, and abnormally fatty stools.

Relief Measures/Foods and Nutrients

Fluid extract of echinacea or goldenseal root (50 drops four times daily in between meals beneath the tongue) is advised. Chaparral tea (4 cups daily) may also be necessary.

Drink with every meal a little (1 cup) of papaya or mango juice. Take some Wakunaga Kyo-Dophilus (2 capsules) also (see Appendix). Pantothenic acid C 200 mg.) and B-6 (100 mg.) are also important. Consume foods such as buttermilk, kefir, and yogurt. See under **DIABETES** for more information.

PARKINSON'S DISEASE

Symptoms

Parkinson's Disease or the shaking palsy is a degenerative disease affecting the nervous system. Its cause is unknown, but symptoms appear when there is an imbalance of two chemicals, dopamine and acetylcholine, in the brain.

Scientists discovered a deficiency of the former in certain brain cells. Dopamine carries messages from one nerve cell to another. When the brain is not able to manufacture dopamine, Parkinson's Disease results. Malnutrition is believed to be a major underlying factor.

Symptoms of this disease include muscular rigidity, drooling, loss of appetite, a stooped, shuffling gait, tremors that include a characteristic pill-rolling movement of the thumb and forefinger as they rub against each other, impaired speech, and a fixed facial expression. The disease may commence with a shaking of the hands while at rest. The body eventually assumes a more rigid position as time passes.

Relief Measures

Maria Treben, an Austrian herbalist of considerable renown, stated that the freshly picked leaves of wood sorrel are good for this. They should be picked, washed and put into a juice extractor. Then 10 drops of the juice should be added to a cup of warm yarrow tea. This should be taken every couple of hours throughout the day. Also fluid extract of thyme rubbed on to the skin or hot packs of thyme tea applied every five minutes, will help to loosen stiff limbs.

Maria also recommends rubbing some Swedish Bitters on stiff limbs and joints as well. And to take a tablespoonful of the same every few hours. To make this solution, she suggests combining equal parts of powdered wormwood, myrrh, senna, rhubarb, cinnamon, eucalyptus, camphor and angelica together in a two-quart canning jar. (Equal parts would mean one heaping tablespoonful of each of these herbs.) Then add one pint of rye whiskey or vodka and seal with a lid. Leave standing in a window where it can get plenty of sunshine. Shake daily for two weeks. After this, the liquid should be strained and then put in smaller bottles, well stoppered, and stored in a cool place. This way it will keep for many years. The longer they stand the more effective the solution in them becomes. Shake well before using.

Foods and Nutrients

The diet should consist mostly of raw foods, especially seeds, whole grains and nuts. Calcium (800 mg.), magnesium (1,600 mg.), GABA (gamma-amino butyric acid) (2 capsules/tablets daily), lecithin (2 tbsps. daily), L-Glutamic acid (2 capsules/tablets daily), L-Tyrosine (1 capsule/tablet daily), vitamin B-complex (600 mg. daily), extra vitamin B-6 (900 mg. daily), vitamin C with bioflavonoids (3,500 mg. daily), vitamin E oil (1, 200 mg. daily), and a multi-mineral supplement are all recommended.

PELLAGRA

Symptoms

Pellagra is a vitamin deficiency disease. It's caused by a long-term shortage of B vitamins, especially niacin, riboflavin, and thiamine. It's prevalent in populations subsisting mostly on corn and corn-derived foods (some Southwest and Central American Indian tribes). Symptoms include an inflamed and sore red tongue, loss of appetite, diarrhea, loss of weight, weakness, depression, anxiety, headaches, and dizziness. Itchy dermatitis on the hands and neck is a prominent characteristic of the disease. Symptoms of subclinical pellagra have sometimes been misinterpreted as mental illness. For this reason, schizophrenic and hyperactive problems in children might indicate niacin and vitamin B deficiencies.

Relief Measures/Foods and Nutrients

A high potency B-complex vitamin (four tablets daily) is called for here. Also foods rich in B vitamins: avocados, bananas, broccoli, collards, figs, legumes, nuts and seeds, peanut butter, potatoes, prunes, tomatoes, and whole grain breads and cereals. Likewise skinless breast of chicken and turkey, halibut, salmon, tuna, and swordfish should be consumed regularly. These foods are rich in the amino acid tryptophan which helps the body to manufacture more of its own niacin.

PERIODONTAL DISEASE

See under GINGIVITIS for more information.

PERNICIOUS ANEMIA

See under ANEMIA for more information.

PHLEBITIS

See under BLOOD CIRCULATION (POOR) and VARICOSE VEINS for more information.

PNEUMONIA

Symptoms

Pneumonia is an inflammation in the lungs caused by different bacteria, viruses, and fungi. The tiny air sacs in the lung area become inflamed and fill with mucus and pus. It generally isn't considered to be contagious. Typical symptoms vary with intensity, but include fever, chills, cough, muscle aches, fatigue, sore throat, enlarged lymph glands in the neck, bluish nails, pains in the chest, and rapid, difficult respiration.

Relief Measures

Helga Wurtheimer, a German postal clerk, suffered from lingering pneumonia in her home city of Munich. Attempts to cure it with prescription drugs proved hopeless. She was desperate to find some way out of her terrible medical predicament. Someone told her about Maria Treben's Swedish Bitters, mentioned in detail under PARKISON'S DISEASE.

"I began rubbing some of this on my chest several times each day and at night, covering it with a warm flannel before retiring," she told one of the authors who speaks fluent German. "I also made a strong tea out of some wild thyme, and took a big swig of that every hour on the hour." In addition to these things, Helga informed her interviewer that she also sipped some warm coltsfoot leaves occasionally. But when asked for specific amounts, she couldn't remember. Within a week she was completely over her infection for good.

It's suggested that four cups of thyme and only two cups of coltsfoot tea be taken each day on an empty stomach, separately and not at the same time.

Foods and Nutrients

Pneumonia sufferers should be taking 25,000 lUs each of beta-carotene and fish oil three times daily. Also vitamin C with bioflavonoids (3,500 mg.) twice a day is just as important.

The following foods should be excluded from the diet until recovery is evident: all dairy and egg products, fried and deep-fried foods, white flour and white sugar products, and white vinegar products (catsup, mustard, pickles, mayonnaise). Only raw fruits and vegetables and whole grains should be consumed. A protein drink of some kind is also advised. Herbal (including black and green) teas and coffee are allowed, though, because they actually help improve breathing. Fruit and vegetable juices are also helpful. A very good tonic is fresh lemon juice (1 tsp.) in an 8 fl. oz. glass of Perrier mineral water.

POISON IVY AND OAK RASH

Symptoms

Sap from the poison ivy plant and poison oak tree produce terrible redness, rash, swelling, blistering and intense, persistent itching in sensitive people. Usually the arms, hands, and face are exposed first, but other parts of the body can be affected also when they are scratched. Even the smoke emitted from the burning of such plants or tree leaves can be harmful if inhaled by those highly sensitive to either of them.

Relief Measures/Foods and Nutrients

A vitamin C spray is very helpful for this. Either dissolve some powder or dilute the syrup (1 tbsp. per cup) in distilled or spring or mineral water, put into an empty, plastic spray bottle, and spray a fine mist on to the affected portions of the skin. Do this frequently to prevent infection and reduce the itchiness.

Vitamin C (7,000 mg.) can also be taken internally along wtth zinc gluconate (100 mg.) daily.

Lotions and ointments work superbly to bring relief and expedite the healing process. Look for those which have calamine, zinc oxide, marigold, calendula, comfrey, and aloe vera in them.

Sufficient amounts of vitamin A (50,000 I.U.) and vitamin E (1,200 mg.) are required to boost immunity and strengthen the nerves during this ordeal. The application of lotion or ointment with vitamin E in it helps to prevent scarring.

A nifty little trick which works quite well for poison ivy or poison oak rash calls for soaking a cotton cloth in cold water, putting it on the skin, and then letting a fan blow over it. The cooling/evaporating effects works just the same as calamine lotion does.

It's an interesting phenomena of nature that close by poison ivy you'll nearly always find some jewel weed growing. Crushing some of it in your hands or making a tea out of it and rubbing it over the skin will bring immediate relief. Other herbs which work well for such rashes are echinacea, goldenseal, lobelia, and myrrh, in either tea or fluid extract forms.

POLIO

Symptoms

Polio is a viral infection of the spinal cord which destroys the nerves controlling muscular movement, resulting in paralysis of certain muscles. There are two stages of this disease: the infectious stage, when the virus is quite active, and the noninfectious, or recovery stage. Symptoms of the infectious stage includes fever, nausea, diarrhea, headache, and irritability.

Relief Measures/Foods and Nutrients

Garlic is valuable in destroying the virus which causes polio. Some years ago garlic was tested in mice and rhesus monkeys inoculated with this virus. The herb inhibited close to 78% of the virus. Wakunaga (see Appendix) makes an aged-garlic extract called Kyolic (available in several different varieties) which can be very effective in fighting this infection. Two capsules per day for prevention is recommended, but double or triple this amount if the virus is suspected of being in a person's system.

During the infectious stage, the diet of the polio patient should be high in protein

and potassium (3,000 mg.) to replace that which is lost because of the rapid tissue destruction. Caloric intake should be increased as well because of the increased energy expenditure during fever. Brewer's yeast (2 tbsps.) in juice should be taken in the morning and afternoon. Alfalfa, barley grass, and wheat grass make excellent proteins, as does seaweed algae. Up to ten capsules of any of these can be taken. Wakunaga makes a nice, delicious green chlorophyll powder mix called Kyo-Green (1 tbsp. per 8 fl. oz. glass of water).

Vitamin C (orally up to 10,000 mg. or intramuscular injections of two grams) and calcium (800 mg.) and magnesium (1,600 mg.) are effective in treating this disease.

POLYPS

Symptoms

Polyps are benign growths of varying sizes, but aren't considered malignant. They are found on stalk-like structures growing from the epithelial lining of the large intestine, cervix, bladder, or other mucous membranes. They are common in the rectum and sigmoid colon.

Relief Measures/Foods and Nutrients

Vitamin A (25,000 I.U.) and vitamin C (3,500 mg. twice daily) protect the membranous linings against future polyps and reduce existing ones. Calcium (1, 200 mg.) and magnesium (2,200 mg.) protect colon walls and the rectum from polyps, too. Vitamin E (800 mg.) and Kyolic 105 (which includes vitamins A and E and selenium; 2 capsules) promote a vital chemical process called lipid peroxidation which can reduce the frequency of polyps.

The diet should be relatively high in different types of fiber. The abrasive kind found in whole grain breads and cereals can help to scrub out polyps that are just starting up. While water-holding, fiber found in vegetables and herbs such as cabbage, potatoes, and psyllium help to promote easier bowel movements.

No animal fats, fried or deep-fried foods, highly processed foods, coffee, tea, alcohol, soft drinks, colas, or chocolate should be consumed. Most of these foods somehow contribute to the formation of polyps, although the specifics on how they do haven't been fully investigated as yet.

POSTNASAL DRIP

Symptoms

Postnasal drip is a condition of the nasal passageways in which the mucus turns gluelike, gathers in pools at the back of the nose, and commences dripping out of the nostrils on its own. To be more specific about it, consider this—every day glands lining your nasal and sinus cavities crank out about two quarts of fluid to adequately lubricate the mucous membranes in your sinuses, nose, mouth, and throat. Normally, those secretions flow down the back of your nose and throat, swept there by tiny threadlike cells called cilia that wave back and forth over some of the surface tissue. They help keep the nasal passageways clear of particulate matter.

But in the winter time, the mucus dries out and begins to get kind of "gloppy" in form. This tends to slow down the action of the cilia. A virus can stop the cilia altogether. When the cilia stop waving, secretions pool in the back of the nose. As this consistency thickens, it becomes postnasal drip.

Relief Measures

Blow your nose regularly. This simple act eliminates some excessive postnasal drainage from the front of the nose.

Flush the nasal passageways with some salt water. Dissolve 1/2 tsp. of ordinary table salt into 8 fluid ounces of warm water. Draw the water into an infant-sized aspirator and put the tip of it in your nostril. Now hold your nose straight back and the aspirator at a right angle to your face, parallel to the roof of your mouth. And then breathe in to "suck" the water into your nostril. It may seem unpleasant in the beginning, but be assured it becomes easier the more often you do it. Do the other nostril the same way and spit the water back into the wash basin. Several attempts at this may be necessary before any true relief can be obtained. When you're finished, blow your nose to remove the water discharge. Irrigate your nostrils this way three times a day for a week on an "as need" basis.

Also gargling with some salt water seems to help clear the throat and voice box problems created by excessive post-nasal drainage. Mix 1/2 tsp. of table salt in 8 fluid ounces of warm water. Those who are hypertensive may need to reduce the amount of salt in either case by half.

Emotional, mental and physical stress is a major factor in chronic postnasal drip. This is because the task of warming and maintaining a proper lining for the nose falls to the parasympathetic nervous system, which is very susceptible to stress. Stress can actually drive the process too hard, causing the nasal lining to produce more mucus than it really needs. So learn to relax through soft music, progressive muscle relaxation, meditation, or stretching exercises.

Drinking herbal teas sweetened with some lemon and pure maple syrup assures the postnasal drainage of going down into the stomach instead of having to expectorate it all the time by clearing the throat.

Foods and Nutrients

Avoid drinking milk and curtail the consumption of cheese, butter, eggs, yogurt, and ice cream, as well as foods rich in white sugar. They tend to aggravate postnasal drip. Intake of vitamins A (50,000 I.U.) and C (3,500 mg.) daily is strongly recommended.

PREGNANCY PROBLEMS

Symptoms/Relief Measures/Foods and Nutrients

While pregnancy should be the happiest time in a mother's life between fetal conception and growth and the actual birth some nine months later, there are a number of problems which usually occur along the way to cloud some of this joy. Most of them

transpire because of hormonal changes within a mother's body, nutritional deficiencies, or a shift in weight distribution due to sudden weight gain.

BACK PAIN. To minimize this, a mother should always wear flat shoes and never those which are high-heeled. She should also never do any forward bending or strong upward stretching. Soak a towel in equal parts (1 cup each) of plain vinegar and tincture of witch hazel. Squeeze off the excess liquid and lay down in bed on your side. Spread the towel directly across your back. Relax in this position for about half-an-hour.

BLEEDING GUMS. Brush the teeth daily with a wet, soft bristle toothbrush that has the emptied contents of one capsule of white oak bark spread evenly on top. Also massage the gums daily with your clean forefingers that have been dipped into a little tincture of witch hazel. Calcium (1,200 mg.), vitamin C with bioflavonoids (3, 500 mg.) and extra rutin (300 mg.) is advised.

CONSTIPATION. The diet should consist of prunes, raisins, figs, seven-grain bread, buckwheat pancakes, cooked oatmeal, carrot or orange juice, and ripe avocados. They are guaranteed to move the bowels nicely. Pregnant women, however, should avoid taking any of the harsh herbal laxatives while in the first 4 or 5 months of their pregnancies, as these herbs are apt to induce early labor and possible miscarriages.

Walking every day for a while helps in setting a steady pace for routine bowel movements.

DIZZINESS. An expectant mom's blood pressure may suddenly plunge due to the pressure of the uterus on major blood vessels, causing instant dizziness. She shouldn't change positions too quickly. Drinking some warm catnip or chamomile tea will help to dispel such dizziness.

GAS (INTESTINAL). Not chewing her food properly will cause a pregnant mother to emit intestinal gas later on in the day, also, the wrong food combinations. She should never combine acidic and alkaline foods together at the same time, and try to consume her proteins separately from the acidic substances. She should eat five small meals a day instead of the standard three big ones. Drinking chamomile, peppermint or spearmint teas with a meal or taking 2 capsules of Wakunaga's Kyo-Dophilus (see Appendix) will help eliminate gas problems.

GESTATION EXTENSION. According to *Science News* for May 16, 1992 (p. 334), fish oil capsules taken during the third trimester of pregnancy could very well extend gestation. Danish scientists gave 266 healthy women in their third trimester daily capsules containing omega-3 fatty acids. A control group of 136 other women got daily capsules containing olive oil. Pregnancies in the fish-oil group lasted an average of four days longer than those in the olive-oil group, the researchers discovered. Fish-oil babies also averaged about 107 grams heavier than their olive-oil counterparts did. These fish-oil babies put on the weight simply by staying in the womb longer, scientists asserted.

Some day in the very near future, the article speculates, doctors may very well prescribe fish-oil supplements or recommend a fish-nish diet for pregnant women at risk of delivering a premature baby. Expectant mothers who think they might run such risks,

are advised to take 2-3 capsules of omega-3 fish oil each day, and to include fish such as salmon, tuna, halibut, trout, and bass in their diets often.

GROIN SPASM. This is usually felt as a "stitch" on the right side. The round ligaments connecting the corners of the uterus to the pubic area will kink and go into a type of spasm. In the advanced months of pregnancy, lower groin pressure could develop. To relieve this, try taking a number of short walks every day. Also remember to breathe deeply during a spasm and bend toward the point of pain in order to permit the ligament to relax. Rest in bed on one side until the spasm finally passes.

HEARTBURN. Heartburn occurs more often during pregnancy due to the re-entrance of stomach fluids into the esophagus because of the expanded size of the uterus. Avoid consuming spicy or greasy foods, alcohol, coffee, baking soda, or antacids. One cup of cool papaya juice or catnip or yarrow tea will soothe the stomach. So will 2 capsules of Kyo-Dophilus (see Appendix under Wakunaga).

HEMORRHOIDS. If an expectant mother has piles, she should increase her intake of fiberous foods such as raw vegetables, fruits, dried fruits and whole grain breads and cereals. And decrease her intake of refined and processed foods. The feet and legs ought to be elevated on a footstool while going to the toilet. This helps to move the bowels by relaxing the anal muscles. Soak some cotton balls in witch hazel and insert between the cheeks; this will help to shrink the hemorrhoids.

INSOMNIA. Drinking some warm milk or some warm herbal teas (chamomile, lavender, lemon balm, hops or catnip) and taking a high-potency B-complex (3 tablets daily) and two capsules of valerian root before retiring, should help bring on a good night's rest.

LEG CRAMPS. See elsewhere in this book under the same heading for more information.

MISCARRIAGE. Some women just can't carry a baby to full term and often experience a miscarriage or spontaneous abortion. There are numerous reasons why such a thing happens—emotional grief, malnutrition, general malaise, infection, and glandular dysfunctions. Women can increase their calcium (1,200 mg.), magnesium (2,400), B-complex (4 tablets), C with bioflavonoids (3,500 mg.) and E (800 mg.) to help prevent this. Also taking capsules of powdered alfalfa (4 daily), marshmallow (4 daily), yarrow (2 daily), and horsetail or shavegrass (2 daily) seems to help as well.

MOOD CHANGES. See under HYPOGLYCEMIA elsewhere in this book for more information.

MORNING SICKNESS. See under NAUSEA elsewhere in this book for more information.

NOSEBLEEDS AND NASAL CONGESTION. See under NOSEBLEEDS and BREATHING DIFFICULTIES elsewhere in this book for more information.

SCIATICA. See elsewhere in this book under the same subject heading for more information.

SKIN PROBLEMS. See elsewhere in this book under the same subject heading for more information.

SORENESS IN THE RIB CAGE. This soreness usually clears up in the last six weeks of pregnancy, once the baby has dropped into position to be born. When experiencing this problem, an expectant mom should just change her sitting or laying positions often enough.

STRETCH MARKS. Stretch marks are wavy reddish stripes appearing on the abdomen, buttocks, breasts, and thighs which gradually turn white. They are caused by excessive and rapid weight gain typically associated with pregnancy, and appear when the skin becomes overstretched and the fibers in the deep layers tear.

They can be prevented by applying the following remedy to those places on the skin in which they commonly appear. Combine in a blender 1/4 cup aloe vera gel, 1/2 cup pure virgin olive oil, 1 tsp. vitamin E oil, and 1/2 tsp. cod liver oil. After thoroughly mixed, pour out into a Mason pint jar, seal with lid and refrigerate. Apply daily as needed.

SWEATING. During pregnancy, the mother's body readjusts its own temperature to suit the baby's normal development. The mother should dress accordingly by wearing loose fitting clothing that is light and comfortable. Nothing that is tight or constricting should be worn during this period. Also hot tubs and saunas should be avoided as well? because they send the unborn infant into fetal distress.

SWELLING OF THE HANDS AND FEET. Some swelling is to be expected during pregnancy as estrogen levels in the body increase. But too much swelling can indicate serious infection and demands a doctor's immediate attention. An expectant mom should remove all rings from her fingers when they start getting a little puffy and swollen. Highly-processed foods should be avoided. No diuretics should be taken either. Clothing to be worn should be comfortable fitting. Daily walks should become routine as they tend to hold swelling down.

URINATION (FREQUENT). Urinating frequently is a part of the pregnancy process. It's also great preparation for the mother when she will have to be making nightly trips to her infant's room. An average of 6-8 glass of fluid a day should be consumed, without any curtailment of this.

VARICOSE VEINS. See elsewhere in this book under the same subject heading for more information.

The following drugs should be *avoided* during pregnancy:

Alka-Seltzer, antihistamines, Di-Gel, estrogens, cold pills, cough remedies, Dratil, decongestants, Gelusil, Maalox, mineral oil, Pepto-Bismol, Rolaids, Tums, Tylenol, Dilantin, pheno-barbital, ampicillin, tetracycline, aspirin, Accutane, and Tegison. The following foods should also be avoided during pregnancy: anything with Nutra-Sweet (asparatame) in it, anything with phenylalanine in it, anything with caffeine in it, junk food, highly seasoned food, fried foods, and alcohol. All of these drugs and foods can cause a variety of problems, both

in the development of the fetus as well as in the final delivery of the newborn.

An expectant mom should take the following nutritional supplements each day:

Wakunaga's Kyolic Garlic	(3 capsules)
Wakunaga's Kyo-Green	(1 glass)
Wakunaga's Yeast-Gard	(1 tablet)
Wakunaga's Kyo-Dophilus	(1 capsule per meal)
folic acid	(800 mcg.)
high-potency B-complex	(3 tablets)
vitamin C with bioflavonoids	(3,500 mg.)
rutin	(300 mg.)
magnesium	(1,400 mg.)
calcium	(700 mg.)
alfalfa powder	(8 capsules)
beet powder	(4 capsules)
vitamin A	(25,000 I.U.)
vitamin E	(800 mg.)
red raspberry leaf tea	(1 glass taken hot every few hours just prior to expected delivery)

squawvine	(3 capsules)
licorice root	(2 capsules)

PREMENSTRUAL SYNDROME

Symptoms

Premenstrual syndrome (PMS) is a disorder that affects menstruating women one or two weeks before the menstrual cycle starts. Symptoms can include any or all of the following: irritability, depression, cramps, water retention, skin eruptions, headaches, bloated abdomen, backache, breast swelling and tenderness, insomnia, fatigue, nervousness, joint pain, fainting spells, and insomnia.

Relief Measures/Foods and Nutrients

Dorothy L. was 35 years of age and in considerable pain. She was fighting her PMS miseries with everything she could muster, but no end to her suffering seemed in sight. Until one day, she went to a wellness convention and heard a female practitioner who specialized in PMS cases, explain what she used to treat her many patients with. "My life just sort of turned around after that," Dorothy informed one of the authors in her Secaucus, New Jersey home sometime ago.

Here is the program she put herself on for the next three months. It resulted in a complete reversal of all of her PMS troubles.

magnesium	2,000 mg.
calcium	1,000 mg.

Efamol evening primrose oil,	3 capsules daily.

(See Appendix under Nature's Way.)

ENAX 2 and RELEAF,	2 capsules of each.

(See Appendix under Wakunaga.)

Schiff high-potency B-complex	4 tablets daily.
an amino acid complex	3 tablets daily.
S dong quai herb	2 capsules daily.
vitamin C with bioflavonoids,	3,500 mg. daily.
vitamin B-6	50 mg. daily *with* rutin, 300 mg.

She also curtailed her intake of coffee, red meat, greasy and sugary foods, soft drinks, colas, and alcohol. She also drank one water of spring or distilled water daily, beginning a week prior to her menstrual period and ending one week after it was finished.

PROSTATITIS

Symptoms

Prostatitis, common in men of all ages, is the acute or chronic inflammation of the prostate gland. The usual cause is a bacterial infection from another area of the body which has invaded the prostate. Prostatitis can partially or totally block the flow of urin out of the bladder, resulting in urine retention. This causes the bladder to become distended, weak, tender, and susceptible to infection as a result of the increased amount of bacteria in the retained urine. Infection in the bladder is easily transmitted up the ureters to the kidneys.

Symptoms of acute prostatitis are pain between the scrotum and rectum, fever, frequent urination accompanied by a burning sensation, and blood or pus in the urine. Symptoms of chronic prostatitis are frequent and burning urination with blood in the urine, lower back pain, and impotence. As prostatitis becomes more advanced, urination becomes more difficult.

Relief Measures

Goldenseal root is especially effective in reducing the infection: tea (three half cups every 4 hours); fluid extract (15 drops three times daily); or capsules (2 every 5 hours). So is chaparral tea (1 cup twice daily); fluid extract (10 drops 3 times daily); or capsules (4 daily).

Anti-inflammatory herbs such as yarrow or marshmallow will bring down pain and burning sensations: tea (2 cups daily); capsules (4 of either daily).

Exercise is also very important. Walking in warm, pleasant weather is the best, but don't jog or bicycle.

Foods and Nutrients

Drink plenty of liquid chlorophyll. In a home juice machine, make up vegetable juices consisting of Romaine lettuce, parsley, and celery. Or drink one glass of Kyo-Green every day (see Appendix under Wakunaga).

Use cold-pressed oils such as sesame seed, safflower, or olive oils to obtain much needed fatty acids. Eat mushrooms, raisins and pumpkin seeds to get more zinc into your system, if you're a man suffering from prostatitis. Also take zinc (100 mg.) and fatty acid (6 capsules daily) supplements as well.

Consume more nuts and seeds, raw vegetables, fruits (avoiding citrus and other very acidic types), fresh juices, dried beans, peas, and brown rice. Stay away from refined carbohydrates, coffee, strong tea, and alcohol. All of these have been linked to cancer of the prostate. Too much fat in the diet causes an increase of free radicals within the body. And these scavenger molecules are believed to play a role in the development of this cancer.

PSORIASIS

Symptoms

Psoriasis usually shows up on the skin as patches of silvery scales or red areas on the legs, knees, arms, elbows, scalp, ears, and back. The toes and fingernails lose their luster and develop ridges and pits. Often hereditary, it's linked to a rapid growth of cells in the skin's outer layer. It may result from a faulty utilization of fat. Psoriasis is most common between the ages of 15 and 25, and isn't infectious. Attacks can be triggered by nervous tension and stress, illness, surgery, cuts, poison ivy, several viral and bacterial infections, sunburn, or various drugs. Only the scales and skin debris, which are quite itchy, can be removed. Presently there is no known cure for it. The disease appears to lessen during the warm summer months, but cranks up again in severity as winter and cold weather approaches. It may go away of its own accord, but can always return later on. Once you have psoriasis, it seems to stay with you for the rest of your natural life.

Relief Measures

Certain herbs make an excellent tea to take internally and to also wash the skin for this problem. The great French herbalist Maurice Mességué recommends this particular combination, which he claims has helped hundreds of his patients to, at least, "live tolerably well with psoriasis." In a quart of hot water, add "2 pinches of chamomile, 2 pinches of lavender, 2 pinches of sage, 2 pinches of thyme, and 2 teaspoonfuls of lime juice." Stir, cover and let everything steep for 40 minutes. Drink 1 cup 3 times daily and also bathe the skin frequently with it.

Foods and Nutrients

Stay away from fats, sugar, processed foods, white flour and citrus fruits. Fish oil and evening primrose interfere with the production and storage of arachidonic acid, a natural inflammatory agent that makes the lesions of psoriasis turn red and swell. Avoid red meat and dairy products because they contain a lot of arachidonic acid, which can only further aggravate psoriasis. Consume a 50% raw foods diet. Oils

made from sesame seeds, flaxseed, or soybeans are helpful. Fresh and salt-water fish should also be added to the diet. Bake, poach or steam it, but avoiding frying or broiling.

Season your fish and other foods with some Adolph's Meat Tenderizer. It contains papain from papaya leaves and latex. This important proteolytic enzyme stimulates protein synthesis and repair of injured skin tissue. So does bromelain, another such enzyme, found in pineapple and pineapple juice. Slippery elm tea (2 cups daily) or capsules (6 daily) is especially helpful here.

The authors also recommend vitamin A divided between vegetable beta-carotene (50,000 I.U.) and fish oil (50,000 I.U.). A high-potency B-complex (3 tablets daily) is in order, too. Vitamin C with bioflavonoids (3,500 mg.) contributes to collagen and connective tissue formation. And horsetail or shavegrass, with its rich silicon content, is vital to take (2 capsules daily) for such a disease.

Vitamins D (400 I.U.) and E (800 I.U.), lecithin (1 tbsp.) and zinc gluconate (100 mg.) taken together every day, promotes similar healing benefits.

PYORRHEA

See under **CAVITIES, GINGIVITIS,** and **TOOTHACHE** for more information.

QUARTAN

See under **FEVERS** for more information.

QUINSY

See under **TONSILLITIS** for more information.

RABIES

Symptoms

Rabies is a highly fatal infectious disease that may affect all species of warm-blooded animals, including man. It is transmitted almost exclusively by the bite of carnivorous animals, and is caused by a neurotropic lysavirus in the central nervous system and the salivary glands. The symptoms are characteristic of a profound disturbance of the nervous system, such as excitement, aggressiveness, and madness, followed by paralysis and death if left unattended.

Relief Measures

Rabies is one of those life-threatening situations which demands *prompt medical attention*. Some homeopathic remedies, though, may be efficacious here in conjunction with prescribed drugs. The *Materia Medica, Pharmacy and Therapeutics*, authored by Samuel O. L. Potter, M.D. (10th Edition) listed belladonna, stramonium, and nicotine as being very useful for the treatment of rabies back in 1906. However, because these herbs are all rather potent, it's advisable to seek the advice of a competent and qualified homeopathist before taking any of them.

Dr. Potter also recommended "baths, warm and hot, to produce calm" in the victim. Two small cuts made on either side of the rabid animal bite will permit the blood to flow more freely, thereby eliminating some of the poison from the system. Other herbs such as goldenseal and echinacea would also be helpful here as well.

Foods and Nutrients

The patient should be kept on juices and not given solid food during recovery. Vitamins A (100,000 I.U.) and C (20,000 mg.) are definitely called for to fight the infection.

RASH

See ALLERGIES, DIAPER RASH, ECZEMA, HIVES, and PSORIASIS for more information.

RAYNAUD'S DISEASE

Symptoms

Raynaud's Disease affects the circulatory system and results in hands and feet that are hypersensitive to the cold. The small arteries that supply the toes and fingers become very sensitive to cold and suddenly contract. Lack of oxygenated blood causes the fingers or toes to become a whitish or bluish hue. Symptoms come on quickly and result in the affected area's shrinking. Ulcers form, damaging the tissues, and resulting in chronic infection under and around the fingernails and toenails. Gangrene can result from prolonged contraction of the arteries.

Relief Measures

Condition yourself to overcome chills. You can do this by placing your hands in a container of warm water for 5 minutes. Then open your freezer and put some warm water in there and again dip your hands in it for another 5 minutes, leaving the freezer door open. Normally, the cold would make the peripheal blood vessels constrict, but instead, the sensation of the warm water keeps them open. Repeat this procedure until you've countered the constriction reflex common to Raynaud's victims without the benefit of the warm water.

Always be sure to dress warmly, even in cool weather. The hands and feet especially should be covered with cotton material of some kind, and the head with a suitable hat.

Don't allow yourself to become stressed by aggravating situations. Stress creates the same reaction in Raynaud's victims as cold does. Blood is pulled from the hands and feet to the brain and internal organs to enable you to think and react more quickly. Try to calm down through simple breathing exercises, focusing the mind on other matters, gently massaging your forehead, temples, neck, and hands, meditation or taking a walk.

Avoid second-hand smoke. Cigarette smoke cools the body in two ways. It helps form plaque in the arteries and the nicotine from cigarettes produces some constriction of the small blood vessels.

Foods and Nutrients

Herbs such as butcher's broom, red pepper, Kyolic garlic, ginkgo (in the Wakunaga combination of ginkgo and garlic called Ginkolic), and red clover are helpful. Two capsules daily of any of these is advised.

Eat a hot, hearty meal first thing in the morning, and again at noontime. Hot oatmeal or cooked millet for breakfast, and a hearty bowl of soup for lunch are recommended. These will keep your hands and feet toasty even in the worst weather.

But stay away from alcohol and coffee as they tend to constrict blood vessels. And this is the last thing that is needed by those who have Raynaud's syndrome.

Coenzyme Q-10 (60 mg. daily), vitamin E (800 I.U.), Wakunaga's Kyo-Green (1 glass daily), liquid lecithin (2 tbsps. daily), and a high-potency B-complex (4 tablets daily) round out the supplement program nicely.

RESTLESS LEGS SYNDROME

Symptoms

Restless Legs Syndrome (also known as Ekbom Syndrome) is more of a chronic annoyance than a serious neurological disorder. It is usually characterized by an irresistible urge to move the legs, a certain "jumpiness" of the legs, and deep creeping or crawling sensations of the legs.

Relief Measures

One of the easiest and simplest ways to get rid of this nuisance is just to get up and walk around for awhile. Another trick is to take a brief stroll or short walk just before retiring, since the problem tends to strike at night.

Soak the feet in hot water for a couple of minutes, then in cold water for the same length of time. Alternating this back and forth for about ten minutes should help.

Massaging the legs with a hand-held vibrator really helps to dissipate the "jumpiness"; so does some mild yoga stretching exercises.

Foods and Nutrients

Increase your intake of red pepper and ginger root (2 capsules each daily). Also powdered beet root (4 capsules daily). They all help to promote better circulation.

Stop drinking caffeinated beverages, as there seems to be a connection between them and this syndrome.

Eat more iron-rich foods such as blackstrap molasses, fish, liver, and eggs. A deficiency in this mineral is apt to produce Restless Legs Syndrome more often.

RHEUMATIC FEVER

Symptoms

Rheumatic Fever is an infection, caused by streptococcal bacteria in the body, which occurs most often in children between the ages of 4 and 18. It affects one or more of the following body parts: joints (showing up as juvenile arthritis), brain (showing up as chorea), heart (turning up as carius), tissues (producing nodules), and skin (manifesting itself as erythema marginatum). Residual heart disease is a likely complication.

Relief Measures

Tea made from the bark or leaves of the birch tree helps to reduce the pain. And catnip tea is great for reducing the accompanying fever. Two cups of each a day on an empty stomach is recommended for the sick youngster.

Foods and Nutrients

Kyolic garlic (2 capsules daily), Kyo-Dophilus (3 capsules daily, one per meal), vitamin C (1,500 mg.), calcium and magnesium combination (2 tablets daily), kelp (2 capsules daily), and cod liver oil (1 tsp.) should be given to the child.

Plenty of fresh juices and distilled water, as well as yogurt, cottage cheese, and clear soup should constitute the diet. No solid foods should be given until improvement is evident.

RHEUMATISM

Symptoms

Rheumatism is a general term referring to acute and chronic conditions characterized by stiffness of muscles and pain in the joints. Rheumatism includes such conditions as arthritis and bursitis, as well as other diseases.

Relief Measures

Yucca and alfalfa (3-6 capsules daily) taken internally, and a salve containing eucalyptus or a few drops of peppermint oil rubbed on to the surface of the skin bring immediate relief. After rubbing the herbal solution on, cover with hot, wet hand towel or heating pad for a few minutes. This allows the herbal oils to penetrate more deeply and quickly.

Foods and Nutrients

Vitamin A (25,000 I.U.), C (3,500 mg.), D and E (800 I.U. each), calcium (800 mg.), thagnesium (1,200 mg.), phosphorus (1,000 mg.) and potassium (2,000 mg.) are all needed here.

See also under **ARTHRITIS** for more information.

RHEUMATOID ARTHRITIS

See under **ARTHRITIS** for more information.

RICKETS & OSTEOMALACIA

Symptoms

Rickets is primarily a childhood disease of malnutrition in which there is a deficiency of vitamin D, calcium, and/or phosphorus. The main symptoms of rickets is an inability of the bones to retain their calcium. In turn, they become soft, which results in deformities when the bones are called upon to support weight that they are too weak to support. Such deformities include bowlegs, knock-knees, protruding breastbone, narrow rib cage, and bony beads along the ribs.

The adult form of rickets is known as osteomalachia. It's most apt to occur at times of bodily stress such as pregnancy or during breastfeeding. Its causes may be due to a kidney dysfunction or disease, a mineral (calcium or phosphorus) deficiency of some kind, or an inability for the body to proper utilize its vitamin D. It can occur in people who get little exposure to sunlight or in those on diets so low in fats (extreme weight loss programs) that inadequate bile is made and vitamin D isn't totally absorbed.

In addition to the symptoms of rickets, aching of joints and generalized weakness usually occur.

Relief Measures/Food and Nutrients

Foods rich in calcium (milk, cheese, molasses, and yogurt) as well as extra calcium (1,600 mg.) and magnesium (800 mg.) should be consumed every day.

Vitamin D (800 I.U.), phosphorus (800 mg.), boron (3 mg.) and the herb horsetail or shave grass (2 capsules) for its silicon content, should all be taken as well.

RINGWORM AND ROUNDWORM

See under WORMS for more information.

RUPTURE

See under HERNIA for more information.

SCARRING

Symptoms

Scarring occurs after a wound or an incision of some type has been made into the skin and the healing process commences soon thereafter. A wound which heals quickly and neatly is less likely to develop a scar than a wound or cut which is allowed to fester.

Relief Measures

Make sure the wound or incision is properly cleaned. Hydrogen peroxide makes a fine cleanser for this; so does alcohol if nothing else is available.

Unless very large in size, such a cut or wound should only be lightly dressed so as to allow the circulation of air around it which expedites healing.

Vitamin E oil can be rubbed over a wound or newly formed scar with some Q-tips or cotton swabs. Aloe vera gel is also very useful, too. Liquid aloe vera (1/2 cup twice daily) can be taken internally; this will often prevent the formation of scar tissue inside a recent surgical incision, but won't work for old ones.

Avoid picking or scratching a scab, which only leaves behind a very visible scar before the healing process is completed.

Foods and Nutrients

Take some vitamin E (800 I.U.) and zinc (100 mg.) internally until the wound or cut is finished healing.

SCHIZOPHRENIA

Symptoms

Schizophrenia is one of two types of mental illness (the other being mood disorders). While those suffering from the latter appear normal between episodes, those with the former seldom ever behave normally between episodes. The symptoms of Schizophrenia are tension, depression, personality problems, fatigue, mental derangement, and hallucinations.

The niacin-deficiency disease, Pellagra, has been linked to Schizophrenia. Sometimes undiagnosed Celiac Disease may produce symptoms very similar to this mental illness. Sometimes high copper levels in the body tissue can bring on Schizo-phrenia.

Schizophrenia usually develops during late adolescence or early adulthood, but this wide-ranging disruption of thought and emotion occasionally turns up in children. Research at UCLA School of Medicine suggests that Schizophrenic children suffer from attention and memory problems that undermine their ability to communicate with others.

UCLA doctors also noticed that during mental tests, the brains of Schizo-phrenic children produce a weaker version of a specific type of electrical activity associated with focused attention among healthy children and adults. Tasks that typically spark surges in electrical activity in one or the other brain hemisphere have no such effect among Schizophrenic kids. For some reason, the right and left hemispheres of the brain don't seem as finely specialized in these children as they do in normal ones.

Relief Measures/Foods and Nutrients

Tom L. of Storrs, Connecticut suffered from one of the mildest forms of Schizophrenic disorder known as Paranoid or Schizotypal Personality. His nutritional-minded therapist placed him on the following regimen. Within just 3 months he was declared "normal" and devoid of any symptoms.

Wakunaga's Gingko Go (Gingko biloba and Kyolic Garlic)

(see Appendix) 4 capsules

Germanium (175 mg. daily)

Niacin (500 mg. daily)

Vitamin B-6 (300 mg. daily) and L-Glutamine (3 grams daily)

Vitamin E (1,200 I.U.)

Evening Primrose Oil (3 capsules daily)

Lecithin (1 tbsp.) and Magnesium (1,600 mg.)

SCIATICA

Symptoms

Sciatica is a condition of severely painful spasms occurring along the sciatica nerve of the leg. This nerve runs from the back of the thigh, down the inside of the leg, to the ankle. Among the possible causes of sciatica are trauma or inflammation of the nerve itself, sprained joints in the lower back, rupture of a disk between the spinal bones, or neuritis.

Relief Measures

Mary H. of Locust Grove, Virginia treated her sciatica by placing applications of hot, wet hand towels upon her affected leg for immediate relief of pain and inflammation.

Foods and Nutrients

She also took a high-potency B-complex vitamin (3 capsules daily), manganese (50 mg.) rutin (300 mg.), magnesium (1,200 mg. daily), zinc (50 mg. daily) and vitamin E (800 mg. daily).

SCLERODERMA

See under ARTHRITIS, BLOOD CIRCULATION (POOR), and RAYNAUD'S DISEASE for more information.

SCOLIOSIS

Symptoms

This is lateral curvature of the spine, discernible mostly through a physical checkup or if the person is wearing a blouse or shirt made of flimsy, see-through fabric of some type.

Most common in adolescence, it is usually noticed between 10 and 18 years of age, in girls 9 times as often as in boys. The spine bones grow faster on one side than the other; no one really knows why this happens.

Relief Measures

Certain physical exercises are the very best therapy for trying to correct this problem at an early age when it first becomes noticeable. Some Indian yoga and Chinese tai chi quan stretching exercises, which require the person to sit or lay on the floor while doing them, is highly recommended. These tend to make back muscles more supple and allow them to grow straighter than they otherwise would.

Denise P. of Youngstown, Ohio, developed a mild form of scoliosis at age 15. She took up ballet dancing and discovered within a year's time that her posture had returned to normal. Denise credits her many hours of practice at dancing for instilling in her good posture habits.

Chiropractic treatments may be advisable from a qualified practitioner. However, one should check around and ask a lot of questions before picking just any doctor. Not every chiropractor is able to deal with this type of problem.

Frequently massaging the back seems to help some people with scoliosis. Doctors recommend the wearing of a brace to help develop more correct posture. Sleeping at night on a firm mattress with a sheet of 3/4-inch plywood underneath may be necessary to guarantee straightness of the spine.

Foods and Nutrients

Essential bone-building minerals are necessary here: calcium (1,200 mg.), magnesium (1,800 mg.), and phosphorus (800 mg.). Also plenty of vitamins D and E (800 I.U.s for both.)

SCRATCHES

Symptoms

Scratches result whenever something sharp scrapes or digs into the epidermal layer of the skin, causing a deep mark that may or may not draw blood. This can range from fingernails or cat claws to a rose bush thorn or a rusty nail.

Scratches usually aren't taken very seriously, and in many instances are often neglected because in the person's mind they don't seem life-threatening. However, the sensible thing to do is to treat them at once to prevent complications from setting in later on.

Relief Measures

Rosa Garcia of Brownsville, Texas told one of the authors awhile ago that when her pet cat playfully scratched the back of her hand, she immediately took care of it. She went to the bathroom and opened a bottle of hydrogen peroxide and poured a tiny amount on each scratch. Within minutes the itching and inflammation disappeared, and she was not bothered any more by them.

Placing some aloe vera gel or vitamin E oil from the cut end of a single capsule on to a scratch will expedite healing considerably.

Foods and Nutrients

A common treatment in the Mexican Yucatan among the Maya is to cut a sour orange or lime in half, and squeeze some of the juice on to a scratch, to stop infection.

Taking vitamin C (3,500 mg.) and zinc (100 mg.) internally helps also.

SCURVY

Symptoms

Scurvy is a malnutrition disease more common in Third World countries than it is here in America. The problem is caused by a diet that is entirely deficient in vitamin D. Symptoms of adult scurvy include swelling and bleeding of the gums, tenderness of joints and muscles, rough, dry, discolored skin, poor healing of wounds, and increased susceptibility to bruising and infection. Because vitamin C facilitates the absorption of iron, scurvy may be complicated by anemia.

Relief Measures/Foods and Nutrients

Scurvy responds dramatically to the daily administration of vitamin C (500-1,000 mg.), vitamin D (800 I.U.), calcium (800 mg.) and magnesium (1,200 mg.). Certain foods such as citrus fruits and juices, milk, nuts, and seafood will supply the body with these and other important nutrients. Adequate sunlight is also a great supplier of vitamin D.

SEASONAL AFFECTIVE DISORDER (SAD)

Symptoms

Seasonal affective disorder or SAD is a distinctive type of depression and malaise suffered by some people during the short dark days of winter. Only since the 1980s, however, has this disorder gained widespread scientific credence. Enough so, in fact, to be included in the psychiatric bible, the *Diag-*

nostic and Statistical Manual of Mental Disorders.

SAD sufferers tend to sleep longer, be less productive at their jobs, become more easily fatigued in recreation and sex, and generally feel down in the dumps for no apparent reason. They tend to eat more (especially sweets and starches) which, together with a low toxicity level, generally leads to winter weight gain.

Nobody knows how common SAD is, but researchers believe that it probably affects as many as 5% of the American population. And many more experience some of these same symptoms, though more mildly or less consistently—sometimes merely because they work in dark or windowless offices. The farther north you are, the more prevalent SAD is. SAD affects four times as many women as it does men. It occurs most often in people in their twenties to forties and tapers off in the elderly. It seems to run in families, leading scientists to think there is a definite genetic connection somewhere. The SAD months are November through March, depending on how far north you live, with January and February being the worst time to cope with this disorder.

Relief Measures

If you think you may suffer from SAD or a mild form of seasonal depression, here are some initial steps you can take to improve your situation:

- Make your house bright. Trim bushes around S your windows and keep the curtains open. Use bright colors on walls and uphositery.

- If you work in an office, ask if you can work near a window.

- Try to take part of your vacation in the winter, instead of taking it all in the summer. Common sense obviously dictates for choosing a sun destination.

- Exercise outdoors. Skiing, for instance, is an excellent way to get lots of light. If you exercise indoors, try to do so near a window or light box.

Light therapy is also recommended. Studies from a number of different countries have demonstrated that SAD can be easily treated with bright artificial lights. Special light boxes are usually suggested, since they have been tested for this condition and emit a measured "dose" of light at a set distance.

Criteria for good light therapy includes: light entering the eyes; must be bright (regular indoor lighting unacceptable for this); must be the right wavelength, (full-spectrum fluroscent bulbs recommended over tanning lamps or plant lights); must be used long enough (about 3-4 hours a day); must be timed just right (morning exposure works best).

Foods and Nutrients

A complete amino acid (3 tablets daily) and vitamin- mineral (4 tablets daily) supplements is necessary. Additional supplementation of vitamin 3-6 (100 mg.), vitamin D (800 I.U.) and magnesium (1,200 mg.) may be needed.

SEBORRHEA

See OILY HAIR AND SKIN for more
information.

SEIZURES

See EPILEPSY for more information

SENILITY

See ALZHEIMER'S DISEASE,
AMNESIA, and MENTAL RETARDA-
TION for more information.

SEXUALLY TRANSMIS-
SIBLE DISEASES

(See also AIDS, CANDIDIASIS, and
HERPES for additional information.)

Symptoms

Sexually transmissible diseases (or
STDs) are those that are passed on during
sexual intercourse or other intimate contact
with the sex organs. The two most common
types of sexually transmitted diseases are
gonorrhea and syphilis. However, there are
many other STDs that include chancroid,
lymphogranuloma venereum, granuloma
inguinal, genital herpes, chiamydia,
trichomoniasis, candidiasis, and AIDS.

In women gonorrhea is generally
asymptomatic. This means that when there

are symptoms, they include frequent and
painful urination, vaginal discharge,
abnormal menstrual bleeding, acute inflammation in the pelvic area, and rectal itching.
Men quite often experience symptoms of
gonorrhea, which include a yellow discharge
of pus and mucus from the penis and slow,
difficult, and painful urination. Symptoms in
both sexes generally show up a week to three
weeks after sexual contact has been made. If
left untreated, gonorrhea can spread through
the bloodstream and enter bones, joints,
tendons and other tissues. A new strain of
gonorrhea identified since 1985 is resistant to
some antibiotic drugs.

Syphilis is caused by a bacterium
called Treponema pallidium. This STD is
often contracted through physical contact
such as kissing and through oral, anal, and
regular sex. In the first stage a sore or
chancre appears, followed later on by a rash
and patches of flaking tissue in the mouth or
genital area. In the final stage, brain damage,
hearing loss, heart disease, and/or blindness
might take place.

Relief Measures

Antibiotic herbs will definitely work
here. A brief list has been prepared of them
and the forms in which they work best:

Chaparral	Tea (2 cups daily)
Echinacea	Fluid Extract (15 drops 3x daily)
Goldenseal	Capsule (twice daily)

Pau d'arco	Fluid Extract (20 drops twice daily)
	Tea (3 cups daily)
Red Clover	Tea (4 cups daily)
Sarsaparilla	Tea (4 cups daily)
Wild Oregon Grape	Capsules (6 capsules daily)
Yellow Dock	Tea (3 cups daily)

Foods and Nutrients

A combination of Wakunaga's Kyolic garlic Formula 101 (4 capsules daily), Kyo-Dophilus (3 capsules daily), and Kyo-Green (1 glass daily) form a nifty trio to rebuild the immune system. They should be accompanied with vitamins A (50,000 I.U.) and C (3,500 mg.) and the minerals germanium (150 mg. daily) and zinc (100 mg. daily).

A complete amino acid complex (3-4 capsules or tablets) per day is suggested. Because these diseases are terribly contagious, most doctors strongly encourage the use of condoms during sexual intercourse. Ministers, priests, and rabbis, however, preach abstinence of sexual indulgence outside of marriage, not only because they deem it sinful but also as a sensible safeguard.

SHINGLES

See HERPES for more information.

SHINSPLINTS

See RESTLESS LEGS SYNDROME and TENDONITIS for more information.

SHOCK

Symptoms

A shock of any kind is a state of profound mental and physical depression consequent upon severe physical injury or an emotional disturbance. Shock can come from a sudden announcement that a loved one has just been killed in a horrible accident. Or from an electrical current passing through the body. Or produced by bacterial endo-toxins, especially of E. coli, in the circulating blood plasma. Or resulting from acute hemorrhaging. Or from an allergic reaction to a bee sting. Or from the administration of insulin for diabetes in which profound hypo-glycemia can occur. These are just a few things which can induce a variety of shocks.

Relief Measures

The most efficacious treatments for any type of shock are the Bach Flower Remedies. Developed by a London bacteriologist, Edward Bach in the 1930's, from wild flowers, bushes, and trees, they are prescribed, not directly for the physical complaint itself but more according to the sufferer's state of mind, based on his or her moods of fear, worry, anger, or depression.

Of the 38 separate remedies he developed, his Rescue Remedy (sometimes called "the 39th Remedy") is the most popular with practitioners and patients alike. Five individual remedies comprise the Rescue Remedy:

Star of Bethlehem, for shock,

Rock Rose, for terror and panic,

Impatiens, for mental stress and tension,

Cherry Plum, for desperation,

Clematis, for the bemused, faraway, out-of-the-body feeling which often precedes fainting or loss of consciousness.

To make up the Rescue Remedy, purchase from any large health food or herb store, one bottle each of the above five other remedies. Then add just two drops from each of them to *an ounce* (30 cc) bottle filled with fine brandy; cork well, label Rescue Remedy and store in a cool, dark place.

When it has to be used, add three drops of the Rescue Remedy to a 6 fl. oz. glass of distilled water. The patient should sip this frequently. As he or she becomes noticably calmer, it should be taken every 15 minutes and then every 30 minutes. If the patient can't sip the water, or is unconscious, rub some of it on his or her lips, on the gums, behind the ears, and also on the wrists. If no water is readily available, use the *undiluted* Rescue Remedy to moisten the lips, gums, or tongue. When used as a medicine over an extended period of time, give the usual 3 drops in a teaspoonful of water 4 times daily. The Rescue Remedy can also be applied to external injuries. It can be used to bathe a painful area; it can also be used as a cold compress or a hot fomentation. Six drops to a pint of water is the usual amount.

Foods and Nutrients

High-potency vitamin B-complex (6 tablets), lecithin (3 teaspoons), magnesium (1,800 mg.), and valenian root (4 capsules) form a good nutritive program for shock.

SIDE STITCHES

Symptoms

A stitch or catch in the side is caused by a spasm of the diaphragm and produces instant, sharp but temporary pain. It occurs when your diaphragm, a muscle between your chest and your abdomen, can't get the oxgyen it requires. If one isn't breathing evenly, he or she can get side stitches when they're running or walking or laughing.

Relief Measures

When the pain commences, cease whatever you might be doing. Relaxation is necessary to calm this twitching muscle. Using three fingers, press on the area where the pain is the worst until the aching stops. Or, use those three fingers to gently massage the painful area. Most often this is all that is required to release the pain.

Another method to get rid of side stitches is this: as you begin to knead the cramp out of your diaphragm, take a breath, purse your lips and then blow it out as hard as you can. Repeat the process several times until the pain is gone. Breathing from the belly instead of the chest cavity will help to prevent side stitches. The key here is to inhale and exhale *slowly and deeply*.

Certain aerobic activities, such as swimming, bouncing on a mini-trampoline, bicycling, jogging, playing tennis, or dancing helps to get rid of side stitches, too.

Foods and Nutrients

Some warm peppermint or catnip teas (1 cup) is useful. So is papaya juice (1 glass).

SINUSITIS

Symptoms

Sinusitis is an inflammation of the nasal sinuses that accompanies upper respiratory infection. Better than half of all cases of it are caused by bacteria. The sinuses affected by this infection include those above the eyes, inside each cheekbone, behind the bridge of the nose, and in the upper nose.

Acute sinusitis is frequently caused by colds or bacterial and viral infections of the nose, throat, and upper respiratory tract. Chronic sinusitis problems may be caused by small growths in the nose, injury of the nasal bones, smoking, and irritant fumes and smells. Allergenic sinusitis may be caused by hay fever and food allergies, especially allergies to milk and dairy products.

Symptoms of sinusitis include headache, earache, toothache, facial pain, cranial pressure, loss of sense of smell, tenderness over the forehead and cheekbones, and sometimes an elevated fever. Once in awhile sinusitis produces a swollen face followed by a stuffy nose and thick discharge of mucus.

Relief Measures

Humidity is the key to keep minute nasal hairs called the cilia working, the mucus flowing, and the sinuses drained. Twice a day stand in a hot shower for a few minutes. Or lean over a pan full of steaming peppermint or yarrow or chamomile tea with a towel draped over your head, creating a steam tent. Inhale the vapors as they waft up toward your nostrils.

If you become congested during the daytime, a cup of hot coffee, black or green tea, or clear chicken or beef bouillon soup is not only good to drink, but also to inhale. Cup your hands over the top of the mug, place your face down over them, and sniff the warm vapors for several minutes.

Flushing out stale nasal secretions helps to remedy sinusitis. Mix a small teaspoonful of table salt with two cups of warm distilled water and a pinch of Arm & Hammer baking soda. Pour it into a shot glass, tilt your head back, close one nostril with your thumb, and sniff the solution with the open nostril. Then blow your nose gently with a Kleenex tissue. Repeat on the other side.

Drink extra liquids—both hot and cold—throughout the course of the day. Liquids thin out the mucus and keep it flowing. Sipping hot anise, fennel, lemon balm, or sage teas helps clear out more of this mucus.

Foods and Nutrients

Eating foods generously flavored with certain spices may help to bring sinus relief through, of all the places, the stomach. Garlic, horseradish, jalepeño peppers, marjoram, oregano, onion, and cajun spice mixture are all highly aromatic and tend to make the eyes water or nose run once they're inside the gut. These aggravating reactions will naturally burst through even the most stubborn sinus blockage.

A fairly effective product is Breathe Free (3 tablets on an empty stomach). (See Appendix under Trace mineral Research.) More importantly are Kyolic aged-garlic extract (3 capsules) and goldenseal root (1 capsule) to be taken daily. (See Appendix under Wakunaga.) Be sure to add pantothenic acid (300 mg.) and vitamin C (3,500 mg.) to this regimen.

SKIN CANCER

See CANCER for more information.

SKIN PROBLEMS

See under their individual listings for more information:

ACNE, BOILS, CHICKENPOX, HERPES, HIVES, MEASLES, MUMPS, OILY HAIR & SKIN, POISON IVY & OAK, PSORIASIS.

SLEEPWALKING

Symptoms

Sleepwalking or somnambulism is a disorder of sleep involving complex motor acts which occurs primarily during the first third of the night but not during rapid eye movement sleep. In this form of hysteria, the purposeful behavior is forgotten when the subject awakens. This anxiety or excitement phenomena is more common in children than it is in adults.

Relief Measures

Norman S. from Yonkers, New York suffered from periodic sleepwalking. He went to a sleep specialist and was given some simple instructions. His doctor told him to take a hot shower *before* he went to bed, to drink some hot milk, and to dress comfortably in some loose-fitting flannel pajamas.

The physician said to Norman: "The warmer your body is when you retire at night, the longer you'll sleep without interruptions."

Norman followed his advice and in less than a month his sleepwalking problem was entirely solved.

Foods and Nutrients

His physician also mentioned that the amino acid tryptophan was very good for inducing drowsiness. He had his patient eat more milk, cheese, eggs, beef, and salmon, which are high in it.

SMOKING DEPENDENCY

Symptoms

Smoking dependency is a habitual addiction to nicotine, which can only be properly satisfied through the frequent puffing on many cigarettes. Nicotine works much like heroin, cocaine, and alcohol in its effect upon the brain. In fact, when nicotine was intravenously administered to volunteers, many of them could not tell the difference between the effects of nicotine and cocaine. Nicotine produces pleasurable sensations and physical dependency because it operates through the central nervous system. Unpleasant withdrawal symptoms often occur when smokers refrain from cigarettes. They usually feel grouchy, depressed, frustrated, and anxious, and tend to experience a phlegmy cough, stomach cramps, and headaches. These symptoms, however, generally last no longer than half-a-month.

Tobacco smoking in the 1990's caused one-third of all cancer mortalities and a quarter of all fatal heart attacks in the U.S. and Canada. A number of respiratory problems are directly related to the act of smoking *and to second-hand smoke* as well. In fact, *second-hand smoke* has now become just as serious a health threat for non-smokers as it is to smokers.

Relief Measures

A fluid extract of common oats appears to decrease the craving for nicotine in smokers. An interesting report about this appeared in the October 15, 1971 issue of *Nature* journal (233:496).

While in India in 1967, C. L. Anand met a practitioner of the ancient Ayurvedic medicine who successfully used a decoction of common oats to cure the opium habit. While using an alcoholic extract of the plant on a group of opium addicts, he noticed that several patients reported a loss of interest in smoking altogether.

Returning to his native Scotland, Mr. Anand decided to test this for himself on some smokers. He used 1.5 parts of the crushed whole, *fresh* plant in 5 parts of 90% ethyl alcohol, kept at room temperature with frequent shaking for 3 days, after which the contents were filtered into another container.

Twenty-six cigarette smokers, including healthy volunteers and chronic patients in the chest wards of Ruchill Hospital in Glasgow, including tuberculosis patients, participated in the trial study. The total duration of their smoking and the average number of cigarettes smoked per day in the preceding six months were recorded.

They were told that a drug was being tested which might affect their smoking, and that they were not to make any conscious effort to alter their smoking during the trial.

Each patient kept a daily record of cigarettes smoked, commenting on any changes in the craving for cigarettes. By random allocation, 13 patients received the drug and the others received placebo for almost a month. The alcoholic extract (1 ml.) was diluted to 5 ml. and each oral dose given just beneath the tongue for faster absorption was 5 ml. of this dilution 4 times a day. No psychotherapy was used. Nor were any patients permitted other medications which could affect smoking. The patients in both groups were comparable in age, sex, and smoking history.

The results of this trial are presented in the table below:

Number of Cigarettes Smoked during Trial

Group I (Oats)

Cigarettes per day before trial	Cigarettes per day after trial
20	20
25	10
10	0
12	0
11	0
9	0
35	3
25	7
22	0
20	7
25	7
20	10
20	10
Av. 19.5	5.7

Group II (Placebo)

Cigarettes per day before trial	Cigarettes per day after trial
22	19
30	28
18	18
14	14
18	17
17	18
17	18
8	18
18	18
20	18
15	14
10	9

8	8
16.5	16.7

The results of the trial were certainly very interesting by way of comparison. In the group taking the fluid extract of fresh oat plant, the total daily consumption by 13 patients was 254 cigarettes; at the end of the experiment it was down to just 74. Five had stopped smoking, seven had reduced it to less than 50% and in one no change had occurred. In the placebo group, the total daily consumption at the start was 215, at the end it was 217. Smoking had been stopped by none of the participants, reduced to above 50% by six, and increased by 3; 4 report no change at all.

In the fluid extract of oats group, various degrees of loss of craving for cigarettes were reported. The herbal preparation appeared to have reduced the number of cigarettes smoked per day, along with diminished craving for smoking. Moreover, the reduction in smoking seems to have persisted even 2 months after the termination of the pilot study.

Catnip tea (2 cups) or valerian root extract (15 drops 3 times daily) or capsules (4 at a time) or hops tea (2 cups) have all been effective in curbing nicotine addiction for short periods of time.

Foods and Nutrients

One of the authors remembers an experience he had with an executive secretary working in a high-rise building in the downtown business district of Jakarta, Indonesia. Josephine Hetarihon, aged 35, related how she overcame her own smoking dependency:

It was on Sept. 26, 1979 that I finally managed to quit smoking. I had been smoking 2 packs a day of Dunhill before this.

I started smoking when I was in junior high school at the age of 15. A friend suggested that I use carrots to help me quit because they were sweet and a good substitute for the nicotine craving.

It took me about a month on this carrot program until I saw results. I would eat 2-3 carrots a day, mostly nibbling on them in the form of carrot sticks. After this all desires to smoke left me.

Avoid the consumption of acid foods and instead opt for more alkaline staples. Research shows that smokers who eat junk food are apt to have more cigarettes in a day than those who supplement their diets with more fresh fruits and vegetables. Sugar and fat tend to flush nicotine out of the body more quickly, thereby creating more frequent cravings, whereas alkaline foods high in potassium cause a longer retention of nicotine in the system, which enables addicts to smoke fewer cigarettes.

Lecithin (1 tsp. daily), vitamin E oil (1,200 mg. daily), B-complex (4 tablets daily), and magnesium (1,800 mg. daily) form a good supplement program to help the body withstand any withdrawal symptoms once a smoker decides to quit the habit.

SNAKEBITE

Symptoms

Snakebite occurs when an individual is bitten on some part of the body by a venomous or non-poisonous snake. Classic symptoms include swelling, skin discoloration, a rapid pulse, weakness, shortness of breath, nausea and vomiting, and sometimes unconsciousness. *Prompt medical attention is desirable!*

Relief Measures

If medical help isn't readily available, apply a constricting band 2-4 inches above the bite. Keep calm and immobilize the affected area, keeping below heart level if possible. Cold therapy like an ice pack isn't advisable. If rapid swelling or severe pain should occur, a half-inch incision should be made directly below the fang marks, and suction should be performed at once. The cut should be made along the long axis of the limb with a sharp, sterilized blade just through the skin, and suction should be done for 30 minutes with a suction cup or with the mouth (spit out the blood!). Never, never make cuts on the head, neck, or trunk! Major veins are located here and doing such could become even more life-threatening than the snakebite itself is.

Echinacea (5 capsules or 30 drops of fluid extract), goldenseal root (4 capsules or 20 drops of fluid extract) or yellow dock tea (2 cups) or capsules (5) or sarsaparilla root (6 capsules) every 1.5 hours is suggested until the symptoms disappear.

Poultices of white oak bark leaves and bark, comfrey root or leaves, or powdered slippery elm bark can be very useful. Plantain poultice, plantain salve, or comfrey salve can also be used.

Foods and Nutrients

Protein-rich and refined carbohydrate foods seem to expedite the assimilation of venom from a poisonous snake or spider into the system more quickly. Consequently, meat, white bread, pastries, and soft drinks and colas should be totally avoided until symptoms have passed.

Massive doses (up to 100,000 mg.) of vitamin C, given orally and intramuscularly should save the life of someone who has been bitten by a deadly viper or spider.

It is also recommended that calcium gluconate (500 mg.) be given every couple of hours, as well as pantothenic acid (500 mg.) every few hours for a couple of days.

SNORING

Symptoms

Snoring is an extremely common problem, afflicting more than half of everyone over 50, especially men. Anything that restricts airflow in the throat and nasal passages can cause it. Mostly, it's due to a loss of muscle tone in the back of the throat—a natural consequence of getting older or gaining extra weight—which tends to make the tissue there hang in loose folds. As you inhale and your breath rushes past, these folds vibrate, somewhat like the reed in a woodwind instrument, resulting in the decidedly unmusical buzzsaw noises or staccato blasts of snoring.

Other conditions that can disrupt normal breathing and thus cause snoring are: nasal polyps, a deviated septum, chronic rhinitis (nasal inflammation), adenoids, enlarged tonsils, a cold, or allergies. Likewise, any sedative—including tranquilizers, alcohol, or even antihistamines that induce drowsiness—can relax muscles enough to lead to snoring. Avoiding these before bedtime, if possible might help.

Relief Measures

Try a nasal decongestant spray with oxymetazoline (i.e., short-acting Dristan) at bedtime, to open up air passages. But don't use the spray during the day, too, or it could lead to a "rebound effect," wherein congestion actually gets worse.

Use a humidifier in your bedroom if your nasal passages tend to dry out when you sleep. Moist air seems to help reduce snoring in many people.

Stay away from alcohol and cigarettes. They both can cause inflammation and swelling of nasal mucous membranes.

Try losing weight if you are obese and snore. Reduction of body weight makes it easier for a person to breathe at night while sleeping.

Put a tennis ball into a sock and pin it to the back of your pajamas. Since many people snore only when they lie on their backs, anything that discourages this might solve the problem. Also, elevating the head can help.

If you have chronic sleep disturbances or often experience daytime sleepiness, you might be suffering from sleep apnea, a potentially dangerous condition associated with snoring, in which breathing actually ceases for brief periods, after which the sleeper gasps or snores startingly in the struggle to regain normal breathing. A physician can determine whether you have apnea from a tape recording of your snoring.

Foods and Nutrients

Believe it or not, sneezing and snoring go hand-in-hand as a rule. Snoring can develop due to allergies or head colds. The elimination of white sugar and extremely sweet foods from the diet, will cut allergies in half. (Consult the entry under ALLERGIES for additional information.)

Taking some powdered effervescent vitamin C with a little distilled water just before retiring, has been known to help habitual snorers from not making so much noise when they fall fast asleep. One level teaspoonful to a glass of water is recommended.

SORE THROAT

Symptoms

A sore throat can be caused by anything that irritates the sensitive mucous membranes at the back of the throat and mouth. Serious irritants include viral and bacterial infections, allergic reactions, dust, smoke, fumes, very spicy foods or drinks, tooth or gum infections, and abrasions.

Chronic coughing and excessive loud talking also irritate the throat. Hoarseness is a common side effect. The 1992 Democratic Presidential candidate Bill Clinton repeatedly found himself with a sore throat due to voice overuse. On several different occasions doctors had to insist that their patient cease all public speaking appearances in order to give his larynx and vocal cords much badly needed rest.

Relief Measures

If your throat happens to be sore because of viral infections, try sucking on some medicated lozenges containing phenol. Phenol kills surface germs and its mild anesthetic action numbs raw nerve endings so your throat doesn't feel as scratchy.

Also sucking on Hall's brand cough drops containing eucalyptus is of value. As well as horehound cough drops orhorehound herb candy. Chewing on a short piece of licorice root (available from some health food stores) and slowly letting the saliva produced trickle down the throat helps immensely.

One of the nicest remedies for quick relief is to squeeze some drops of 40% bee propolis tincture from Montana Naturals (see Appendix) down the back of the throat. At first it may burn a little, but the relief it gives lasts for hours.

Foods and Nutrients

A winning trio of supplements helps to relieve even the worst sore throat. First, take 3 Kyolic garlic capsules (see Appendix under Wakunaga). Then follow this up with the equivalent of 1,500 mg. of effervescent vitamin C mixed with water or juice. Finally,

suck on a zinc gluconate lozenge every 1.5 hours until pain is sufficiently relieved.

Another popular remedy among some European opera singers is to repeatedly gargle with some hot lemon juice or tea, flavored with a little wild honey or molasses. Sometimes a pinch of sea salt is added. Another variation on this same idea is to substitute equal pinches of powdered horse-radish and ground cloves for the salt.

SPINAL MENINGITIS

See MENINGITIS for more informa-tion.

SPIDER BITE

Virtually the same remedies, dietary applications and nutrients previously given for SNAKE BITE apply here as well.

SPRAINS

Symptoms

A sprain occurs when the ligament connecting bone to muscle is stretched beyond its capability and sometimes tears in the process. The soft tissue surrounding the joint may become sore, swollen, and bruised. The joints most often injured are the ankles, back, fingers, knees, and wrists. Sprains may result from unexpected movement or twisting of the affected area or from a hard fall. Such injuries are common to athletes.

Relief Measures

One of the simplest yet most effective methods of reducing the symptoms attending any sprain is with the aid of hot and cold water. But as simple as this seems, it's terribly ironic how so many people are virtually ignorant of it.

Some years ago one of the authors visited some friends of his then residing in Springville, Utah. They had a 15-year-old son named Hans. He had just come home from the doctor's office after sustaining a badly sprained ankle in his physical education class playing basketball. The doctor prescribed some heavy duty aspirin to take away the pain, and said the foot would get better in a couple of days.

This author had the mother get two five-gallon plastic white food storage buckets, and fill one of them a quarter full of boiling water. He then went to a local supermarket and purchased a large plastic bag of ice. He put most of this into the other bucket and then had her pour just a little boiling water over the ice to quickly melt it down but not enough to warm it.

He then instructed her son to sit down on a chair, roll up his blue jeans pant leg and stick his foot into *the cold water first,* leaving it there for several minutes. With some encouragement from his mom, the kid reluctantly did this and shivered when his swollen foot made contact with the icy water. After 2 minutes, he was told to plunge it into the other bucket containing the hot water. This he did and left it there for the same

amount of time. This back-and-forth procedure was kept up for about 20 minutes or until the water in both buckets had lost their heat and chill.

It was explained to both of them that this simple treatment worked upon the circulatory system in much the same way as the ocean waves do upon a beach. Impressions left in the sand are quickly washed away with each incoming and outgoing tide. The hot-and-cold water treatment sends the blood to and from the injured site, reducing tissue inflammation and nerve pain.

By the next morning the boy's ankle was only one-fourth the size of what it had been the night before, and looked a lot better in terms of reduced skin discoloration. Several more treatments the second day cleared the problem up entirely.

Foods and Nutrients

The spice called turmeric, which is one of the chief ingredients in curry powder and used in many Indian dishes, is good for reducing muscle tissue inflammation. Combine 1/2 level teaspoon in 1.5 cups of warm water and drink slowly.

Mullein (3 cups) and yarrow (2 cups) teas consumed each day when warm, offer additional relief for sprains and strains. The same can be said for ginger root (4 capsules) as well.

Papain (4 tablets daily) or regular papaya juice (1 glass) destroy those scavenger molecules known as free radicals which are released during injury and cause cell deterioration.

An amino acid supplement (6 capsules or tablets daily), vitamin B-6 (50 mg.), calcium gluconate (1,000 mg.), magnesium (1,800 mg.), potassium (2,000 mg.), manganese (50 mg.), and silicon from horsetail or shave grass herb (2 capsules) all help to expedite the healing of sprains, strains, and other muscle and joint injuries.

STAINED TEETH

Symptoms

The natural color of the teeth is more of a light yellow to light yellow-red than an actual white any dentist will tell you. But they can become discolored when colas, black or green teas, soft drinks, citric juices, highly pigmented foods such as beets, and smoke from cigarettes, cigars, or pipes slosh past them many times each day.

Stains can also be caused by prescription antibiotics and water high in natural fluoride. Chewing tobacco stains them further. And the older we get, the more our teeth are apt to darken.

Surface enamel cracks and erodes, exposing dentin, the less dense substance inside of the tooth, which absorbs food color. Stains also latch onto the plaque and tartar buildup on teeth, finding anchorage among the nooks and crannies. There are different kinds of stains. Those of the coffee and cigarette variety are easier to remove in between professional Scleanings than those attributed to old age or medications.

Relief Measures

Brush your teeth after *every* meal with a natural brand of toothpaste devoid of chemical additives and sugar. One of the most popular sold in health food stores is Tom's Toothpaste. Then once or twice a week spend some time polishing your teeth. Mix baking soda with enough hydrogen peroxide to make a toothpaste, then brush those stains away. Or substitute powdered black walnut for the baking soda.

Occasionally rinse with a disclosing solution that will indicate where any plaque might remain on your teeth after brushing and flossing. Those are the areas where stains are the most likely to occur unless your brushing technique is improved. Be sure to rinse any food particles remaining inside your mouth after every meal or snack. One of the authors has been in the habit of doing this for years, even in public eating places which, admittedly, has drawn some bewildered looks from curious people around him.

Studies have shown that an electric toothbrush can remove more stain-collecting plaque from the teeth than an ordinary toothbrush can. But don't scrub your teeth too hard, because excessive brushing can cause just as much wear on tooth enamel as some abrasive toothpastes.

Foods and Nutrients

Calcium-rich foods such as milk, cheese, yogurt, almonds, and dark leafy green vegetables can help to preserve the natural color of the teeth longer. However, acidic, sugary, and greasy foods tends to stain them a lot more quickly.

STINGS

Symptoms

Bees, wasps, hornets, and yellow jackets inject venom into the skin tissue of their unlucky victims when they sting. This action leads to considerable pain, immediate swelling, and a lot of redness at the site of the sting. Such discomforts can last from a few hours to a full day or more, depending, of course, on what and how many of them have stung you.

Relief Measures

Properly identifying which insect injured you is essential to the type of treatment to be employed. A honeybee, for instance, can only sting once. This is due to its barbed stinger which remains imbedded in the skin, causing the bee to die. On the other hand, bumblebees, wasps, hornets, and yellow jackets, have smooth stingers that can repeatedly injure you. The so-called "killer bees" from Africa which were imported to Brazil years ago and some of which escaped, eventually have made their way northward and now appear in Texas and other southern states. These bees are highly aggressive in nature and vicious enough to attack an animal or human in swarms, inflicting hundreds of stings in a matter of minutes, often leading to death. And if a yellow jacket is squashed, its crushed venom sac releases a chemical signal that notifies other yellow jackets nearby to attack immediately.

Removing the stinger from an injury inflicted by a honey-bee as quickly as possible is imperative, otherwise the venom sac attached to it will continue to pump for up to 4 minutes, driving the stinger and its poison deeper into the flesh.

But be careful not to squeeze the stinger or the sac—doing so will release more poison into your body. Scraping the stinger out is by far the best approach. Use your fingernail, a nail file, or even the edge of a plastic credit card to gently scrape under the stinger and flip it out.

Because such insects are known to collect around dung heaps and garbage piles, it's not unusual to find bacteria mixed in with their venom. So remember to wash the sting well with soap and water or a good antiseptic to prevent infection.

After doing this, you'll want to do something which will relieve the throbbing pain very quickly. Placing an ice pack or even an ice cube over the injured site can reduce swelling and prevent the venom from spreading out further. Also, some mashed cucumber slices placed over it works well. Even wetting the surface of the injury a little and then sprinkling some Adolph's meat tenderizer or plain alum over it, and then gently rubbing into the skin will bring relief. The meat tenderizer contains papain, a proteolytic enzyme from papaya latex, and alum has aluminum salt in it, both of which manifest analgesic actions.

One of the simplest and most effective remedies is to crush a tablet of Bufferin or Excedrin, dribble some saliva on to the sting site, and then rub this powder in. The aspirin neutralizes certain inflammatory agents in the venom.

Believe it or not, heat can also make the injury feel a lot better by neutralizing one of the chemicals that produces inflammation. A hot pack placed over the swelling and changed every few minutes when it becomes cool with a fresh one does the trick.

If nothing else is available, try using a little household ammonia to relieve the pain promptly. Mr. Clean or Lysol may not be items you have in mind for first-aid kits, but they *do* work. Just soak a cotton ball with a little of either solution and dab it on the skin.

A paste made from powdered activated charcoal is useful for drawing the poison out rapidly so the injury won't swell or become painful. Carefully open a few charcoal capsules and remove the powder. Moisten it with water and apply to the sting. Cover with gauze or Saran wrap. The purpose in this is because the charcoal works best when it remains moist.

If nothing else is available, plain, ordinary mud will suffice. Make sure that it's "clean," however. By this we mean that the soil doesn't come from a barnyard, toxic waste site, or garbage dump, but from a field, meadow or similar place where man-made or animal pollution isn't evident. Follow the same procedures as you would for charcoal and cover with either a bandage or handkerchief.

Avoiding getting stung is more important than treating the injury itself. Wearing white clothing tends to keep such insects at a comfortable distance, but anything dark, colorful or too gaudy is bound to attract them. That's probably why beekeepers generally wear khaki, white, or other light colors.

Avoid wearing perfume, after-shave lotion, and any other fragrance that will lead a bee or wasp to confuse you with a nectar-bearing flower.

Foods and Nutrients

Several days before making a trip into the outdoors, go on a mild food fast and cleansing program in order to detoxify the system of excess sugar. Mosquitos, bees, wasps, and the like are instantly attracted to persons who's sweat glands generate moisture that is sweet-smelling. Consume only alkaline foods that are non-acidic and not sweet, in order to make your body perspiration more bland and slightly salty.

Taking 100 mg. of zinc each day for a week in advance of your contemplated trip helps to prevent insect stings.

STRAINED MUSCLES

See under SPRAINS for more information.

STREP THROAT

See under SORE THROAT for more information.

STRESS AND ANXIETY

Symptoms

Stress is from the Latin *strictus*, which means "to tighten" or from "stringo" which is "to draw together." Stress is the reaction of the body to forces of a harmful nature, infections, and various abnormal states that tend to disturb its normal physiologic equilibrium.

Anxiety is from the Latin "anxius" or "distressed" or from "ango" which is "to press tight," or "to torment." Anxiety is the apprehension of danger and dread accompanied by restlessness, tension, rapid heartbeats, and shortness of breath, all of which are unattached to a clearly identifiable stimulus.

Stress can result from many things: a high-pressure job, relationships, loneliness, crowds, noise, and traffic jams. Anxiety of the mind is due more to things with an element of uncertainty about them: floundering marriage, potential job layoff, impending litigation, IRS tax audit, bank foreclosure, and so forth.

Long-term stress usually occurs when the situation that produces anxiety isn't relieved. For instance, a person who must care for and live with a family member who is physically or mentally ill experiences stress on a daily basis. Families whose economic status is far below what they need, who must worry about where the next meal will come from or where they will sleep that night, suffer from extreme stress.

Even those who are better advantaged economically, educationally, and healthily, can experience some stress and anxiety in their own lives. For example, one of the authors knows of a wealthy dowager living in the heart of Manhattan, who, quite literally, "has money to burn." Yet in spite of all her jewels, furs, stocks and bonds, penthouse suites in New York and London, fabulous art collection, and expensive rugs and furniture, she went through a stressful period of almost half-a-year some time ago.

It didn't have to do with the death of her late husband or some other close relative or friend, but rather with the demise of her Scottish terrier named Chuckles. This animal meant more to her than her own hubby did. She bawled all the time, and carried on as if it were the end of the world for her. "Oh, what's the use of living any longer without my pet," she moaned and groaned in the author's presence one day.

To most readers, her case may seem extreme and quite laughable. But, in fact, the very purpose of her existence hinged on that one mutt. No material things could ever take away the pain she was then feeling, and no soft-spoken, well-intentioned words could ever comfort the heartaches she must have felt. It took a great deal of psychiatric therapy to finally bring her back to a reasonable state of normalcy.

Not everyone who experiences stress can handle it responsibly. The body is able to cope with a certain measure of it, and most of us fare well enough because of this innate ability. But beyond an unspecified point (different for each of us), there is a limit to such capabilities. Once that range has been exceeded, the body begins to break down.

Many of us attribute our stress-related symptoms to "nerves," and, in fact, stress first affects the parts of the body that are related to the nervous system, especially through the digestive and intestinal systems. Initial symptoms of stress-related digestive disorders may be an ulcer attack or colitis. Irritability, hypertension, headaches and neckaches, diarrhea, dizziness, and loss of appetite are other disorders precipitated by stress. If the stress that produces these symptoms is not handled properly, more serious illness can result.

Scientists believe that when the brain is under stress and anxiety for any duration, it produces an abundance of the hormone ACTh. This hormone inhibits the manufacture of white blood cells so vital in combatting disease. Accumulating evidence suggests a direct "mind-body" link between the way we think and how we feel physically.

Relief Measures

Relaxation is paramount to easing mental and emotional tensions. Think of stress as a strung bow, all taut and ready to shoot arrows at a target. Then imagine it unstrung, and that's relaxation. Ordinary stress is much easier to alleviate than more deeply rooted anxiety.

Often times mechanical things can go a long ways in resting the body from tension—i.e., a good massage, soft music, sitting in a rocking chair, reclining on a couch or in a hammock, petting a cat or dog, watching a favorite movie or TV program, reading a good book and so on.

But because anxiety involves the mental perception of fear and may even be deeply centered in the soul as well, other approaches must be taken to adequately cope

with the problem. By turning the focus of that dread to something else more cheerful in nature, the dark cloud of anxiety can be lifted from the mind.

The action is similar to a two-way jacket one of the authors has. When the darker-colored side became dingy from considerable wear, he simply turned it inside out and wore the lighter color instead. This reaching in, if you will, to your own anxiety, grabbing a hold and turning the thing inside out might be termed "reverse focusing." But the idea works and can be successful if properly done.

The key here is to first consider the present anxiety itself. Examine it from all sides, and then ask yourself the simple question: "What could be worse than this?" As one lady told one of us some time ago, "I was despondent over my husband's unemployment and not being able to make ends meet with the meager public assistance we were getting, until I met a friend who had lost her home, car, furniture, and savings account to an Internal Revenue Service seizure for her husband's unpaid back taxes. Then all of a sudden, things didn't look so bad for us after that!"

Then alternate this view of despair with an outlook that is filled with hope and the strong possibility of becoming fulfilled. Hope is the antidote to anxiety and replaces fear with a surge of confidence in the tormented soul.

One of the best ways of dealing with short-term stress is to get adequate rest. At first this might seem rather impossible to do, considering how stress can keep you up part of the night. But sleep does wonders for the nerves, brain, and heart. Upon awakening the next morning, one feels invigorated and imbued with a renewed sense of trying again. Things look and feel a lot better than they did the night before.

Interrupt your hum-drum routine by taking time off to do the things you enjoy doing. It's bad enough to do that which you don't like but have to do. So allow yourself lots of little mini-vacations to go places you've never been or attempt things you've only dreamed about but never quite gotten around to trying.

Develop hobbies for yourself. They are a great way of relieving stress and anxiety. They not only take your mind off of that which is negative and depressing, but also buoy up your spirits and relax your body. With most hobbies one has to concentrate on that which is enjoyable, thereby directing personal attention away from those things which are burdensome and troubling.

Foods and Nutrients

There seems to be a commonality in some symptoms between candidiasis or yeast infection, chronic fatigue syndrome, and hypoglycemia. A sensible diet devoid of sugary things and too many refined carbohydrates is called for here. Colas, fired foods, junk foods, white flour products, and so forth create a kind of "nutritional stress" within the system. Whereas raw food creates life and vitality! You'd be amazed just how much of a drag a lousy diet can be on the mind and emotions!

A high-potency B-complex (4 tablets daily) supplemented with extra vitamin B-6 (100 mg.) and pantothenic acid (300 mg.) is

important. So too is calcium (1,000 mg. daily) and magnesium (1,800 mg.). The amino acid L-Tyrosine (500 mg. taken with 50 mg. of B-6 twice daily) relaxes the nerves and enables the body to rest more soundly at night.

Stress and anxiety have a way of depleting the anti-stress hormones manufactured by the adrenal glands. Vitamin C (3,500 mg.) and bioflavonoids taken separately (100 mg. each of rutin and hesperidin) is suggested for normal adrenal functions.

Lecithin (1 tablespoon) and vitamin E oil (800 mg.) on a daily basis helps the nerves.

STROKE

See under HEART ATTACK for more information.

SUDDEN INFANT DEATH SYNDROME (SIDS)

Symptoms

Sudden infant death syndrome (SIDS) or crib death is the abrupt and inexplicable death of an apparently healthy infant. The termination of life usually comes when the baby is soundly asleep. This remains one of the major killers of infants from one month to one year of age in the U.S. and Canada.

Various theories have been advanced to explain such deaths; i.e., sleep-induced apnea, laryngospasm, overwhelming infectious disease, and so forth. But none of them have been generally accepted or demonstrated at autopsies.

Relief Measures

Two very controversial possibilities have been posed by some pediatricians as the likely cause of SIDS. Both seem to hold equal merit for being plausible, although there is virtually a dearth of evidence to actually support such claims. Still, they are well worth considering in the light that they just might possibly save a few infant lives if implemented.

Some doctors have noticed that those babies who are given the DTP vaccines appear to be at greater risk for SIDS, than infants who have *not* been immunized at all. Doctors have found that there is a correlation between pertussis (whooping cough) immunization in the early months of life, and the risk of SIDS. They have advised parents to forego the DTP vaccination because of this uncanny coincidence. And parents who have listened to these doctors, have usually been spared the heart-wrenching agonies of seeing their babies die for no apparent reason.

Foods and Nutrients

The second, equally radical hypothesis put forth by a handful of pediatricians is that *bottle*-feeding newborns cow's milk or infant formula is likely to *increase* the risk of SIDS. Whereas moms who breast-feed their infants with their own body milk, substantially reduce the chances of this ever happening.

The problem here is that these doctors don't know if it's the bottle feeding itself or the solution inside or both. So they have made the broad-sweeping assumption that both of them may increase the risk of SIDS.

SUNBURN

Symptoms

Sunburn is caused by excessive exposure to ultraviolet rays, which actually burn up surface skin and later the lower cells. The amount of exposure to ultraviolet rays which causes burning depends basically on four things: the individual, the place, the time, and atmospheric conditions.

Caution should be used in exposing oneself to the sun for extended periods of time between 10:00 A.M. and 2:00 P.M., when most of the ultraviolet rays are present. Reflections from water, metal, sand, or snow may double the amount of rays one absorbs.

Burns can be categorized three different ways. First-degree sunburn produces reddening of the skin and possibly slight fever. Second-degree sunburn causes reddening of the skin accompanied by water blisters. Third-degree sunburn causes lower cell damage and the release of fluid, resulting in eruptions and breaks in the skin where bacteria and infection can enter.

Relief Measures

Brew up a quart of mullein and yarrow tea (equal parts of both herbs or one handful apiece). Let it cool. Then soak a clean cotton terry towel or cloth in the solution, lightly wring out excess liquid, and apply over the afflicted parts of the skin. Leave on for half-an-hour.

Follow this up by massaging some aloe vera juice on the sunburned area. Reapply every hour on the hour.

Foods and Nutrients

A reasonable supplement program for sunburn recovery should include: potassium (2,000 mg. daily), magnesium (1,000 mg. daily), phosphorus (800 mg. daily), calcium (600 mg. daily), an amino acid (3 capsules or tablets daily), vitamin A (25,000 I.U.), vitamin E (1,000 I.U.), vitamin C with bioflavonoids (3,500 mg. daily), and zinc (100 mg. daily).

Diet is critical for repairing skin tissue in second and third-degree burns. Eat high-protein foods and drink plenty of fluids (up to 8 glasses a day).

SWEATING EXCESSIVELY

Symptoms

In the adolescent years, there is normally a great increase in the development and activity of the sweat glands, and an alteration in the odor of the sweat itself. However, when it persists into adulthood, it can be potentially embarrassing.

Excessive sweating can be due to a number of different factors: the consumption of spicy foods, confinement to an overheated room for very long, wearing too many

clothes, a thyroid gland disorder, a fever, or menopausal hot flashes.

Relief Measures

Do *not* use commercial body deodorants as they contain aluminum compounds, which can enter the pores of the skin and poison the bloodstream. Instead use tincture of witch hazel or apple cider vinegar to reduce sweat gland flows.

Wear loose-fitting clothing which is cool and comfortable. Remain calm and collected; any duration of stress is apt to start the beads of perspiration pouring out of you.

Foods and Nutrients

Liquid chlorophyll is especially helpful for controlling excessive sweating. One glass of Kyo-Green each day is advised (see Appendix under Wakunaga).

One of the authors who is an anthropologist has spent considerable time in the tropical regions of the earth. There he has noticed that in spite of the unbearable temperatures, the natives seem to get along nicely with minimal discomforts. An investigation into their diets revealed a frequent intake of certain spices, particularly cayenne pepper. Capsicum does appear to at least slow the rate of perspiration flow, but more importantly it helps to keep the body cool in spite of its thermonuclear qualities. Foods can be seasoned with cayenne pepper or it can be taken in capsule form (2 daily). Beware, however, that capsicum is hypoglycemic and may not be tolerated very well by those who have low blood sugar.

SWIMMER'S EAR

See EAR DISORDERS under Otitis Externa for more information.

SWOLLEN GLANDS

Symptoms

Swollen glands is a term often applied to enlargement of the lymph nodes, or glands of the neck, on both sides of the throat. Technically, though, it can also describe enlargement of any of the lymph glands, such as those located in the armpit or groin. The enlargement of lymph glands is generally a sign of an impending infection about to occur in the area, because the lymph glands function to filter out microscopic material, such as bacteria, in order to prevent the spread of infection.

Symptoms include enlarged or swollen glands that may be hard or soft. These symptoms may be accompanied by heat, tenderness, and reddening of the overlying skin, and fever. Swollen glands may simply mean a localized infection has set in or could be a symptom of a more serious disease. Swollen gland conditions may develop with such illnesses as measles, mumps, chickenpox, sexually transmissible disease, cancer, and tuberculosis.

Relief Measures

Two of the finest herbs for treating swollen glands due to childhood diseases or an infection, are mullein and yarrow. Make a tea by adding two tablespoonfuls of each in a quart of boiling water. Cover, remove from the stove, and simmer 40 minutes. Strain, and drink warm, one cup every two hours. Also, soak a cotton terry cloth hand towel or piece of linen cloth in the same solution, gently wring out excess liquid, and apply to the sides of the neck and throat, while somewhat hot. Cover with a heavier towel. When it turns cool, remove and repeat process. These teas help to take the swelling down rapidly.

Foods and Nutrients

Infections can be cleared up by ample dosages of vitamins A (50,000 I.U.) and C (10,000 mg.), B-complex (3 tablets daily), germanium (150 mcg.) and zinc (100 mg.).

SYSTEMIC LUPUS ERYTHEMATOSUS

See under LUPUS ERYTHEMATOSUS for more information.

SYPHILIS

See under SEXUALLY TRANSMISSIBLE DISEASES for more information.

TACHYCARDIA

(Also see ARRHYTHMIAS)

Symptoms

Tachycardia, or more specifically paroxysmal atrial tachycardia is the medical terminology for any rapid heartbeat that exceeds 90 beats per minute. Tachycardia is normal following exercise, big meals, emotional upset, and monthly periods. Some substances such as tobacco, alcohol, coffee, tea, and belladonna can induce this state, too.

A much more serious and life-threatening type of rapid heartbeat is ventricular tachycardia in which the electro-cardiogram reading shows a steady irregularity in bursts of 5 to 20 *rapid* beats interchanged with some slow ones.

Relief Measures

A racing heart should serve as a flashing red semaphore in the intersection of life that real danger lies ahead if you don't slow down and rest! Another way to slow rapid heartbeat is to breathe deeply and then bear down, as if you were sitting on the toilet about ready to have a bowel movement.

Have your doctor show you where your right carotid artery is located, and the correct amount of pressure to use on it. Then gently massage as far underneath the jaw as you can, right where this artery is connected in the neck.

When sea mammals dive into icy waters, their heart rates automatically slow. You can mimic this peculiar diving reflex yourself by filling a basin with ice-cold water and then plunging your face into it for a few seconds at a time to interrupt the tachy-cardia.

Doctors have observed that people who are perfectionists, upwardly mobile, and success-oriented tend to suffer from tachy-cardia more. By and large, they're the same individuals who also experience migraine headaches. They've allowed their adrenal glands to overproduce adrenalin, which in turn, throws the regular rhythm of the heart completely out of whack. They need to compensate for this by learning to not be so fussy in every minor detail, and to not let ambitions ruin their lives or their health. They need to become more serene and calm in a tranquil setting of some kind. Finding inner peace should be a lot more important to them than material concerns.

Foods and Nutrients

Calcium (800 mg.), magnesium (1,600 mg.) and potassium (2,000 mg.) are all important for the heart. They help to prevent tachycardia if taken regularly in the suggested amounts.

TAPEWORM

See under WORMS for more information.

TARDIVE DYSKINESIA

Symptoms

Tardive Dyskinesia is a serious movement disorder characterized by involuntary twitches, jerks, and grimaces that develop in about 20% of those taking an antipsychotic medication.

Relief Measures/Foods and Nutrients

Symptoms of tardive dyskinesia decreased sharply among 9 of 16 psychiatric patients treated for 8-12 weeks with large daily doses (1,200 I.U.) of vitamin E, reported Lenard A. Mier of the Dept. of Veterans Affairs Medical Center in New York City. Only 1 of 12 psychiatric patients with the same disorder treated for the same time period with placebo pills showed comparable improvement. During the trials, patients took prescribed doses of an antipsychotic medication and other drugs. (Science News 141:351, May 23, 1992). Lecithin (1 tbsp. daily) should be included, too.

TARTAR AND PLAQUE BUILDUP

Symptoms

Plaque is a white, brown, or yellow-brown sticky film of living and dead bacteria that grows at or below the gingival gum margin of your teeth. When this plaque isn't removed, it can harden - 50% within 48 hours, becoming rock hard after only two weeks. That tough crust is commonly known as tartar. Combined, both make your teeth look, feel and taste pretty awful. Even worse

dental problems can result if they're left on long enough: gingivitis and periodontal disease.

Relief Measures

Tartar is next to impossible to remove alone. It's the equivalent to sailors trying to scrape away barnacles from their ship's sides and bottom. You need the services of a professional dentist for this.

But plaque can be removed, which in turn will prevent a buildup of tartar. Regular and proper brushing is the key here. Up and down or back and forth isn't the correct way of doing it. What you need is to turn your toothbrush so the bristles are at a 45-degree angle to the area where your tooth and gum meet (the gum around the tooth). Now, slowly work your brush around in small circles, covering one or two teeth at a time.

Most of us worry about the smile areas of our mouths and give the rest of the teeth a quickie brushing. But the majority of brushing time—at least 3 minutes—needs to be focused on the back of your lower teeth where plaque is most apt to concentrate. Brush at night before retiring.

The *way* in which a toothbrush is held determines just how successfully or unsuccessfully accumulated debris can be swept away from your teeth and gums. Dental researchers in Finland discovered that when a toothbrush is held much like a writing pen would be instead of the more common tennis racket grip, less gum abrasion was noticed and healthier gums and greater plaque removal was observed.

Flossing immediately after brushing controls the formation of plaque even better than correct brushing does. Here's how to floss correctly. Break off 1 1/2 feet of floss and wind one end around the middle finger of one hand and the other end around the same finger on the other hand, leaving a couple of inches between them. Employing a gentle, back and forth motion, pass the floss between two teeth at a time. When the floss gets to the gumline, curve it in a C against one tooth and slide the floss between the gum and tooth until you can feel some resistance. Now, curve it around the other tooth the same way. Scrape floss downward on upper teeth and upward on lower teeth.

An herbal scrub for your chompers that really whitens them up, consists of the following several ingredients: 1 tsp. of Arm & Hammer baking soda, 1/4 tsp. of sea salt, 1/4 tsp. of granulated kelp, and 1/4 tsp. of black walnut powder. Mix everything together in a cup. Then wet your toothbrush, dip it in this mixture, and scrub your teeth and gums good.

After every meal remember to give your mouth a good oral flushing with plenty of water. This will help to remove most of the debris in between the teeth until they can be properly brushed later on.

Studies have shown that Listerine antiseptic mouthwash is very good for the reduction of plaque. An experiment in Baltimore, Maryland demonstrated that people who rinsed with Listerine reduced their own plaque almost 25% and their gingivitis nearly 30%. You can make an effective mouthwash of your own right at home. Bring a pint of water to a boil, and add one tablespoonful of dried, coarsely cut thyme herb. Remove from heat, cover with a lid, and steep an hour or until cool. Strain into another cup, and add 2 tbsps. of 3% hydrogen peroxide solution.

You can test the amount of plaque residue on your teeth at any given time by buying some special tablets at any local drugstore. These tablets contain a dye that will stain any plaque remaining on your teeth after you've brushed them. Chew the tablet, then look in the mirror and inspect your teeth. The color will be darkest near the gums where plaque is the thickest. Brush again, and be sure to especially concentrate on those areas where plaque shows up.

Or you can make your own plaque spotter right at home. Just coat your lips with some Vaseline to avoid staining. Then put a level teaspoonful of food coloring into your mouth, swish it around, and expectorate into the wash basin or sink. Rinse with tap water. Then, standing in front of a mirror, observe carefully for plaque, stained by the dye. Brush those areas good where plaque remains.

Foods and Nutrients

Studies have shown that aged cheddar cheese will somehow eliminate the acid production necessary for plaque buildup. It is thought by some that the enzymes which went into making the cheese, also act as buffering agents to prevent plaque formation. So nibbling on a little cheese every few days won't hurt a bit.

If your schedule doesn't always permit the convenience of brushing, then chew a stick of sugarless gum for about half-an-hour. As you chew away, your saliva will rinse your teeth and neutralize the acid in plaque before it does any serious damage. Moving the gum around in your mouth with your tongue can also dislodge food which sometimes gets stuck in between teeth.

TEETHING

Symptoms

Teething in an infant actually commences even before birth by several months. Tooth buds, in fact, appear as early as the 6th week in the developing fetus. By the time the baby is born, all 20 of his or her primary teeth that will be sprouting over the next couple of years are already in place and accounted for in the jawbone.

When those initial teeth start pushing the baby's gums some months later, ear and tooth pain and inflammation occur because both share the same nerve. Excessive dribbling is also common. The infant can become quite irritable and restless.

Relief Measures/Foods and Nutrients

One of the niftiest remedies to provide a baby relief with is to refrigerate a clean teething ring. Or even a damp, ice cold wash cloth for that matter will do. The cold acts as an anesthesia of sorts to stop numb pain and tender soreness.

Another trick is to wrap a small gauze pad around your forefinger, then lightly moisten it with some previously chilled tincture of witch hazel, and then very gently massage the baby's gum pads with this.

Another favorite is to take a small slice of cold apple and wrap it in a wet, child-size washcloth. Most of the teething rings sold on the market today lack taste and have a bland flavor to them. But the sweetness of a ripe, delicious, cold apple will be very appealing for the infant to chomp down on.

TEMPEROMANDIBULAR JOINT SYNDROME (TMJ)

Symptoms

Temperomandibular joint syndrome (TMJ) or myofacial pain-dysfunction syndrome is a dysfunction of the chewing apparatus related to spasm of the muscles of mastication. This is usually brought on by one of several different factors: dysharmony of the back grinding molars; alteration in the vertical dimensions of the jaws; frequent emotional outbursts characterized by considerable screaming or shouting; and the grinding of teeth.

Symptoms include pain which starts in the jaw muscles and joints and radiates outward to the face, neck, and shoulders; muscle tenderness; a popping noise in the tempomandibular joint itself; and obvious limitation of jaw motion.

One of the authors knows of an instance where TMJ was caused by a dentist. Some friends of his who reside in Plain view, Texas sent their oldest daughter to a local dentist some years ago for the usual dental work. Without realizing it, the dentist had his patient open her mouth wider than she was capable of, and kept her in that very uncomfortable position for longer than was normal to do.

As a result of this, two very unfortunate things happened. The young lady was plagued with migraine headaches and pain for many years thereafter, due to her dentist-induced TMJ. The other equally sad thing was that their two youngest sons, John and Joe (who are now grown young men) never received the necessary dental work their crooked teeth demanded. Both the mother and especially the father, were adamantly opposed to ever trusting any of their other children's dental care needs into the hands of any dentist because of this one mistake. Which just goes to show how a simple error by one person can affect the lives (and looks) of others not directly connected with that fault.

Relief Measures

Rubbing some fluid extracts of valerian root, hops, passion flower, or a nervine formula on the inside back jaw hues of the mouth as well as on the outside skin directly behind each jawbone, and on the temples of the head, will help to relieve some of the pain caused by TMJ. Some chiropractic manipulation of the head, neck and jaws may be especially helpful in such instances.

Foods and Nutrients

Calcium (1,000 mg.), magnesium (2,000 mg), zinc (150 mg.), vitamin E (800 I.U.), and pantothenic acid (300 mg.) afford relief. Stay away from junk foods and hard-to-chew items.

TENDONITIS

Symptoms

Tendonitis is a condition in which any tendon can become inflamed; also, more specifically, inflammation of the Tenon's capsule or the connective tissue within Tenon's space (located behind the eyeball).

Tendonitis is brought on mainly through overuse of a particular muscle tendon, be it in the knee, heel (Achilles' tendon), elbow, wrist, or shoulder.

Relief Measures

The most obvious thing to do is to stop using that particular part of the body and give the injured tendon a chance to rest and recuperate. But this isn't easy in every case to do. Some professions such as window-washing, professional tennis and golf, and writing, demand that some of these body parts be constantly used, even when tendonitis may be apparent.

One of the authors periodically has this problem in his wrists and finger joints, because of the vast amount of typing he does on a word processor (he averages two full-length books and numerous articles every year).

He has discovered that by simply massaging the sore wrist or finger joints for a few minutes every hour on the hour, helps to improve the blood circulation, which, in turn, seems to diminish the pain somewhat. Occasionally, he might even resort to rubbing a little Ben-Gay or Mentholatum Deep-Heat Rub on his wrist or finger joints, which gives penetrating comfort because of the eucalyptus oil present in such liniments.

Whirlpool baths or just soaking in some warm bathwater helps to raise your body temperature and increases blood flow, which tends to decrease tendon soreness. Tendonitis of the knee can be alleviated by placing a thin towel over the knee first, and then placing a heating pad over that. This prevents the skin from being burned accidentally.

Stretching exercises such as those common to Indian yoga or Chinese tai ji quan, prevents the shortening of muscles and tendons that goes along with excessive physical activity. It also promotes greater circulatory flow of the blood as well.

After exercising, ice is terrific for holding down both the swelling and pain of tendonitis. But people suffering from coronary artery disease, sugar diabetes, or circulatory disorders should exercise caution about using ice, because it constricts the blood vessels and, in their particular conditions, might cause serious health problems.

Simply wrapping your tendonitis in an Ace bandage is another alternative for reduction of the pain and swelling. But be sure you wrap it a little loose and don't leave it on too long.

Foods and Nutrients

A great combination of nutrients for doing a fantastic job of curing your tendonitis, are these, taken on a regular basis together at the same time: calcium (800 mg.), magnesium (1,600 mg.), chromium (300 mcg.), zinc (150 mg.), yarrow herb capsules (4), and pantothenic acid (300 mg.).

TENNIS ELBOW

Symptoms

Tennis elbow or epicondylitis (it's proper medical term) is when the elbow tendons, or serve or forehand tendons, of tennis players develop microscopic tears because of repeated stress placed upon them during a vigorous game. Sports medicine specialists think it's not the vibration that causes the tears but excess torsion—for example, when the ball hits off center, the racquet twists your arm. Pain on the lateral side of your arm (the side your thumb is on) is 10 times more common than pain on the other (medial) side.

Tennis elbow eventually sidelines about half of all amateurs who play tennis at least 3 times weekly. A too-heavy racquet or poor playing technique can dispose players to this disorder. A recently published roundtable discussion with orthopedists revealed that the backhand may be the main culprit causing this problem, because during the backhand the muscles that extend the wrist undergo an eccentric contraction—that is, they lengthen during activation. But the hand can also develop this condition as well.

Relief Measures

The old age "an ounce of prevention is worth a pound of cure," seems to apply to the game of tennis. Changing racquets and wearing braces may help, but they won't clear up any residual muscle weakness you may have. Half the tennis-elbow sufferers in this country have some major strength deficits in the shoulder and upper back, sports medicine doctors note. The key therefore is to restore strength, endurance, and flexibility to the arm, shoulder, and back.

There are two simple forearm exercises to get you started in this direction. Lay your forearm on a table with your hand hanging over the edge and your palm up. Holding a 5-lb. weight, slowly flex your wrist 10-20 times. Then turn your hand over so the palm faces down and repeat. Switch arms and do the same exercise over again. The second is to lay your forearm on a table with your hand hanging over the edge and your palm down. Using your other hand, push the hand up into a vertical position; hold for 10 seconds and repeat 10 times. Then push the hand down so that the fingers point towards the floor; hold for 10 seconds and repeat 10 times. Switch arms and repeat. A third forearm strengthener is to simply squeeze a ball 40-50 times with your arm extended horizontally in front of you.

If you're just starting to play, remember that your technique and conditioning are far more important than your racquet in preventing tennis elbow. Power your serve and backhand with your legs, body, and shoulders, not your wrist and forearm. Beginners should learn a two-handed backhand stroke. If you aren't sure about your form, get some professional advice.

Racquets can aggravate tennis elbow. Try a mid-sized racquet, which has a bigger sweet spot and absorbs vibration better than a small one. It plays softer and gives more power, so you don't need to swing as hard. An oversized racquet, in contrast, can increase the risk of the racquet over-twisting if you hit the ball off center.

Choose a flexible racquet - one that is injection-molded or that contains a high proportion of fiberglass—which will dampen shock well. Composite racquets with an increased ratio of nylon matrix, as opposed to epoxy resin, are good shock stoppers.

An increased grip size can also help. Too small a grip can lead to arm muscle fatigue from overtightening. But too large a grip may put you at a strength disadvantage.

Lower your string tension to dampen shock—usually 2-3 pounds less than the manufacturer's low-range suggestion. Higher string tension does give more control, but also increases the shock to your arm after ball impact.

Braces can be of definite help in correcting tennis elbow. In one study of 2,633 tennis players who suffered from this condition, 84% of them claimed an elbow brace improved their problem considerably. The brace recommended by most health professionals is called a counterforce brace. This is different from the elastic braces you may find in sporting goods stores—elastic doesn't give enough support.

The counterforce brace (trade name: Count'R-Force), designed in the early 1970s by Dr. Nirschl, is a nonelastic padded girdle that fits the contour of the forearm and is held in place by two small buckles and velcro straps. It functions as a constraint against muscle contraction and excessive movement of the tendons, thus reducing force and overload on the soft tissues of the elbow. When a muscle contracts, it tends to expand, and the nonelastic brace controls the expansion and thus reduces the forces developed by the muscle. A counterforce brace, however, won't interfere with your game because it does not prevent motion, as would a brace with metal supports (such as a knee brace). Another type of counterforce brace is the Aircast band, which is also nonelastic, but contains an air bubble. This brace also has been shown to be effective at reducing muscle activity. You can obtain a counterforce brace through your physician; some sporting-goods stores also carry them. There is one brace that can be used for lateral, medial, and posterior elbow pain (the brace extends back over the elbow bone), and a smaller brace for lateral pain only. Don't strap your brace too tightly. You should feel its pressure only when the forearm muscle contracts and expands.

Foods and Nutrients

There are certain foods which can be consumed frequently to give the muscle tendons greater elasticity and tensile strength. These are foods which are rich in the trace element silicon and help the body to produce more of its own special lubricant, a unique substance called hyaluronic acid. Silicon plays a crucial role in the production of this slippery substance which oils the joints, gives muscle tendons greater elasticity, protects delicate tissues in the eyes, and helps the skin to stretch and bend.

According to a back issue of the *American Journal of Botany* for October, 1978, silicon occurs in the following plants and herbs: tomato, radish, green onion, Chinese cabbage, alfalfa, wheat and barley grass, horsetail or shave-grass, red clover tops, comfrey root and leaf, and marsh-

mallow root. Most of these items are readily available from the produce section of any major supermarket or from the herb section of any health food store. The cereal grasses can be mixed with water or juice (one teaspoon to 6 fl. oz.), and the herbs can be taken in capsules (2-3 daily).

TETANUS

See under BLOOD POISONING for more information.

THRUSH

See under CANDIDIASIS for more information.

TICS, TREMORS, AND TWITCHES

See under MULTIPLE SCLEROSIS and NERVOUSNESS for more information.

TOOTHACHE

Symptoms

The manifestation of a toothache is readily discernible - a painful throbbing occurs which doesn't seem to go away and focuses all of your attention on trying to get rid of this awful misery somehow. In reality, though, a toothache could be a symptom of several things. The pulp of your tooth or the gums surrounding it could be infected. There might be decay inside a back molar. You could have a cracked bicuspid. Or you might have been smacked in the mouth. Or the ache could be something as simple as a piece of food caught between two teeth. Or even a backlash from a serious sinus problem.

Only your dentist can tell for sure, however, exactly what is causing it.

Relief Measures

One of the authors was down in New Orleans over a decade ago attending the National Health Federation convention at which he was a speaker. One of his amalgam fillings dropped out by accident while he was lunching on some catfish. This particular tooth immediately started hurting him.

He managed to get several wedges of a garlic clove from the waiter in the restaurant at which he was dining. He peeled two of them, and with the bottom of a very heavy glass ashtray which sat on the table, he mashed them into pulp. He then put this crushed mixture inside his mouth, being careful to insert it inside the cavity space.

He left it there overnight and didn't drink or eat anything else after this. By the next morning, his pain had almost subsided to the point that it was tolerable to bear until he could get back home and visit his family dentist to have the problem fixed.

Also, placing a cold ice cube inside the mouth adjacent to the aching tooth, will serve as an effective analgesic in relieving the pain very quickly. But it's only temporary, and after it has melted away, the pain will eventually return. So something more permanent like garlic or clove oil is needed instead.

Most drugstores sell small bottles of oil of cloves, which contains eugenol, a great anodyne for pain. Holding 2 or 3 cotton Q-tips together, or a cotton ball, dip them into this oil and then rub them next to the ache itself. In the case of the cotton ball, it should be saturated and packed inside the mouth between the offending tooth and the cheek pouch and left there for several hours.

Another effective way to relieve toothache, is to swirl a mouthful of salt water around inside and hold for several minutes before spitting out.

Don't do a lot of talking if you have a toothache because cold area rushing inside will make it hurt worse.

Foods and Nutrients

Don't eat anything hard or crusty or which requires a lot of chewing. For nourishment, try cool juices or canned pears or a ripe banana.

Take pantothenic acid (300 mg.), vitamin E oil (800 I.U.), cooper (4 mg.), and zinc (100 mg.) to help relieve pain.

TRAVELER'S DIARRHEA

See under DIARRHEA for more information.

TRIGLYCERIDES (ELEVATED)

Symptoms

Until recently "bad" cholesterol (low-density lipoproteins) was blamed for causing hardening of the arteries. Now new information suggests that triglycerides may be even worse in promoting arteriosclerosis of the heart.

High triglyceride levels are generally associated with very low levels of "good" cholesterol (or high-density lipo-proteins). Unlike "bad" cholesterol, which is *directly* linked to clogged arteries, having too many triglycerides in your circulating blood plasma isn't that clear cut. Hence, one could infer that triglycerides are an important *secondary* factor in coronary and vascular diseases, but not the primary cause as is the case with "bad" cholesterol.

Normal triglyceride levels can run from 40-250 mg. per deciliter of blood (mg/dl), which is a fairly broad range. Levels of 250 mg/dl to 500 mg/dl are considered "borderline elevated," while levels over 500 mg/dl are considered "high." The safest bet is to keep your triglyceride levels below 150.

As stated before, triglycerides *and something else* become life-threatening, but not them alone. A friend of one of the authors by the name of Bruce A., who works for the Marriott Corp. in Salt Lake City, went to Cottonwood Hospital several years ago to have his cholesterol and triglyceride levels checked. His cholesterol reading was 225 mg, but his triglyceride count was *over 1,000* mg/dl to the astonishment of the doctor and nurses who reviewed the results with him.

Nothing of significance occurred with his health until June, 1992 at which time he suffered a major heart attack and required temporary hospitalization. His physician informed him that not only did he need to reduce his whopping triglyceride count, but also he had to reduce the level of job stress along with it. This is illustrative of what was noted earlier: triglycerides and other factors bring imminent danger to one's state of health, and must be effectively dealt with in the appropriate ways.

Relief Measures/Foods and Nutrients

For most people, a diet low in fat and calories and high in complex carbohydrates is ideal for lowering all blood fats, including triglycerides, the chief form of fat used and stored by the body. However, simple carbohydrates or those foods high in sugar, should be cut down because they pose an added risk to the heart.

Some people with high triglycerides have a specific genetic defect that makes it difficult for them to process calories from refined carbohydrates and alcohol. For this reason, a low-fat diet rich in unprocessed, high-fiber carbohydrates from whole grains, fruits, legumes, and vegetables, with strict limitations on empty calories from alcohol and sugars, is strongly recommended.

Although the types of food consumed usually contribute to how a lipid profile reads, elevated triglycerides may not always be diet-related. Blood-pressure medications, oral contraceptives and estrogen supplements can raise blood fats, as can diabetes, kidney disease, infections and stress. These factors should be taken into account when determining the possible causes of a high triglyceride count.

Certain spices such as garlic, onion, and chili peppers seem to cut cholesterol and triglyceride levels in half or more. Consequently they should be employed frequently in the preparation of those many foods which call for their wonderful flavoring properties. Also individual supplements of Kyolic aged-garlic extract (3 capsules daily) and powdered cayenne pepper (2 capsules daily) should be taken with meals as an extra health precaution.

TUBERCULOSIS

Symptoms

Tuberculosis is a very contagious disease caused by bacterial infection. A person ordinarily has some defense against the bacteria, which lurks in most of us anyway (40% by the age of 21, and 95% by the age of 50)—only the scars remain to be seen by X-ray. The majority of the population acquires a gradual immunity which protects them from further infection.

However, when the system becomes weakened or rundown, because of disease, improper hygiene, poor diet, and social stress, its susceptibility to infection dramatically increases. This is evident in A.I.D.S. patients, poor people who live on the streets, and corporate workaholics. Tuberculosis usually affects the lungs, but it may also involve other organs and tissues.

Many tuberculosis patients may exhibit mild symptoms from which they recover completely. This usually means that the body has successfully controlled the bacteria. Mild symptoms of the disease include fatigue and appetite and weight loss. As the disease becomes more severe, symptoms include fever, increased perspiration, and rapid loss of weight and strength. Coughing up blood is often the first indication of a severe form of the disease.

Tuberculosis patients were once confined to sanitariums, away from the rest of society. But in hard economic times such as those we're now living in, more victims of TB are out in public mingling with the rest of us, and rapidly spreading their own deadly bacteria around those whom they come into contact with. So it's not only necessary to treat existing cases, but also to find preventative measures for healthy people to avoid contracting it.

Relief Measures

Because early signs of TB often resemble influenza, it is especially important that you fortify your body with adequte nutrients (listed below in the other section), good food, and plenty of rest. These few measures will almost certainly guarantee that you do not pick up the bacteria.

Next in line is to keep these several organs of the body in good shape—the kidneys, intestines, spleen, and liver. Goldenseal root and gotu kola herb both are good antibiotics for the spleen; buchu leaves and uva ursi are fine for the kidneys; garlic is ideal for the intestines; and dandelion root is splendid for the liver. One or two capsules of each herb every other day with meals is recommended.

Flushing the organs regularly with lots of liquid in the form of water, juices and herbal teas is important, too.

Sunshine and fresh, dry air are especially beneficial for infected lung tissue. A place like Arizona or Southern California has proven to be the ideal climate for TB patients to fully recover in. An industrial engineer one of the. authors is personally acquainted with, contracted the disease while working in San Francisco.

The company for which he worked sent him over to the small nation of Yemen, located at the bottom of the Saudi Arabian Peninsula. The huge construction project he was in charge of while there lasted approximately 27 months. During this time, he became completely cured of his TB. He attributed it to the "dry climate and hot weather."

The fluid extracts of echinacea and pau d'arco (25 drops of either twice daily) are excellent for treating existing forms of tuberculosis.

Foods and Nutrients

The diet should consist of at least 50% raw fruits and vegetables. Investing in a good juice machine is worthwhile doing. Eat two fertilized eggs daily. Also consume yogurt, buttermilk (and all soured forms of milk), fish, fowl, raw cheese, raw seeds and nuts, and whole grains.

Take four capsules of Kyolic-EPA garlic daily, along with 3 capsules of Kyo-Dophilus and 1 glass of Kyo-Green (mixed according to the directions on the label). (See Appendix under Wakunaga.)

Also include the amino acids, L-cysteine and L-methionine (1,000 mg. of each daily), selenium (200 mcg. daily),

vitamin A (50, 000 I.U.), vitmain B-6 (200 mg. daily), vitamin C (7,000 mg. daily), vitamin E (800 I.U. daily), germanium (200 mcg. daily), and a calcium-magnesium supplement (2 tablets daily).

TUMORS

See under CANCER for more information.

TYPHOID & TYPHUS

See under FEVERS for more information.

ULCERATIVE COLITIS

See under COLIC and COLITIS for more information.

ULCERS

Symptoms

Ulcers occur along the gastrointestinal tract, especially in the stomach (gastric ulcer), duodenum, and colon. Ulcers may also appear as bedsores or on the legs of diabetics.

An ulcer results when, during moments of periodic stress, the body's defense of the lining of the stomach is damaged and the stomach cannot secrete sufficient mucus to protect it against the strong acid essential for digestion. The ulcer is aggravated by the level of anxiety of the individual before eating.

The varied symptoms of an ulcer can include stomach pain, lower back pain, headaches, choking sensation, and terrible itching.

Relief Measures

Certain mucilaginous herbs make excellent teas for the stomach on account of their slick and slimy properties, which have a soothing, healing effect. They are marshmallow root, comfrey root and leaves, slippery elm bark, and fenugreek seed. Others include German chamomile, yarrow, catnip, and peppermint. Cayenne pepper is very good for peptic ulcers, in spite of its fiery properties, while licorice root is very beneficial for gastric and duodenal ulcers. One cup of tea twice daily with meals of any of the foregoing herbs is advised. Or 2 capsules twice daily with meals of any of them.

Foods and Nutrients

Hydrochloric acid (hcl) is essential for the breakdown and digestion of many things you eat. You can determine if you need hydrochloric acid with a very simple test. Take a tablespoon of apple cider vinegar or lemon juice. If this makes your heartburn go away, then you need more stomach acid. If it makes your symptoms worse, then you have too much hcl and you shouldn't take enzymes that contain hcl. If it helps the symptoms, though, then sip a diluted mixture of apple cider vinegar (two tablespoons) in some water (one cup) with every meal.

Don't smoke or take aspirin. Try to relax and avoid stressful situations. Don't drink milk, even though it neutralizes stomach acid. The calcium and protein in milk stimulates the production of more acid; milk has a rebound effect. Choose almond or cashew nut milks instead. They can be made by adding some of these slivered or chopped nuts in a food processor with a little water, and let them mix for about 3 minutes. Don't eat fried food. Don't drink coffee, colas, or soft drinks. Stay away from salt, chocolate, and red meat.

Do eat small and frequent meals instead of three large ones as most of us are in the habit of doing each day. Consume cooked millet, rice, oatmeal, raw goat's milk, avocados, bananas, squash, potatoes, yams, and steamed broccoli and carrots.

Take L-glutamine (500 mg. daily on an empty stomach), vitamin E (800 I.U.), aloe vera juice (1 cup), digestive enzymes (2 tablets), Wakunaga's Kyo-Dophilus (2 capsules), Wakunaga's Kyolic-EPA (2 capsules), vitamin A (50,000 I.U. fish-oil), and zinc (100 mg.) supplements on a regular basis.

UNDERWEIGHT

Symptoms

Being underweight usually occurs when more calories are utilized by the body than are consumed. Underweight without a lack of nutrients may or may not be serious, depending upon the degree of underweight. The thin person is probably less apt to suffer from heart diseases and certain other ailments and will live longer than someone else who is overweight.

Malnutrition occurs when an individual is deficient in the nutrients essential for life. Individuals with this problem are very susceptible to infections, lack nutrient reserves for times of stress and become easily fatigued.

When underweight and malnutrition are severe, there is starvation, the body's stores of nutrients and fats are depleted, and muscle tissue is broken down to provide energy for bodily functions.

Symptoms that may accompany underweight are weakness, fatigue, sensitivity to cold, hunger, dizziness, and loss of ambition. Underweight may be caused by poor eating habits, a nervous condition, overactivity, illness, heredity problems, or poorly functioning digestion and absorption processes.

Relief Measures

Certain herbs will assist a thin person in putting on much badly needed weight. Powdered slippery elm bark (6 capsules daily), alfalfa (4 capsules daily), fenugreek seed (3 capsules daily), and guar gum (4 capsules daily), when taken together for a 6 week period have been known to add as much as 8 pounds to some people's frames.

Foods and Nutrients

Underweight can be easily treated by removing those underlying factors which brought it about in the first place. Also improvement of the diet is critical. Foods intended for consumption should be well-balanced, of considerable variety, and unrefined for the most part.

Starchy vegetables like potatoes and beans, grains, fowl, fish, eggs, avocados, olive oil, safflower oil, raw cheese, raw nuts and nut butters, and raw seeds should form part of these. Also use soy-based cream soups that are non-dairy. Purchase soy milk from any health food store and use it in place of regular cow's milk. These cream soups are much higher in protein content, as a rule, than broth soups and can be well tolerated. Bananas and cabbage are good for weight gain in the young and elderly alike.

Stay away from junk foods, as they tend to put on the *wrong* kind of weight. Eat in relaxed surroundings and never eat a meal if you're upset or high-strung.

Vitamin B-complex (3 tablets daily), vitamin E (800 I.U.), magnesium (1,000 mg.), iron (25 mg.), digestive enzymes (2 tablets daily), zinc (75 mg. daily), and liquid lecithin (one tablespoon every morning) are good supplements to take for putting on extra weight.

VAGINITIS

See under CANDIDIASIS for more information.

VARICOSE VEINS

Symptoms

Varicose veins are veins that have become enlarged, twisted, and swollen. They may be found anywhere in the body, but seem to be most concentrated in the legs.

Factors that inhibit blood circulation, such as obesity, certain hereditary conditions, tight clothing, crossing of legs, and a sedentary occupation, can increase susceptibility to varicose veins. A pregnant woman or a woman who has had several pregnancies is often more inclined to develop varicose veins than are most other women, because pregnancy tends to increase pressure on the legs with the added weight carried in the womb.

These prominent, bluish, bulging veins are often accompanied by dull, nagging aches and pains. Swelling, leg sores, leg cramps, and a feeling of general heaviness in the legs are characteristic of varicose veins.

Though some may not realize it, hemorrhoids are actually varicose veins of the anus or rectum. See under **HEMMORHOIDS** for further details.

See under **BLOOD CIRCULA-TION (POOR)** for additional data.

Relief Measures

If you are plagued with varicose veins, you should never be sitting for long periods of time. Instead, you should be up and moving around to promote good circulation. Take rest periods several times each day to elevate your legs. Avoid crossing them, doing any heavy lifting, and putting unnecessary pressure on them. Wear loose clothing and stockings which won't restrict blood flow. It may be a good idea for women to wear supportive elastic stockings, however, as they offer support to such veins and prevent them from swelling further.

Soaking in a whirlpool bath or a tub of warm water to which has been added some Epsom salts can be very therapeutic. Bathe the legs twice each day with strong solutions of *warm* white oak bark to help stimulate blood flow. Raw potato suppositories and garlic enemas help heal hemorrhoids and relieve pain. Peel the spuds and cut them so that they are shaped like small cones for easier insertions.

Butcher's broom as a tea (1 cup daily) or capsules (2 daily) and uva ursi (same amounts) are highly recommended.

Foods and Nutrients

Regulate your diet carefully. Your diet should be low in fat and refined carbohydrates. You should include plenty of fish and fresh fruits and vegetables. Stay away from red meat, processed and refined foods, sugar, ice cream, fried foods, cheeses, peanut butter, junk foods, alcohol, and salty snacks. Make sure that your diet includes a lot of fiber. If you have a juice machine and are into drinking lots of juices, make sure you add some pulp (a level tablespoonful) of whatever was juiced to every glass you drink.

Also include vitamin C (3,500 mg.), rutin and hesperidin (150 mg. of each), liquid lecithin (one tablespoon daily), a high-potency B-complex vitamin (3 tablets), vitamin E (800 I.U.), potassium (1,000 mg. daily), and zinc (100 mg.), and yarrow capsules (4 daily) taken together.

VENEREAL DISEASE

See under **SEXUALLY TRANSMISSIBLE DISEASE** for more information.

VERTIGO

Symptoms

Vertigo is a faint or unsteady feeling often referred to as giddiness or dizziness. But true vertigo implies disorientation in space, or a sensation of movement, often rotatory, either of objects which are actually stationary, or of the individual. In severe cases, the person may swag, stagger, or even fall.

It is a disturbance of the balancing mechanism within the inner ear, either direct or through a temporarily inadequate supply of blood to the brain. The great film director, Alfred Hitchcock entitled one of his suspense-action movies, "Vertigo," because the lead character suffered from a fear of heights and became very disoriented if subjected to being very many feet off the ground.

Some authors have attributed at least 20 different reasons for vertigo, but these can be simplified down into just a few of the more important considerations:

Sudden paroxysms, accompanied by ringing in the ears and deafness, nausea, vomiting, and pallor; typical of such might be Ménière's disease.

Coming on after lying down or prolonged stooping.

Usually occurs in those over so, or in convalescents. There is a delayed readjustment of circulatory arrangements for the upright position, so that the brain is temporarily short of blood.

Hardening of the arteries makes them less efficient, rather like rusted pipes, and this commonly produces a decrease in the blood supply to the brain and certain spinal nerves, which may temporarily become inadequate.

Variations in blood pressure, head injuries, mental and emotional stress, neurological disease, and atmospheric changes in air pressure are some of the other causes of vertigo.

Relief Measures

When the sensation of vertigo strikes unexpectedly, the person should sit down and bend forward, or lie flat on the floor if possible. In about ten minutes, he or she may get up *slowly*.

A person with frequent occurrences of vertigo should never turn his or her head very quickly. Nor should such an individual make sudden changes in body position. Everything ought to be done *gradually*.

Foods and Nutrients

Stay away from tobacco, coffee and colas, salty snacks, and greasy foods of any kind. They are hard for the stomach to digest, and will only contribute to the queasy feeling which comes with vertigo.

Herbs should be taken for the liver, as this organ's state of health is often involved in vertigo to some extent. Dandelion root tea (2 cups daily) or capsules (6 daily), organic beet root powder (one level tablespoonful in 8 fl. oz. of water), peach leaf tea (2 cups daily) or bark (2 capsules daily), and Wakunaga's goldenseal root (2 capsules daily) are all good for liver improvement.

Nutritional supplements should include niacin (150 mg. daily), vitamin B-6 (150 mg. daily), vitamin C (3,500 mg. daily), vitamin E (800 I.U. daily), calcium-magnesium (2 tablets daily), and fluid extract of ginkgo biloba (20 drops daily beneath the tongue).

VIRAL INFECTION

See under INFECTION for more information.

VITAMIN AND MINERAL DEFICIENCIES

Symptoms/Foods and Nutrients

You don't have to live in a struggling Third World nation or impoverished ghetto neighborhood somewhere to suffer from nutritional deficiencies. Even the most affluent families, who can afford to eat a wide variety of the best foods money can buy, suffer from the same malady, but obviously not as severely as millions of economically disadvantaged folks do.

A number of factors are responsible for causing nutrient shortages within the system. Bad social habits such as smoking, drinking, and using illicit drugs take their toll. Many of the wonderful technological advances we've surrounded ourselves with today create unusual stresses, which our pioneer forefathers didn't even have in their time. Our great-grandparents may have had to fight off Indians, grizzly bears, buffalo stampedes, and rattlesnakes, but they certainly didn't have to cope with the low-levels of radioactivity or electromagnetic waves emitted by many of these gadgets in our homes, offices, cars, trucks, and boats.

Pollution now is a thousand times worse than it was just a century ago. Not only is our water and air more foul, but we're currently faced with big gaping holes in the earth's fragile ozone layer, through which harmful ultraviolet rays from the sun are shooting down in increasing amounts. And then there is the food we eat—processed to death and embalmed with just about every conceivable chemical additive allowed by law. No wonder we can sit down to what appears to be a nourishing meal, eat our fill, and afterwards still feel somewhat lifeless and without much vitality to speak of.

Different lifestyles, health situations and age groups demand different amounts of vitamins, minerals, amino acids, and enzymes. Athletes, for example, need higher dosages of some nutrients to give them energy and stamina. Patients recuperating from surgeries or recent illnesses, require larger amounts of some things in order to regain their health back. Children and teenagers, as a rule, don't seem to need supplements as such. But the middle-aged and especially the elderly sure do, because with the advancement of years comes a general deterioration of the body as a whole.

Vitamin and mineral deficiencies aren't always evident on the surface. In fact, most deficiencies take time to develop and only become noticeable when a health crisis suddenly arises. For instance, a woman may be suffering from a gradual loss of valuable bone calcium, but won't notice it for years until she falls and breaks a leg or hip and suddenly discovers she has had osteoporosis all this time. Or, a man may coast along for quite awhile consuming too many refined carbohydrates, and all of sudden wake up one morning to find out he has diabetes, because his chromium and zinc levels are nearly bankrupt.

The following list, while by no means complete, offers the reader some general information with respect to each nutrient considered important for the body's health. Food as well as supplement sources are presented in the hopes of encouraging well-rounded and varied diets with lesser

dependency on health products for nutritional support.

VITILIGO

Symptoms

Vitiligo (or leukoderma) is a skin condition marked by white patches surrounded by a dark border. In such an instance, the skin is unable to produce the skin pigment known as melanin. A dysfunctioning thyroid gland is believed to be the chief cause of this.

Relief Measures/Foods and Nutrients

Jill K. of Bozeman, Montana started noticing white patches turning up on the backs of her hands and arms. At first, she laughingly referred to it as being due to "all the bleach I use doing laundry for my ten kids." But when it moved to her throat and neck six months later, she began taking the problem a lot more seriously.

Jill read in a national health magazine that vitiligo responds well to the use of the B-complex vitamin, para-amino-benzoic acid or PABA, and the mineral magnesium. So she started on a supplement program of 100 mg. of PABA three times a day and 1,800 mg. of magnesium with it. She also bought some skin cream containing PABA and rubbed it on those areas where the pigment had faded away. She also took 1,400 I.U. of vitamin E oil internally, and rubbed some of the oil on these white patches of skin. About two weeks later, she added Efamol brand of evening primrose oil, taking 6 capsules a day.

Within 2.5 months time, Jill later reported to one of the authors, her vitiligo had ceased, and about 50% of the melanin had returned to her neck, arms, and hands.

VOMITING

See under NAUSEA AND VOMITING for more information.

WARTS

Symptoms

Venereal or genital warts are single or clusters of soft, cauliflower-like growths found in and around the vagina, anus, penis, groin, or scrotal areas. They are caused by the human papilloma virus (HPV). There are more than 35 kinds of HPV, and two have been associated with cancer of the cervix and genital area.

Common warts, however, aren't as serious and usually may be found on the hands, fingers, feet, forearms, neck, face, back and chest. They range in size from a pinhead to a small bean. They can also occur in the larynx and cause hoarseness sometimes. They are rough, irregular skin growths, and are caused by a virus. Highly contagious, they can be spread by picking, trimming, biting or touching them. They can also be spread on the face by the simple act of shaving. Ordinary warts like these occur most often on skin that is frequently exposed to friction, trauma, or abrasion. They may be flat or raised, dry or moist, and have a rough and pitted surface that is either flesh-colored or darker than the surrounding skin. They typically do not cause pain or itching and can be left to disappear on their own unless they become bothersome.

Relief Measures

Clifton L., a retired carpenter from Vernal, Utah, discovered a handy cure for getting rid of his own warts right in his wife's kitchen. "I just took one of her garlic cloves, peeled the thing, and then pounded it to a pulp with the flat end of my claw hammer. After which I then placed it directly on my warts, covering it with some duck tape to hold it in place. The next evening I changed it again. Some blisters formed where the garlic was put, but about a week later all of my warts just fell off by themselves," he told one of the authors confidently.

Matthew Midcap, M.D., a plastic surgeon residing in Morganstown, West Virginia, told one of the authors how he came about his own unique cure for warts over a decade ago:

"I first read about this banana treatment in the December, 1981 issue of the *Journal of Plastic Reconstructive Surgery*. A short article by an Israeli physician from the city of Safad related how he treated a single patient – a 16-year-old girl with painful plantar warts—with just ripe banana peels. The doctor in Wheeling, West Virginia with whom I was working in a clerkship capacity while still a medical student then, decided to join me in conducting further experiments based on this one recorded episode. His name is Dr. Phillip Polack.

"One of our very first patients was a male Caucasian, 48 years old. He's a prominent banker in Wheeling and loves to play golf. But a cluster of plantar warts on the bottom of one foot, about 2 inches in diameter, prevented him from enjoying his favorite sport. By the time he came to us, he had tried all the standard medical therapies available: acid therapy, cryotherapy where they freeze it off, surgery and even radiation. But nothing seemed to work, they just kept coming back. I cut a piece of ripe banana skin and applied the inside white mushy part against the warts, taping it down good with some adhesive tape.

I instructed him to keep it on, removing only when bathing or showering. After which, he was to dry his foot well and apply another ripe peel. He came in each week to have us scrape away the old, dead wart tissue. Within less than a month we could see his warts were definitely getting smaller. In six months he was not only completely cured, but has never experienced another recurrence of them since then. He has been golfing a lot since then without any pain that I know of."

Foods and Nutrients

Camille Thurston, R.N. works at a major metropolitan hospital in California. For her venereal warts, she decided to try the nutritional approach first, before going the drug route later on. She took one table-spoonful of brewer's yeast in milk every morning, 7,500 mg. vitamin C, 25,000 I.U. of vegetable beta-carotene and 25,000 I.U. of fish oil vitamin A, two tablets of L-Cysteine (a sulphur amino acid), 1, 200 I.U. of vitamin E, and 100 mg. of zinc every day for a month.

With this, she added 3 capsules of Kyolic aged-garlic extract, one capsule of Wakunaga goldenseal root, and two capsules of chaparral every day. (See Appendix under Wakunaga.) Within two months her venereal warts had disappeared, much to her satisfaction and delight.

WORMS

Symptoms

Worms are tiny parasites which live in the gastrointestinal tracts of man and beast alike. They are more common in children than in adults, however. Types of worms include tape-worms, threadworms, hookworms, pinworms, or roundworms. They can cause loss of appetite and weight, diarrhea, anemia, colon disorders, and rectal itching. Worm infestation also results in poor absorption of essential nutrients from the gastrointestinal tract. Causes include improper disposal of human waste, walking barefoot on contaminated soil, and ingestion of eggs or larvae from uncooked or partially cooked meat. Because the worms tend to come outside of the anus in the warmth of the bed, check this area of the child after he or she is sound asleep if you suspect him or her of having worms.

Relief Measures

Mahalia P. is of African-American descent and resides in Lafayette, Louisiana. She grew up around a tradition of herbal healing, having lived with her grandmother for a number of years. Mahalia is a social worker and works with many low-income families. In her line of work she often sees the results of poor hygiene and bad diets in the homes she visits every month.

A number of the single-parent families she calls on, have kids of varying ages who have intestinal parasite problems. Mahalia has taken it upon herself to recommend certain herbs to the mothers of such youngsters, which she remembers her grandma using years before for the very same thing.

For tapeworm, she tells the mother of one nine-year-old to have her daughter chew some pumpkin seeds. For another seven-year-old child afflicted with round-worms, she informs the mother to give her three capsules of black walnut bark every day until the problem has cleared up. For a boy troubled with hookworms, she suggests that his grandmother with whom he is staying, give him half cupfuls of wormwood tea twice daily on an empty stomach.

Foods and Nutrients

Mahalia recalled for one of the authors how her grandmother used to recom-mend salty snacks like potato chips, pig skins, pretzels, and roasted peanuts for pinworms. Somehow, she said, "them worms don't like salt very much."

Those who have worms of any kind should not be eating very much meat, and definitely not pork by any means! Meats that are consumed, though, should be fully cooked and thoroughly refrigerated.

Kyolic garlic and zinc are two of the very best supplements for getting rid of any kinds of worms. Take two capsules 4 times a day on an empty stomach. And each time you do so, take 25 mg. of zinc with them.

YEAST INFECTION

See under CANDIDIASIS for more information.

ZITS

See under ACNE VULGARIS and BLACKHEADS for more information.

Vitamins	*Dosages*	*Food Sources*
A	50,000 I.U.	fish, fish liver oil, green and yellow fruits and vegetables, milk products
B-1	50 mg.	blackstrap molasses, brewer's yeast, brown rice, fish, meat, nuts, organ meats, poultry, wheat germ, lobster
B-2	50 mg.	blackstrap molasses, brewer's yeast, eggs, fruit, green leafy vegetables, legumes, nuts, organ meat, poultry, tongue, whole grains
B-6	50 mg.	avocado, banana, blackstrap molasses,brewer's yeast, cabbage, dessicated liver, fish, green leafy vegetables, meat, organ meat, peanuts, prunes, walnuts, raisins, wheat germ, whole grains
B-12	300 mg.	beef, eggs, fish, milk products, organ meats, pork, cottage cheese, liver
Biotin	300 mg.	brewer's yeast, egg yolk, legumes, organ meats, whole grain, roasted peanuts
Choline	100 mg.	brewer's yeast, egg yolk, fish, lecithin, legumes, organ meats, soybeans, wheatgerm
Folic Acid	400 mg.	citrus fruits, eggs, green leafy vegetables, milk products, organ meats, seafood, whole grains
Inostol	100 mg.	blackstrap molasses, brewer's yeast, citrus fruits, lecithin, meat, milk, nuts, organ meats, vegetables, whole grains
Niacin	100 mg.	eggs, lean meats, milk products, organ meats, peanuts, poultry, seafood, whole grain breads and cereals, roasted peanuts in the shell
Pantothenic	100 mg.	brewer's yeast, eggs, legumes, mushrooms, organ meats, salmon, wheat germ, whole grains
Para Amino-benzoic Acid (PABA)	25mg.	blackstrap molasses, bran, brewer's yeast, eggs, liver, milk rice, organ meats, wheat germ, whole wheat

B-15 Pangamic Acid	50 mg.	brewer's yeast, lentils, bengal gram chickpea, brown rice rare meat, eggs, seeds (sunflower, pumpkin, sesame), whole grains organ meats
B-17	300 mg.	Bitter almonds, peach pits, apricot kernels Amygdalin Laetrile
C	3,500 mg.	fresh fruits and vegetables, sunlight
D	400 I.U.	egg yolks, organ meats, sunlight
E	400 I.U.	butter, dark green vegetables, eggs, fruits, nuts, organ meats, vegetable oils, wheat germ
F	400 I.U.	vegetable oils (safflower, soy, corn)
K	500 mcg.	alfalfa, wheat grass and barley grass, green leafy vegetables, safflower oil and herb, blackstrap molasses, yogurt, cayenne pepper, kelp, stinging nettle
P	500 mg.	fruit (skin and pulp) of apricots,
Rutin	150 mg.	cherries, grapes, grapefruit,
Hesperidin	150 mg.	lemons, limes, plums
"X" oxide Dismutase and other antioxidant enzymes	5 million units	barley grass, wheatgrass, broccoli, Brussel sprouts, Super-cabbage, cauliflower, kale, kohlrabi, garlic, onion, rosemary, thyme, sage

Minerals	*Dosage*	*Food Sources*
Boron	3mg.	leafy vegetables, seaweed, fruits, nuts, cereal grains
Calcium	1,000 mg.	milk, cheese, yogurt, salmon, sardines, shrimp, green leafy vegetables, alfalfa, almonds, asparagus, blackstrap molasses, brewer's yeast, broccoli, cabbage, carob, collards, dandelion greens, stinging nettle, dulse, figs, filberts, kale, kelp, mustard greens, oats, parsley, prunes, sesame seeds, tofu, turnip greens, whey
Chromium	150 mcg.	dark foreign beers and stout ales, hops, brewer's yeast, brown rice, dark breads (pumpernickel, rye), cheese, meat, dried beans, chicken, corn and corn oil, cow and goat milk, calves liver, mushrooms, potatoes
Cobalt Cobalamin (B-l2)	1 mcg.	beef, eggs, fish, milk products, comfrey root and leaf, organ meats, pork, goose liver, trout, Brazil nuts
Copper	3 mg.	almonds, chocolate, carob, avocados, barley, beans, beet root, blackstrap molasses, groccoli, dandelion greens, garlic, lentils, liver, mushrooms, nuts, oats, oranges, organ meats, pecans, radishes, raisins, salmon, lobster, shrimp, oysters, soybeans, green leafy vegetables, black pepper
Fluoride	———	many city water supplies, seaweed, shrimp, lobster, clams, swordfish, halibut
Germanium	25 mg.	aloe vera, comfrey root and leaves, aged garlic extract and garlic, onion, prickley ash bark, pau d'arco bark, shiitake mushroom, suma herb
Iodine	225 mcg.	kelp, lobster, shrimp, saltwater fish, asparagus, dulse, Irish moss and carrageenan, white deepwater fish, garlic, lima beans, mushrooms, sea salt, sesame seeds, pinenuts, soybeans, summer squash, Swiss chard, kale, turnip greens
Iron	18 mg.	eggs, fish, liver, meat, poultry, green leafy vegetables, whole grains, and enriched breads and cereals, almonds, avocados, beets, blackstrap molasses, brewer's yeast, dates, dulse, egg yolks, kelp, kidney and lima beans,

		lentils, milet, parsley, peaches, pears, dried prunes, buck wheat, pumpkins, rice, raisins, wheat bran, sesame seeds, rice bran, soybeans
Magnesium	1,800 mg.	milk, butter, cheese, salmon, lobster, oysters, trout, apples, apricots, avocados, bananas, berries, blackstrap molasses, brewer's yeast, brown rice, figs, garlic, kelp, lima beans, millet, nuts, peaches, black-eyed peas, sesame seeds, tofu, green leafy vegetables, buckwheat, oats, wheat
Manganese	4 mg.	avocados, Brazil nuts, cashews, sunflower seeds, blueberries, boysenberries, raspberries, egg yolks, legumes, dried peas, pineapple, spinach, leafy green vegetables
Molybdenum	30 mcg.	beans, cereal grains, legumes, peas, dark green leafy vegetables, white oak bark, black and green teas, cran berry juice, buchu leaves, juniper bark
Nickel	---	carrots, parsnips, burdock root, yellow dock root, sarsparilla root, potatoes, turnips, seeds
Oxygen	---	Ocean air, mountain air, air by waterfalls and turbulent rivers (white water), peppermint, spearmint, lemon balm
Phosphorus	600 mg.	Carbonated soft drinks, asparagus, bran, brewer's yeast, corn, dairy products, eggs, fish, dried fruit, garlic, legumes, nuts, sesame, sunflower and pumpkin seeds, meats, poultry, salmon, whole grains
Potassium	1,800 mg.	apricots, avocados, bananas, blackstrap molasses, brewer's yeast, brown rice, dates, figs, dried fruit, garlic, nuts, potatoes, raisins, winter squash, wheat bran, goat's milk, tofu, lamb, yams
Selenium	200 mcg.	Brazil nuts, cashews, almonds, pinenuts, brewer's yeast, broccoli, savoy cabbage, schizandra berry, hawthorn berry, brown and wild rice, chicken, duck, goose, goat's milk, garlic, liver, blackstrap molasses, onion, salmon, shark, swordfish, tuna fish, lobster, shrimp, crab, vegeta-vegetables, wheat germ, rye, millet, buckwheat, amaranth, whole wheat

288

Minerals	Dosage	Food Sources
Silicon	––	alfalfa, amaranth, beet tops, brown and wild rice, horse tail or shave grass, mother's milk, goat's milk, green bell peppers, taco shells, sour oranges, limes, soybeans, leafy green vegetables, marshmallow root, fenugreek seed, slippery elm bark, whole grains
Sodium	400 mg.	Virtually all manufactured foods contain varying amounts of sodium; and nearly all seafoods and seaweeds do, too.
Minerals	*Dosage*	*Food Sources*
Strontium (and Barium)	–	Bone marrow, turtle soup, crabs, lobsters, ocean fish, seaweed, plantain flowers, red clover blossoms, coltsfoot leaves and flowers, slippery elm twig and leaves, birch buds, black elder twigs and leaves, hawthorn twigs and leaves and berries, rose hips, dandelion root and flower, stinging nettle leaves and flowers, white willow twigs and leaves, sunflower seeds
Sulphur	––	blackstrap molasses, garlic and aged garlic extract, leeks and onions, Brussel sprouts, cabbage, kale, kohlrabi, radishes, cauliflower, turnips, soybeans, watercress, mustard greens, turnip greens, fertilized eggs, ocean fish (especially shark), catfish, lobster, crab, dried beans, lentils, almonds, dried fruit, dried meat or beef jerky, certain amino acids: L-cysteine, L-lysine, L-cystine, L-methionine
Tin	––	Mother's milk, dill weed, pickles, organ meats (especially beef heart, brain, liver, and tripe or cow's stomach lining), thymus glandular supplement
Vanadium	10 mg/kg body weight	Trout, halibut, salmon, catfish, perch, flounder, vegetable oils (olive, sesame, sunflower), Brazil nuts, pecans, walnuts, snap beans, dill weed, red radishes, green onions, almonds, peanuts, whole grains, veal
Zinc	50 mg.	Brewer's yeast, egg yolks, lamb chops, veal, lima beans, liver, mushrooms, pecans, pumpkin seeds, sardines, seeds, soy lecithin, soybeans, sunflower seeds, raisins, trout, salmon, turkey, chicken

APPENDIX

A GUIDE TO COMPANIES AND THEIR PRODUCTS

Company	*Products*
Alta Health Products 1983 East Locust St. Pasadena, CA 91107 (818)-796-1 047	Alta Sil-X Silica Pau d'arco Fluid Extract
Brooks Appliance Co. Brooks Building Marshall, MI 49068	Hernia trusses and belts
Custom-Made Formulas PO Box 1623 Salt Lake City, UT 84110-1623	CIR (Circulation Formula) Herbal formulas individually made for specific health needs.
Great American Natural Products, Inc. 4121 16th Street North St. Petersburg, FL 33703 1-(800)-323-4372	Essential Oils AquaVite
Montana Naturals 1994 Hwy. 93 Arlee, MT 59821	40% Propolis Tincture

Company	*Products*
Montana Naturals 1994 Hwy. 93 Arlee, MT 59821	40% Propolis Tincture
Nature's Sunshine Products, Inc. PO Box 1000 Spanish Fork, UT 84660	Bach Flower Remedies Rescue Remedy
Nature's Way Products, Inc. 10 Mountain Springs Springville, UT 84663	Alfalfa Buchu Efamol Evening Primrose Oil Sinustop Thisilyn
Old Amish Herbs 4141 Iris St. North St. Petersburg, FL 33703	Calendula Dairy Salve Green Onion Oil Cabbage Compound
Pines International POB 1107 Lawrence, KS 66044	Organic beet root powder
Sierra Botanicals 2955 Yellowtail Road Reno, NV 89510 Chinese herbal formulas:	Life Enhancer Emperor's Formula Ming VMM Mink Renu Thinyu

Quick Trim
Shangri-La Elixir
Chinese Immune Booster
Lady Ch'eng's Heart Tonic

Wakunaga of America Co., Ltd.
23501 Madero
Mission Viejo, CA 92691
Calif. 1-(800)-544-5800
Nationwide 1-(800)-421-2998

Ginkgolic
Goldenseal root
Kyo-Chrome
Kyo-Dophilus
Kyo-Green
Kyolic aged garlic extract
Kyolic liquid garlic
Kyolic liquid garlic with vitamin B-1
    and B-12
Kyolic 101
Kyolic 102
Kyolic 105
Kyolic EPA
RELEAF
Yeast Gard